Key Topics in Neonatology

Key Topics in Neonatology

Second Edition

Richard Mupanemunda BSc BM MRCP(UK) FRCPCH
Consultant Neonatologist
Birmingham Heartlands Hospital NHS Trust
Honorary Senior Clinical Lecturer
University of Birmingham, UK

Michael Watkinson MB BChir MA FRCP FRCPCH
Consultant Neonatologist
Birmingham Heartlands Hospital NHS Trust
Honorary Senior Clinical Lecturer
University of Birmingham, UK

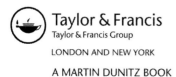
Taylor & Francis
Taylor & Francis Group

LONDON AND NEW YORK

A MARTIN DUNITZ BOOK

© 2005 Taylor & Francis, an imprint of the Taylor & Francis Group

First edition published in the United Kingdom in 1999 by
BIOS Scientific Publishers Limited

Second edition published 2005
by Taylor & Francis, an imprint of the Taylor & Francis Group,
2 Park Square, Milton Park, Abingdon, Oxon OX14 4RN

Tel.:   +44 (0) 20 7017 6000
Fax.:   +44 (0) 20 7017 6699
E-mail: info@dunitz.co.uk
Website: http://www.dunitz.co.uk

Important Note from the Publisher
The information contained within this book was obtained by Taylor & Francis from sources believed
by us to be reliable. However, while every effort has been made to ensure its accuracy, no respons-
ibility for loss or injury whatsoever occasioned to any person acting or refraining from action as a
result of information contained herein can be accepted by the authors or publishers.

The reader should remember that medicine is a constantly evolving science and while the authors and
publishers have ensured that all dosages, applications and practices are based on current indications,
there may be specific practices which differ between communities. You should always follow the
guidelines laid down by the manufacturers of specific products and the relevant authorities in the
country in which you are practising.

A CIP record for this book is available from the British Library.

Library of Congress Cataloging-in-Publication Data

Data available on application

ISBN 1 85996 234 3

Distributed in North and South America by
Taylor & Francis
2000 NW Corporate Blvd
Boca Raton, FL 33431, USA

Within Continental USA
Tel.: 800 272 7737; Fax.: 800 374 3401
Outside Continental USA
Tel.: 561 994 0555; Fax.: 561 361 6018
E-mail: orders@crcpress.com

Distributed in the rest of the world by
Thomson Publishing Services
Cheriton House
North Way
Andover, Hampshire SP10 5BE, UK
Tel.: +44 (0)1264 332424
E-mail: salesorder.tandf@thomsonpublishingservices.co.uk

Composition by Wearset Ltd, Boldon, Tyne and Wear

Printed and bound in Great Britain by TJ International Ltd, Padstow, Cornwall

Contents

[a] Contributed by R. Danha, Specialist Registrar in Anaesthetics, Nuffield Department of Anaesthetics, John Radcliffe Hospital, Oxford, UK.
[b] Contributed by M. Chaudhari, Consultant Paediatric Cardiologist, Freeman Hospital, Newcastle Upon Tyne, UK.
[c] Contributed by H. Goodyear, Consultant Paediatrician, Birmingham Heartlands Hospital, Birmingham, UK.

Preface to the first edition

Neonatology is a relatively new subspecialty in medicine, having largely come into being in the last three decades. This short period has, however, witnessed a dramatic reduction in neonatal mortality, particularly of very small preterm infants, due to the rapid advances in perinatal and neonatal medicine. Many areas of neonatology are still changing as new information becomes available, often leading to new diagnostic and therapeutic techniques. Although large formal neonatology textbooks serve as a very useful resource, they soon become dated as new information becomes available.

This book aims to provide the reader with a very up-to-date summary of the current concepts and practices in neonatal medicine. The field is covered in a series of self-contained, easily read topics set in a unique format which encourages the adoption of a problem-based approach ideal for day-to-day clinical practice. Although some topics reflect our personal clinical practice, the systematic approach to each topic is retained. Reference is made to related topics which allows the reader ready access to the subject matter of their choice unencumbered by extraneous detail.

As such, the text is an ideal revision aid for the neonatology components of the postgraduate paediatric examinations (including MRCP or DCH). It will also serve as a useful reference text for other professionals, both trainees and qualified, who are involved in the care of both well and sick newborns.

We are thankful to our colleagues for reading through various topics, in particular Dr R. Danha who read through most of the topics and was a source of great encouragement. Also our sincere appreciation to Tracey Fantham whose secretarial assistance made this book possible. Finally, we are especially thankful to the staff at BIOS for their helpful guidance from the outset, and their enduring patience despite the many broken deadlines.

We dedicate the book to our own 'ex-prems' Francesca, Grace and Henry.

Richard H. Mupanemunda
Michael Watkinson

Preface to the second edition

Following the long labours of reviewing all the relevant published works in this rapidly changing field, distilling this large body of evidence into compact, and yet clear, topics proved more arduous than we had envisaged. However, the success of the first edition in the face of the wealth of texts now available in neonatal medicine would suggest that our efforts were well received. We have retained the same format in this second edition, updating topics where significant recent developments have taken place, and widening the scope of the text by adding some entirely new topics.

It is our hope that this book will continue to have an important role in the education and training of medical, nursing and midwifery staff in training grades, as well as providing a quick reference text to the trained staff and other health care professionals involved in the care of newborn infants. It remains an ideal revision aid for the neonatology components of the MRCPCH and DCH postgraduate medical examinations. Those training to become advanced neonatal nurse practitioners will find it equally useful.

Once more we would like to thank our colleagues for reading through the entire contents. We would like to express our sincere appreciation to Tracey Fantham for her invaluable secretarial assistance. Finally, our heartfelt thanks to our publisher Alan Burgess and his colleagues at Taylor & Francis for their patience during the preparation of the manuscript.

Richard Mupanemunda
Michael Watkinson

Abbreviations

17-OHP	17-hydroxyprogesterone
25-OHD	25-hydroxyvitamin D
1,25-(OH)$_2$D	1,25-dihydroxyvitamin D
3ß-HSD	3ß-hydroxysteriod dehydrogenase
AAP	American Academy of Pediatrics
A1ATD	α-1-antitrypsin deficiency
AC	abdominal circumference
ACE	angiotensin-converting enzyme
ADH	antidiuretic hormone
ADHD	attention-deficit hyperactivity disorder
ADPCKD	autosomal dominant polycystic kidney disease
AFP	alpha-fetoprotein
AGA	appropriate for gestational age
AIDS	acquired immunodeficiency disease
ALT	alanine aminotransferase
APH	antepartum haemorrhage
ARDS	acute respiratory distress syndrome
ARPCKD	autosomal recessive polycystic kidney disease
ASD	atrial septal defect
AST	aspartate aminotransferase
AVSD	atrioventricular septal defect
BP	blood pressure
BPD	biparietal diameter
BSE	bovine spongiform encephalitis
BT	bleeding time
CAH	congenital adrenal hyperplasia
CAM	cystic adenoid malformation
CBF	cerebral blood flow
CDC	US Centers for Disease Control and Prevention
CDG	carbohydrate-deficient glycoprotein
CDH	congenital diaphragmatic hernia
CF	cystic fibrosis
cGMP	cyclic guanylate monophosphate
CHB	complete heart block
CHD	congenital heart disease
CHF	congestive heart failure
CI	confidence interval
CLD	chronic lung disease
CM	conventional management
CMD	congenital muscular dystrophy
CMV	cytomegalovirus
CNS	central nervous system
CP	cerebral palsy
CPAP	continuous positive airway pressure

CPD	citrate, phosphate, dextrose
CPDA	citrate, phosphate, dextrose and adenine
CPK	creatine phosphokinase
CRP	C-reactive protein
CRS	congenital rubella syndrome
CSF	cerebrospinal fluid
CT	computerised tomography
CVH	combined ventricular hypertrophy
CVS	chorionic villus sampling
DA	ductus arteriosus
DCA	dichloroacetate
dd1	didanosine
DDH	developmental dysplasia of the hip
DHT	dihydrotestosterone
DIC	disseminated intravascular coagulation
DISIDA	di-isopropyl iminodiacetic acid
DMSA	dimercaptosuccinic acid
DNPH	dinitrophenylhydrazine
DORV	double outlet right ventricle
DPPC	dipalmitoyl phosphatidylcholine
DTap	adsorbed diphtheria, tetanus and acellular pertussis
DTwp	adsorbed diphtheria, tetanus and whole-cell pertussis
ECG	electrocardiogram
ECHO	echocardiography
ECM	external cardiac massage
ECMO	extracorporeal membrane oxygenation
EDD	expected date of delivery
EDF	end-diastolic flow
EEG	electroencephalogram
ELBW	extremely low birth weight
ELISA	enzyme-linked immunosorbent assay
EMG	electromyogram
ENT	ear, nose, and throat
EOGBS	early-onset group B streptococcus disease
ET	endotracheal
FBC	full blood count
FBS	foetal blood sampling
FDP	fibrin-degradation products
FFP	fresh-frozen plasma
FISH	fluorescence in situ hybridisation
FiO_2	fractional inspired oxygen concentration
FL	femoral length
FRC	functional residual capacity
G6PD	glucose-6-phosphate dehydrogenase
GABA	gamma-aminobutyric acid
GBS	group B streptococcus
GFR	glomerular filtration rate

GH	growth hormone
GOR	gastrooesophageal reflux
HBeAg	hepatitis B 'e' antigen
HBIG	hepatitis B immunoglobulin
HBsAg	hepatitis B surface antigen
HBV	hepatitis B virus
HCV	hepatitis C virus
HDN	haemorrhagic disease of the newborn
HFJV	high-frequency jet ventilation
HFOV	high-frequency oscillatory ventilation
Hib	haemophilus influenzae type b
HIE	hypoxic-ischaemic encephalopathy
HIV	human immunodeficiency virus
HLHS	hypoplastic left heart syndrome
HNIG	human normal immunoglobulin
HSV	herpes simplex virus
ICD	immune complex dissociation
ICROP	International Classification of Retinopathy of Prematurity
ICH	intracranial haemorrhage
IDM	infant of diabetic mother
Ig	immunoglobulin
IGF	insulin-like growth factor
IGFBP	insulin-like growth factor binding protein
i.m.	intramuscular
IMD	inherited metabolic disease
IPPV	intermittent positive pressure ventilation
IPV	inactivated poliomyelitis vaccine
IQ	intelligence quotient
IRT	immunoreactive trypsin
ITP	idiopathic thrombocytopenic purpura
IU	international units
IUGR	intrauterine growth restriction
IV	intravenous
IVH	intraventricular haemorrhage
IVIG	intravenous immunoglobulin
IVS	intact ventricular septum
IVU	intravenous urography
LA/Ao	left atrial to aortic root ratio
LBW	low birth weight
LCP	long-chain polyunsaturated fatty acid
LGA	large for gestational age
LIP	lymphoid interstitial pneumonia
LP	lumbar puncture
LV	left ventricle
LVH	left ventricular hypertrophy
MAG-3	mercapto-acetyl-triglycerine-3

MAP	mean airway pressure
MAS	meconium aspiration syndrome
MCUG	micturating cystourethrogram
mIU	milli international units
MIS	Müllerian inhibitor substance
MRI	magnetic resonance imaging
MRSA	methicillin-resistant *Staphylococcus aureus*
MSUD	maple syrup urine disease
mU	milli units
NAS	neonatal abstinence syndrome
NEC	necrotising enterocolitis
NICE	National Institute of Clinical Excellence
NICHD	National Institute of Child Health and Human Development
NICU	neonatal intensive care unit
NIPS	Neonatal Infant Pain Score
NKH	non-ketotic hyperglycinaemia
NNU	neonatal unit
NO	nitric oxide
NO_2	nitrogen dioxide
NOS	nitric oxide synthase
NTD	neural tube defect
nvCJD	new variant Creutzfeldt-Jakob disease
OA	oesophageal atresia
OI	oxygenation index
OPV	oral poliomyelitis vaccine
OR	odds ratio
PA	pulmonary artery
$PaCO_2$	arterial carbon dioxide tension
PaO_2	arterial oxygen tension
PAS	periodic acid-Schiff reaction
PBF	pulmonary blood flow
PCA	postconceptual age
PCKD	polycystic kidney disease
PCP	*Pneumocystis carinii* pneumonia
PCR	polymerase chain reaction
PCV	packed cell volume
PDA	patent ductus arteriosus
PE	pre-eclampsia
PEEP	positive end-expiratory pressure
PET	pre-eclamptic toxaemia
PFO	patent foramen ovale
PG	prostaglandin
PHH	post-haemorrhagic hydrocephalus
PI	protease inhibitor
PIE	pulmonary interstitial emphysema
PIP	peak inspiratory pressure

PKU	phenylketonuria
Pl^{A1}	platelet A1 antigen
PLH	pulmonary lymphoid hyperplasia
PM	post-mortem
PMA	postmenstrual age
PNDM	permanent neonatal diabetes mellitus
p.o.	by mouth
PPHN	persistent pulmonary hypertension of the newborn
PROM	preterm rupture of membranes
PS	pulmonary stenosis
PT	prothrombin time
PTT	partial thromboplastin time
PUJ	pelvi-ureteric junction
PVH	periventricular haemorrhage
PVL	periventricular leucomalacia
PVR	pulmonary vascular resistance
RDS	respiratory distress syndrome
rHuEPO	recombinant human erythropoietin
ROP	retinopathy of prematurity
RSV	respiratory syncytial virus
RSVIG	respiratory syncytial virus immunoglobulin
RT	reptilase time
RTA	renal tubular acidosis
RVH	right ventricular hypertrophy
SaO$_2$	oxygen saturation
s.c.	subcutaneous
SCD	sickle cell disease
SCID	severe combined immunodeficiency
SGA	small for gestational age
sGC	soluble guanylate cyclase
SIADH	syndrome of inappropriate antidiuretic hormone
SLE	systemic lupus erythematosus
SMA	spinal muscular atrophy
sPDA	symptomatic patent ductus arteriosus
SRY	sex determining region Y
SVT	supraventricular tachycardia
TA-GVHD	transfusion-associated graft-versus host disease
TAPVD	total anomalous pulmonary venous drainage
TAR	thrombocytopenia with absent radius
TB	tuberculosis
TDF	testis-determining factor
Te	expiratory time
TGA	transposition of great arteries
THAM	tris-hydroxymethyl-aminomethane
Ti	inspiratory time
TMI	transient myocardial ischaemia
TNDM	transient neonatal diabetes mellitus

TOF	tracheo-oesophageal fistula
TORCH	toxoplasmosis, other (particularly syphilis), rubella, cytomegalovirus, herpes
TPHA	*Treponima pallidum* haemagglutination assay
TPN	total parenteral nutrition
TRH	thyrotrophin-releasing hormone
TSH	thyroid-stimulating hormone
TT	thrombin time
U and E	urea and electrolytes
UAC	umbilical artery catheter
UDCA	ursodeoxycholic acid
UDPGT	uridine diphosphate glucuronyl transferase
UTI	urinary tract infection
UVC	umbilical venous catheter
VCV	volume-controlled ventilation
VDRL	Venereal Disease Research Laboratory
VKDB	vitamin K deficiency bleeding
VLBW	very low birthweight
VSD	ventricular septal defect
VT	ventricular tachycardia
VUR	vesico-ureteric reflux
VZV	varicella-zoster virus
VZIG	varicella-zoster immunoglobulin
WBC	white blood cell
WPW	Wolf–Parkinson–White syndrome
ZDV	zidovudine

Abdominal distension

Abdominal distension is one of the commonest physical signs for which a medical opinion may be sought. The causes are legion, varying from physiological abdominal distension through a variety of benign causes to serious acute medical emergencies.

Aetiology

Physiological
- gaseous distension in infants receiving mechanical ventilation or continuous positive airway pressure (CPAP)
- delayed bowel action
- lax abdominal muscles (as in prune belly syndrome)
- urinary retention.

Pathological
- ascites
- Hirschsprung's disease
- intestinal obstruction (as in atresia or volvulus)
- intra-abdominal masses (organomegaly or tumours)
- iatrogenic (such as intraperitoneal extravasation of parenteral infusates)
- intra-abdominal haemorrhage
- imperforate anus
- meconium ileus or plug (associated with cystic fibrosis [CF])
- necrotising enterocolitis (NEC)
- pneumoperitoneum.

Presentation

Abdominal distension may be the sole abnormal physical sign in an otherwise well infant when physiological causes are responsible. On the other hand, pathological abdominal distension may present at birth or later with bilious vomiting, in a sick infant with a shiny, silent, tense and tender abdomen with perforated NEC. In non-ventilated infants, this may be heralded by apnoea and bradycardia or acute collapse. A ventilated infant with a rapidly increasing abdominal girth may have developed a pneumoperitoneum.

Investigations

- abdominal radiograph or ultrasound scan
- water-soluble contrast or barium enema study
- infection screen
- electrolytes.

Management

Infants presenting with meconium ileus or those passing a meconium plug should be screened for CF (immune reactive trypsin or DNA analysis for common CF mutations). Acute and subacute intestinal obstruction is managed by gastric decompression (nasogastric suction) and elective surgery in an appropriate centre. The infant should be in a stable condition prior to surgery. Infants with severe or perforated NEC may require more urgent surgical intervention and should receive adequate analgesia, broad-spectrum antibiotics including anaerobic cover (such as ceftazidime, vancomycin and metronidazole) and, if necessary, mechanical ventilation. Intra-abdominal collections (such as ascites) may be drained with a fine canula to decompress the abdomen and the peritoneal fluid cultured. Adequate analgesia should always be administered where the infant may be in pain (for example, intravenous morphine infusion at 20–40 μg/kg per h for an infant with perforated bowel).

Useful website

www.emedicine.com/ped/neonatology.htm
A part of the largest and most current online clinical knowledge base available to physicians and health professionals.

Further reading

Beasley SW, Hutson JM, Auldist AW. *Essential Paediatric Surgery*. London: Arnold, 1996.

Black JA, Whitfield MF. *Neonatal Emergencies: Early Detection and Management*, 2nd edn. Oxford: Butterworth-Heinemann, 1991.

Clark DA. *Atlas of Neonatology – A companion to Avery's Diseases of the Newborn*, 7th edn. Philadelphia: WB Saunders, 2000.

Fletcher MA. *Physical Diagnosis in Neonatology*. Philadelphia: Lippincott, Williams & Wilkins, 1997.

O'Doherty N. *Atlas of the Newborn*, 2nd edn. Lancaster: MTP Press, 1985.

Philip AGS. *Neonatology: A Practical Guide*, 4th edn. Philadelphia: WB Saunders, 1996.

Related topics of interest

- analgesia and anaesthesia
- feeding difficulties
- Hirschsprung's disease
- necrotising enterocolitis
- neonatal surgery
- vomiting.

Abdominal wall defects

Abdominal wall defects, most commonly gastroschisis and exomphalos, have an incidence of approximately one in 2000 live births. With modern obstetric care it should be possible to identify all major abdominal wall defects during routine prenatal ultrasound evaluation. Furthermore, maternal alpha-fetoprotein (AFP) levels are raised when bowel is exposed to amniotic fluid.

Once an abdominal wall defect has been detected, it is important to identify the type of defect and to perform a detailed level II ultrasound evaluation to assess overall foetal development and rule out other structural malformations. Families then consult with the obstetrician, neonatologist and paediatric surgeon to discuss the diagnosis, prognosis, prenatal management, delivery, and likely postnatal medical and surgical options. An individual management and follow-up plan is then formulated.

Gastroschisis

Gastroschisis results from a failure of the midgut to return to the abdomen by week ten of gestation. The bowel herniates through a small anterior abdominal wall defect (usually located to the right of the umbilicus), a condition which may lead to vascular compromise of herniated gut. Usually only the small and large bowel is eviscerated; rarely, the stomach, liver, or genitourinary system may be involved. The exposed bowel may be thickened and dilated due to exposure to amniotic fluid, leading to intestinal dysfunction.

- Incidence varies from 1:5000 to 1:30000.
- Gastroschisis is associated with young maternal age. Mothers under 20 years are 12 times more likely to have infants with gastroschisis.
- Bowel complications (typically malrotation and segmental atresia) are present in 15% of cases.
- Gastroschisis is rarely associated with other anomalies (cardiac defects in 2%) and is not associated with chromosomal abnormalities (though familial cases have been reported).
- Prematurity (50–60%) and intrauterine growth restriction (IUGR) are common.
- Overall prognosis is good with survival rates of 70–90%.

Management
It is preferable to transfer the mother to a centre offering immediate neonatal surgical expertise. Where in utero transfer is not possible immediately after delivery, place the lower half of the baby in a large polyethylene bag secured around the chest (or wrap the abdomen and exposed gut in several layers of cling film) to minimise fluid and heat loss from the exposed bowel. If resuscitation is needed, do not use mask ventilation, as this will increase the distension of the stomach and bowel. Place a large-bore nasogastric tube and leave on free drainage. Administer fresh-frozen plasma (FFP) or human albumin (20 ml/kg), commence antibiotics and IV dextrose infusion, keep the infant warm, and arrange urgent transfer to a neonatal surgical facility.

Operative repair

Surgical correction can be performed as an immediate primary repair, or a staged repair, depending on the condition of the exposed bowel. The preferred surgical approach, primary repair, entails reduction of the herniated viscera and complete abdominal wall closure in one operation. If this is not feasible, a protective covering of silastic sheeting (a 'silo') is placed around the herniated bowel and sewn to the edges of the abdominal wall defect, and the intestine is gradually reduced into the abdomen over a period of time prior to abdominal wall closure.

Long-term outcome

Although normal intestinal function may resume quite rapidly, it is not uncommon for these infants to be dependent on total parenteral nutrition for weeks or months before satisfactory bowel motility and absorption are achieved to allow oral nutrition. NEC may occur in 18%. Mortality is fairly low at approximately 10%.

Exomphalos (omphalocele)

An exomphalos is a midline defect of the abdominal wall that results in herniation of the bowel and intra-abdominal contents into the umbilical cord. This defect results from a failure of migration and fusion of the cephalic, caudal, and/or lateral folds of the embryonic disc, beginning as early as the week three. Unlike gastroschisis, a membrane limits the bowel contents, and the maternal AFP levels are not elevated. The sac may contain intestinal loops, liver, spleen, and bladder, with the cord arising from the apex of the sac.

- Incidence varies from 1:500 to 1:10 000.
- The incidence of major associated anomalies is 45–55% (cardiac, 20%; gastro-intestinal, 37%, especially volvulus, intestinal atresia, and Meckel's diverticulum), and these anomalies determine the prognosis.
- Chromosomal abnormalities are present in 30%, especially trisomy 13, 18, and 21; triploidy; and Turner's syndrome. Another associated syndrome is the Beckwith–Wiedemann syndrome.
- Prematurity (10–20%) and IUGR are less common than in gastroschisis, but overall mortality is higher (up to 40%).

Management

If resuscitation is needed, do not use mask ventilation, as this will increase the distension of the stomach and bowel. Great effort should be made to maintain the integrity of the sac. Wrap the abdomen in cling film and support the sac. Place a large-bore nasogastric tube and leave this on free drainage. Obtain vascular access and commence an intravenous dextrose infusion to maintain euglycaemia. Provided the sac is intact, emergency surgery is not required.

Operative repair

Treatment depends on the size of the lesion. Small defects can be closed surgically. Large defects may require staged procedures with silastic or prolene sheeting.

Long-term outcome

Associated anomalies determine the outcome. Heart disease has a major impact on the prognosis. In the absence of heart disease, survival is 70%, but when heart disease is present, survival is reduced to 20%.

Bladder exstrophy

Bladder exstrophy results from a failure of mesodermal migration with breakdown of ectoderm and endoderm, leading to the absence of the anterior abdominal wall and bladder wall. It is more common in males. The umbilicus is abnormally low, and the pubic bone is unfused. In males, the penis is epispadic and upturned, while in females the genital tract is often normal, though vaginal stenosis may require surgery later.

Management

Referral to a specialist surgical centre is essential. As reconstruction of the bladder is particularly difficult, many children are treated by urinary diversion in the form of an ileal conduit or ureterosigmoidostomy. In an ileal conduit, the ureters are anastomosed to one end of an isolated loop of ileum, with the other end being anastomosed to the skin and drained into an adhesive appliance. In ureterosigmoidostomy, the ureters are implanted into the sigmoid colon. A major drawback of this procedure is the reflux of faeces from the colon into the kidney.

Family support groups and information

- GEEPS (Gastroschisis, Exomphalos, Extrophies Parents Support) www.geeps.org
- Contact a Family
  209–211 City Road
  London EC1V 1JN, UK
  Tel: 0808 808 3555
  www.cafamily.org.uk
  A UK-wide charity providing support, advice and information for families with disabled children.

Further reading

Curry J, McKinney P, Thornton JG, Stringer MD. The aetiology of gastroschisis. *British Journal of Obstetrics and Gynaecology* (2000) **107:**1339–46.

Langer JC. Gastroschisis and omphalocele. *Seminars in Paediatric Surgery* (1996) **5:**124–8.

Nyberg DA, Mahony BS, Pretorius DH. *Abdominal Wall Defects in Diagnostic Ultrasound of Fetal Anomalies*. St Louis, MO: Mosby-Year Book, 1990: 395–432.

Puri P. *Newborn Surgery*, 2nd edn. London: Arnold, 2003.

Stringer MD, Oldham KT, Mouriguand PDE, Howard ER. *Paediatric Surgery and Urology: Long Term Outcomes*. Philadelphia: WB Saunders, 1998.

Related topics of interest

- congenital malformations and birth defects
- neonatal surgery
- surgical emergencies.

Acid–base balance

In most tissues, the generation of hydrogen ions is linked with the energy production necessary for life, and if the oxygen supply is adequate, most of the excess hydrogen ions are converted to water, and pH changes are minimal. If the supply of oxygen is inadequate to deal with such a load, these hydrogen ions must be inactivated or buffered until they can enter aerobic pathways or be eliminated from the body. Excess acid may also be generated from respiratory failure, decreased renal excretion of acid or the inappropriate renal loss of bicarbonate, enteral or parenteral intake, and other metabolic processes, including inborn errors of metabolism. Hydrogen ions can be lost from the body only through the kidney and the intestine. There are several buffering systems to prevent the buildup of excess acid (especially bicarbonate, haemoglobin, protein, and phosphate). These systems are not fully developed in newborns and particularly preterm infants. Consequently, there is a tendency for newborns to develop acidosis (most commonly mixed acidosis). The acid–base balance is therefore a vital dynamic index of an infant's well-being, and it is best assessed by arterial blood gas analysis. The pH of plasma is 7.36–7.45 (33–44 nmol/l of H^+). An infant is acidotic if the pH is <7.26, and alkalotic if pH is >7.46. If pH is <7.26 and carbon dioxide is high, a respiratory acidosis is present, but if carbon dioxide is normal or low, a metabolic acidosis is present. If pH is >7.46 with a low carbon dioxide, a respiratory alkalosis is present (such as hyperventilation); if carbon dioxide is normal, metabolic alkalosis is present. Metabolic and respiratory alkalosis is uncommon and invariably iatrogenic (excess base administration or hyperventilation). Acidosis, on the other hand, is quite common and may be respiratory (high carbon dioxide), metabolic (low or normal carbon dioxide), or mixed (combination of both) with a negative base excess.

The difference between the total concentration of measured cations (dominated by sodium $[Na^+]$ and potassium $[K^+]$), and that of measured anions (dominated by chloride $[Cl^-]$ and bicarbonate $[HCO_3^-]$) is sometimes called the 'anion gap' (normal value 8–16 mmol/l). The sum of the measured anions, that is $[Na^+ + K^+] - [Cl^- + HCO_3^-]$ is 8–16 mmol/l. A larger anion gap in the newborn suggests the presence of an unmeasured organic acid (such as lactate). The causes and management of various acid–base disturbances are detailed in Table 1.

Problems associated with marked acidosis

- increased pulmonary vascular resistance
- inhibition of surfactant synthesis
- impaired myocardial contractility
- impaired diaphragmatic contractility
- impaired renal excretion of acid load.

Base administration

First check that the blood gases make sense and repeat if necessary, as excess heparin in a blood gas syringe may give erroneous readings. Administer base when pH is

Table 1 Causes and management of acid–base disturbances.

Respiratory alkalosis

Causes	*Management*
Hyperventilation	Reduce ventilatory support if ventilated

Respiratory acidosis

Unventilated

Respiratory failure	Intubation and ventilation

Ventilated

Endotracheal (ET) tube-blockage (raised $PaCO_2$, normal or low PaO_2)	Change ET tube
ET dislodged (raised $PaCO_2$, low PaO_2)	Reintubate
Pneumothorax (raised $PaCO_2$, and low PaO_2)	Aspirate pneumothorax and insert chest drain

Metabolic alkalosis

Causes	*Management*
Excessive gastric losses as in high atresia or pyloric stenosis	Replacement of gastric losses
Excess base administration	Stop base administration

Metabolic acidosis

Causes	*Management*
Hypoxia, anaerobic metabolism	Administer oxygen $\pm$ IPPV
Anaemia	Blood transfusion
Excessive respiratory effort	IPPV
Hypotension and hypovolaemic	Colloid administration $\pm$ inotropes
Renal bicarbonate loss	Bicarbonate replacement
Excess acid administration parenterally	Reduce intake appropriately
Infection	Broad-spectrum antibiotics after all appropriate cultures
Inborn error of metabolism (persistent acidosis)	Assay serum amino acids, lactate, and ammonia, with urinalysis for pH, acetone, ketoacids, and urine amino and organic acids

<7.25 and base deficit is greater than −10 mmol/l. Amount of base (in mmol) is calculated from the following formula: *base deficit (mmol/l) × body weight (kg) × 0.4 (extracellular volume)*.

Give bicarbonate as 4.2% solution (0.5 mmol/ml of solution) as a slow infusion (0.5 mmol/min). In presence of a high $PaCO_2$ or hypernatraemia, THAM (tris-hydroxymethyl-aminomethane) may be preferable. A 7% THAM solution contains 0.5 mmol/ml. THAM, however, may cause apnoea and should preferably be administered to ventilated infants. It is preferable initially to administer an amount of base sufficient only to *half-correct* the calculated base deficit, with repeat gases to reassess the acid–base balance. For persistent acidosis, a constant infusion of base may be required.

Problems associated with base administration

Provided appropriate doses of base are administered slowly, concerns regarding intracerebral haemorrhage associated with base administration may be allayed. However, overcorrection of metabolic acidosis may carry more risks than persistent mild acidosis. Thus, some patients with urea cycle defects may present with mild acidaemia, which should not be corrected, as acidosis protects against NH_4 dissociation and toxicity.

Common patterns of blood gas abnormalities

- respiratory alkalosis (acute): pH raised, $PaCO_2$ reduced, HCO_3^- normal or slightly reduced
- respiratory alkalosis (chronic): pH normal or raised, $PaCO_2$ reduced, HCO_3^- reduced
- respiratory acidosis (acute): pH decreased, $PaCO_2$ raised, HCO_3^- normal or slightly raised
- respiratory acidosis (chronic): pH slightly decreased, $PaCO_2$ raised, HCO_3^- raised
- metabolic acidosis (uncompensated or partially compensated): pH reduced, $PaCO_2$ reduced, HCO_3^- reduced
- metabolic acidosis (fully compensated): pH normal, $PaCO_2$ reduced, HCO_3^- reduced
- metabolic alkalosis: pH raised, $PaCO_2$ raised or normal, HCO_3^- raised.

Table 2 pH and corresponding hydrogen ion concentration.

pH	$[H^+]$ nanomolar
6.9	126
7.0	100
7.1	79
7.2	63
7.3	50
7.4	40
7.5	32
7.6	25

Further reading

Driscoll P, Brown T, Gwinnut C et al. *A Simple Guide to Blood Gas Analysis*. London: BMJ Publishing, 1997.

Seri I. Regulation of acid–base balance in the fetus and neonate. In: RA Polin, WW Fox (eds). *Fetal and Neonatal Physiology*, 2nd edn. Philadelphia: WB Saunders, 1998: 1726–30.

Sessler D, Mills P, Gregory G et al. Effects of bicarbonate on arterial and brain intracellular pH in neonatal rabbits recovering from hypoxic lactic acidosis. *Journal of Pediatrics* (1987) **111**:817–23.

von Planta I, Weil MH, von Planta M et al. Hypercarbic acidosis reduces cardiac resuscibility. *Critical Care Medicine* (1991) **19**:177–82.

Related topics of interest

- acute collapse
- inherited metabolic disease—investigation and management
- mechanical ventilation
- metabolic acidosis
- resuscitation
- shock.

Acute collapse

This is one acute medical emergency where swift and appropriate response can make a major difference to outcome. Irrespective of the cause, the major objectives should be to re-establish adequate gas exchange and maintain the cardiovascular circulation.

Aetiology

- overwhelming sepsis
- pneumothorax
- aspiration of vomitus
- major haemorrhage (intra-abdominal, intrapulmonary or intracranial)
- severe NEC (with or without perforation)
- metabolic and endocrine disorders
- congenital heart disease (as in hypoplastic left heart syndrome or interrupted aortic arch)
- compromised airway in the ventilated infant (blocked or displaced ET tube).

Presentation

Sudden onset of bradycardia, hypotension, pallor, or cyanosis in either a previously well or already unwell infant. There may also be vomitus in the mouth, blood coming from the oropharynx or trachea, abdominal distension, and hypothermia. The infant may look extremely ill with laboured or absent respiratory effort, mottled skin, marked hypotonia, and cold peripheries. Bloody stools may be passed at the same time, suggesting intra-abdominal pathology (NEC). Occasionally, seizures may also be noted.

Investigations

- fibre-optic cold light chest transillumination for pneumothoraces
- chest and abdominal radiographs
- arterial blood gases
- blood glucose
- urea and electrolytes (U and E)
- full blood count (FBC)
- clotting screen
- head ultrasound scan
- infection screen (blood and urine with or without cerebrospinal fluid [CSF])
- metabolic screen (obtain acute blood and urine samples and store accordingly).

Management

Near normal gas exchange, adequate tissue perfusion, and normal pressure should be re-established and maintained as rapidly as possible. If the respiratory effort is inadequate and the infant is not already ventilated, clear oropharynx and commence bag and mask (or T-piece) ventilation with 100% oxygen. Check pulse and peripheral pulses. If absent, commence external cardiac massage (ECM). If the infant is unresponsive after 1 min, intubate and continue ECM with bagging. Ensure that the bag and mask or T-piece setup is connected to oxygen and that it is turned on! Transilluminate the chest wall to exclude a large tension pneumothorax and drain (needle aspiration) if present. If still unresponsive, check ET tube position and administer 0.3 ml 1:1000 adrenaline via ET tube. If this produces a satisfactory response in the pulse and oxygenation (saturations >95%), discontinue ECM and continue with respiratory support and connect to a mechanical ventilator. Check arterial blood gases and blood glucose and adjust ventilation accordingly. Give dextrose and/or base as required. Obtain chest and abdominal radiographs.

Administer colloid if peripheral circulation is inadequate; if necessary, follow this by inotropes (dopamine or dobutamine at 5–20 μg/kg per min). Once infant is stable, work out the most likely cause if not already evident. Consider performing a head ultrasound scan in a newborn where IVH might be a possibility. If a haemorrhage has occurred, check clotting and administer fresh-frozen plasma (FFP) or cryoprecipitate (if fibrinogen is <1 g/l). If sepsis is likely, complete septic screen (with LP if stable) and cover with broad-spectrum antibiotics. If cause is obscure, consider rarer metabolic disorders, especially if there is persistent acidosis, hypoglycaemia, or inordinate neurological depression. Suspect adrenal insufficiency if dehydration, low sodium (<130 mmol/l), high potassium (>5 mmol/l) and ± hypoglycaemia are present. Maintain respiratory support with full monitoring over several hours, and gradually wean according to the status of the infant and the results of the investigations.

If an infant remains unresponsive to full cardiopulmonary resuscitation for 4–5 min, give 1:1000 adrenaline 0.4–1 ml IV and consider giving base if the resuscitation efforts are still unsuccessful by 10 min (3–5 mmol of 4.2% $NaHCO_3$ IV). Needle both sides of the chest in case bilateral pneumothoraces are present. Continue with resuscitation efforts for at least 20 min.

Unsuccessful resuscitation

Always try to obtain consent for a postmortem. A coroner may need to be informed. Where inherited metabolic disease is a possibility, obtain urine (amino and organic acids), blood (amino acids and DNA studies), skin (fibroblast cultures), muscle, and/or liver biopsies. Freeze urine, spin blood, separate red cells and plasma, and freeze separately. Snap-freeze liver and muscle samples in liquid nitrogen or store at 4 °C in tissue culture medium or plain saline, but transfer to most appropriate storage medium at the earliest opportunity.

Further reading

Black JA, Whitfield MF. *Neonatal Emergencies: Early Detection and Management*, 2nd edn. Oxford: Butterworth-Heinemann, 1991.

Burchfield DJ. Medication use in neonatal resuscitation. *Clinics in Perinatology* (1999) **26**:683–91.

Emery JL, Variend S, Howat AJ et al. Investigation of inborn errors of metabolism in unexpected infant deaths. *Lancet* (1988) **2**:29–31.

Kattwinkel J, Denson S, Zaichkin J et al. *Textbook of Neonatal Resuscitation*, 4th edn. Dallas, TX: American Academy of Pediatrics, 2000.

Meerstadt PWD, Gyll C. *Manual of Emergency X-ray Interpretation*. Philadelphia: WB Saunders, 1995.

Reece RM (ed.). *Manual of Emergency Pediatrics*, 4th edn. Philadelphia: WB Saunders, 1992.

Surtees R, Leonard JV. Acute metabolic encephalopathy: a review of causes, mechanisms and treatment. *Journal of Inherited Metabolic Disease* (1989) **12:**42–54.

Taeusch HW, Christiansen RO, Buescher SE. Pediatric and Neonatal.

Willett LD, Nelson RM Jr. Outcome of cardiopulmonary resuscitation in the neonatal intensive care unit. *Critical Care Medicine* (1986) **14:**773–6.

Related topics of interest

- acid–base balance
- inherited metabolic disease
- pulmonary haemorrhage
- resuscitation
- shock.

Anaemia

The cord haemoglobin concentration in term infants averages 17 g/dl (range 14–20 g/dl) and 14 g/dl (range 13–18 g/dl) in preterm infants. Delayed clamping of the cord and holding the infant below the level of the placenta at birth will significantly raise the haemoglobin concentration. After birth, erythropoietin production is switched off by the greater availability of oxygen, reticulocytosis falls from 5% (at birth) to less than 1%, and the haemoglobin level falls to a nadir of 7–10 g/dl by 8–10 weeks, remaining stable for several weeks before gradually increasing. The fall in haemoglobin is more rapid and more marked in preterm infants, with the nadir of haemoglobin concentration varying inversely with gestational age. In term infants, this decline and rise in haemoglobin concentration have been labelled physiological, as the infants are asymptomatic. In preterm infants, the fall in haemoglobin concentration is often so marked that some infants require erythrocyte transfusions; thus, this 'anaemia of prematurity' is labelled nonphysiological. It is characterised by reticulocytopenia, bone marrow hypoplasia, and erythropoietin levels that are low relative to the degree of anaemia.

Anaemia may present at birth or during the first week of life (early anaemia) or later (later-onset anaemia), depending on the aetiology. Anaemia presenting after the first day of life commonly follows haemorrhage or haemolysis (nonimmune) while the anaemia due to impaired red cell production often presents after the first month of life.

Early-onset anaemia

This is a haemoglobin of <13 g/dl (PCV < 40%) during the first week of life. This is primarily a haemorrhagic anaemia resulting from repeated blood sampling during intensive care of very low birth weight infants with small blood volumes.

Aetiology
- twin-to-twin transfusion
- foetomaternal transfusion
- foetal haemorrhage: placenta praevia, abruption, vasa praevia, or placental incision at caesarean section
- foetoplacental transfusion at birth
- chronic or acute foetal haemolysis: rhesus disease and α-thalassaemia
- perinatal neonatal haemorrhage: intracranial, subaponeurotic fractures, ruptured spleen or liver, umbilical cord rupture, or accidents
- iatrogenic losses: repeated blood sampling.

Clinical features
Acute blood loss
- pallor
- hypotension
- poor capillary refill
- tachycardia
- tachypnoea.

Chronic blood loss
- pallor
- tachycardia
- congestive cardiac failure
- hepatosplenomegaly
- jaundice
- hydrops fetalis.

Investigations
- full blood count and film
- blood group and Coomb's test
- maternal Kleihauer test
- coagulation screen
- cranial ultrasonography (intracranial haemorrhage) and/or abdominal ultrasonography (concealed internal haemorrhage)
- exclude red cell abnormalities: haemoglobin eltrophoresis (haemoglobinopathies) and red cell enzymopathies
- serum bilirubin.

Management
Always look for the underlying cause and rectify this if possible. For acute blood loss and shock, rapid resuscitation is paramount. Give blood 10–30 ml/kg (group O rhesus-negative or blood harvested from placenta) at once. Alternatively, give 4.5% human albumin or plasma as volume expanders until blood is available. Repeat colloid administration (albumin or blood) until blood pressure normalises and correct acidosis. For severe hydrops fetalis due to rhesus isoimmunisation (cord haemoglobin <11 g/dl, cord bilirubin >80 μmol/l, or rate of rise of bilirubin >10 μmol/l/h, with positive Coomb's test), carry out an exchange transfusion. The primary aim is to correct the anaemia and raise serum albumin and not removing bilirubin. Remember to maintain the airway and, if necessary, give oxygen.

Later-onset anaemia

This is a haemoglobin of <10 g/dl after the first week of life. This is primarily a hyporegenerative anaemia resulting from the inability of the immature haematopoietic tissue to react adequately to hypoxia.

Aetiology
- anaemia of prematurity: impaired erythropoiesis and reduced red cell survival
- iatrogenic: repeated blood sampling
- chronic haemolysis, which may be subdivided into immune haemolysis (isoimmunisation), congenital red cell defects (morphologic, enzymatic, and haemoglobin abnormalities), and acquired red cell defects (secondary to toxins, drugs, or infection)
- the haemoglobin abnormalities may be synthetic defects (thalassaemia) or structural defects (haemoglobin variants)

- bleeding: intracranial or intra-abdominal haemorrhage, NEC, or disseminated intravascular coagulation (DIC)
- severe infection
- iron deficiency (after 6–8 weeks)
- vitamin E deficiency (haemolytic anaemia)
- other essential vitamin or mineral deficiencies (folic acid, vitamin B_{12}, or copper and zinc deficiencies)
- maternal autoimmune disease (systemic lupus erythematosus or autoimmune haemolytic anaemia)
- failure of red cell production as in Diamond–Blackfan syndrome (autosomal recessive inheritance), characterised by reticulocytopenia (<0.2%) and anaemia but normal leucocyte and platelet production.

Clinical features
- apnoeic attacks
- tachycardia
- poor feeding
- poor weight gain
- increased oxygen requirements in oxygen-dependent infants.

Investigations
- full blood count; film and reticulocyte count
- serum bilirubin (total and conjugated)
- coagulation screen (if actively bleeding)
- serum biotin, copper, and zinc (perioral dermatitis)
- check of stools for occult blood.

Management
Transfuse with packed cells if symptomatic. For oxygen-dependent infants with chronic lung disease, transfuse to raise the haemoglobin to 12–14 g/dl (PCV > 45%). For anaemia of prematurity, transfuse if haemoglobin is <8 g/dl. Give iron (2 mg/kg per day from four weeks until weaned), folic acid (0.1 mg daily orally from day ten until three months post-term), and vitamin E (5–25 IU/day orally).

There are several formulae for estimating the blood transfusion requirements of anaemic infants:

- Transfusion of 3 ml of packed red cells per kg body weight will raise the baby's haemoglobin by 1 g/dl.
- Transfusion of 10 ml of packed cells per kg will raise PCV by 10%.
- Volume of packed red cells (PCV = 80%) to be transfused = desired rise in haemoglobin $\times$ weight in kg $\times$ 3.
- For most infants, a transfusion of 20 ml/kg of packed red cells will suffice.

Prevention
Recombinant human erythropoietin (rHuEPO) has recently been licensed for the treatment of anaemia of prematurity in several European countries (e.g., Recormon®, Boehringer Mannheim, UK). rHuEPO at doses of 750 U/kg per week (given as three

doses of 250 U/kg by s.c. injection [IV shorter half-life] on 3 days per week) with oral iron supplementation at 6 mg/kg per day (initiated at 2 mg/kg per day and gradually increased) from the first week of life for 6 weeks reduces the need for transfusion for later-onset anaemia in infants of <34 weeks' gestation (birth weight 750–1500 g). Some restrict rHuEPO administration to all infants <28 weeks' gestation, but only those of <3rd percentile at 28–32 weeks gestation. Sick ventilated infants or those having daily venesection of >1.2 ml per day may receive a high-dose rHuEPO regimen consisting of 1400 U/kg per week given as 200 U/kg per day by IV infusion, beginning within 72 h of birth and continued for 2 weeks; thereafter, the standard regimen may be continued for the remaining 4 weeks. rHuEPO has been demonstrated to be both safe and cost-effective.

Further reading

Andersen C. Critical haemoglobin thresholds in premature infants. *Archives of Disease in Childhood Fetal and Neonatal Edition* (2001) **84:**F146–6.

Attias D. Pathophysiology and treatment of the anaemia of prematurity. *Journal of Pediatric Hematology and Oncology* (1995) **17:**13–18.

Boulton F. for the British Committee for Standards in Haematology Transfusion Task Force. Transfusion guidelines for neonates and older children. *British Journal of Haematology* (2004) **124:**433–53.

Carbonell-Estrany X, Figueras-Aloy J. Anaemia of prematurily: treatment with erythropoictin. *Early Human Development* (2001) **65** Suppl:S63–7.

Kling PJ, Winzerling IJ. Iron status and the treatment of anemia of prematurily. *Clinics in Perinatology* (2002) **29:**283–94.

Nathan DG, Orkin SH, Look T (eds). *Nathan and Oski's Hematology of Infancy and Childhood*, 6th edn. Philadelphia: WB Saunders, 2003.

Obkaden M, Maier RF. Erythropoietin therapy in preterm infants. In: TN Hansen, N McIntosh (eds). *Current Topics in Neonatology*, No. 2. London: WB Saunders, 1997: 108–24.

Smith OP, Hann IM. *Essential Paediatric Haematology*. London: Martin Dunitz, 2002.

Useful website

www.emedicine.com/ped/neonatology.htm
Part of the largest and most current online clinical knowledge base available to physicians and health professionals.

Related topics of interest

- bleeding disorders
- jaundice
- polycythaemia
- shock
- transfusion of blood and blood products.

Anaesthesia and postoperative analgesia

Ratidzo Danha

Neonates presenting for surgery are usually in urgent need of such treatment. They are also at a period when significant physiological and maturational changes of transition from foetal to extrauterine life are occurring. The special problems related to this age group which may influence anaesthetic management are as follows:

- thermoregulation
- the neonatal airway and respiratory function
- cardiovascular function
- renal function
- glucose homeostasis.

Thermoregulation

Heat loss occurs by conduction, convection, radiation, and evaporation, the major mechanism being radiation. Anaesthesia interferes with heat production by inhibiting shivering and nonshivering thermogenesis. Hypothermia delays recovery from anaesthesia, prolongs the effects of muscle relaxants, and increases oxygen consumption. If heat loss is not minimised aggressively, the anaesthetised neonate readily becomes hypothermic.

Cardiovascular function

The neonatal heart has much less contractile power since the myocardial cell has half as much contractile mass as an adult cell. Augmenting preload does not increase cardiac output, but increasing heart rate does. Sympathetic innervation is incomplete, but parasympathetic innervation is complete, resulting in increased susceptibility to bradycardia. The commonest cause of bradycardia in the newborn is hypoxia.

The neonatal airway and respiratory function

The neonate has a narrow subglottic area, which limits the size of the endotracheal tube. A large abdomen, weak intercostal muscles, and the horizontal configuration of the ribs pose additional mechanical disadvantage. The ability of the neonate to breathe spontaneously is limited, and ventilation should always be controlled. Premature infants less than 45–55 conceptual weeks are at risk of life-threatening apnoea following anaesthesia, and they are more prone to ventilatory dysfunction from the effect of residual anaesthetic agents.

Renal function

Renal function is immature at birth, and this may prolong the effects of drugs administered during anaesthesia. Renal excretion of drugs is influenced by the glomerular filtration, tubular excretion, and reabsorption. In newborns, the glomerular filtration rate is only 20% of that of adults, but this rapidly increases to 50% by day ten of life and approaches adult values towards the end of the first year of life. Both full-term and preterm infants have a limited ability to handle sodium loads, the preterm infant being an obligate sodium loser. A careful selection of both the composition and volume of fluids given intraoperatively is required, since neonatal renal function is limited.

Glucose homeostasis

This is not well developed in the early postnatal period and predisposes the neonate, especially the preterm infant, to the risk of both hyperglycaemia and hypoglycaemia. The stress of surgery and uncontrolled exogenous glucose therapy are the two most important causes of hyperglycaemia in the perioperative period. Normoglycaemia can be maintained by restricting the amount of exogenously administered glucose to 4–6 mg/kg per min and frequent monitoring of blood glucose levels.

Preoperative preparation

This is aimed at stabilising sick neonates so that they can be transported to the theatre and anaesthetised without undue haemodynamic compromise. Adequate intravenous access should be established, and an arterial line should be inserted in critically ill neonates. If the neonate has indwelling umbilical arterial and venous lines, their location should be confirmed radiologically prior to transport.

Preoperative starvation orders

For elective procedures, the last milk feed is allowed up to 4h preoperatively and clear liquid up to 2h preoperatively. In case surgery is delayed, an intravenous infusion with a dextrose-containing solution must be commenced to maintain normoglycaemia.

Transport to theatre

This may pose significant risks especially to the small sick ventilated preterm infant. Monitoring must be continued throughout the period of transfer. The trip to and from theatre involves lifting the infant (and all its attached equipment) into and out of the transport incubator four times within a short space of time. The most commonly encountered problems include:

- accidental extubation
- cold stress (hypothermia)
- dislodging of arterial and venous lines
- dislodging chest drains and surgical drains
- changing ventilator modalities (five ventilator changes in all for a round trip)
- adverse effects of ambulance transportation if surgery is performed off-site.

Intraoperative care

- Full remote continuous monitoring of all vital parameters should be continued during surgery.

- Take meticulous care to avoid hypothermia.
- Monitor fluid balance carefully to avoid hypo- and hypervolaemia.
- Replace significant blood losses intraoperatively (small total blood volume).
- Check blood gases and blood glucose during prolonged procedures.
- High-risk infants (such as those with chronic lung disease [CLD]) undergoing minor procedures such as hernia repair have fewer respiratory complications if the surgery is done under regional anaesthesia (that is, epidural anaesthesia) rather than general anaesthetic.

Postoperative analgesia and pain control

Neonates are often denied postoperative analgesia because they are susceptible to the respiratory depressant effects of narcotics, and they cannot vocalise pain. It is also especially difficult to assess pain in neonates, in particular, ventilated infants. Regional blocks performed intraoperatively provide analgesia during the immediate postoperative period. Systemic narcotics are the most commonly used agents for management of pain, and morphine may be considered the prototype. Neonates requiring postoperative ventilation are ideal candidates for narcotic analgesia. The suppression of respiration due to narcotics promotes synchronous mechanical ventilation. However, greater skill and judgment are required in use of narcotics for pain management in newborns who are not ventilated. The newborn must be observed closely with apnoea monitoring. Equipment and personnel for emergency airway management and treatment with naloxone should be readily available. However, for minor degrees of discomfort or pain, opiates may be avoided, and mild analgesics such as paracetamol (10 mg/kg per dose given every 4 h) may suffice.

Further reading

Alexander SM, Todres ID. The use of sedation and muscle relaxation in the ventilated infant. *Clinics in Perinatology* (1998) **25:**63–78.

Cote CJ, Ryan JF, Todres ID et al (eds). *A Practice of Anaesthesia for Infants and Children*, 2nd edn. Philadelphia: WB Saunders, 1993.

Gavilanes AWD, Heineman E, Herpes MJHM et al. Use of neonatal intensive care unit as a safe place for neonatal surgery. *Archives of Diseases in Childhood Fetal and Neonatal Edition* (1997) **76:**F51–3.

Krishna G, Ernhardt JD. Anaesthesia for the newborn ex-preterm infant. *Seminars in Paediatric Surgery* (1992) **1:**32–4.

Zeigler JW, Todres ID. Intubation of newborns. *American Journal of Diseases of Childhood* (1992) **146:**147–9.

Related topics of interest

- intubation
- neonatal surgery
- sedation and analgesia on the neonate intensive care unit
- thermoregulation.

Apnoea and bradycardia

Apnoea in the neonate is defined as a pause in breathing of more than 20s or a shorter pause associated with bradycardia or hypoxaemia. This condition increases in incidence at lower gestations. Thus, below 30 weeks' gestation, three out of four infants will have recurrent apnoea and bradycardia, the incidence falling to less than one in ten by 35 weeks' gestation and 0.08% in term infants. Apnoea may represent a central disturbance in the regulation of breathing, with airflow and respiratory effort ceasing at the end of expiration (central apnoea). Alternatively, the upper airway may intermittently become totally occluded while the infant continues to make ever-increasing, regular respiratory effort in an attempt to overcome the obstruction (obstructive apnoea). Some infants, however, may have 'mixed apnoeas', which resemble central apnoea initially with cessation of respiration followed by intermittent but ineffective respiratory effort indicative of airway obstruction.

Most apnoeas are of the mixed type with initial central episodes being followed by pharyngeal soft-tissue collapse. Furthermore, upper airway protective reflexes may result in apnoea. Thus, gastrooesophageal reflux or pharyngeal incoordination may also induce apnoea in coordination.

Aetiology

Abnormal airway
- choanal atresia
- micrognathia
- tracheomalacia
- upper airway incoordination (neurologic abnormality).

Central nervous system disorders
- brainstem immaturity
- intracranial haemorrhage
- seizures
- hypoxic-ischaemic encephalopathy
- congenital malformations
- maternal medication during pregnancy and labour
- central hypoventilation syndromes.

Metabolic disorders
- hypoglycaemia
- hypocalcaemia
- hyponatraemia
- inherited metabolic disease.

Systemic disorders
- anaemia
- sepsis

- hypoxia
- cardiac failure.

Miscellaneous
- overheating
- recent general anaesthesia.

Bradycardia often accompanies apnoea but may be unassociated with apnoea and may not be due to central hypoxaemia. Marked bradycardia (pulse of <80/min) may be deleterious and requires therapy.

Investigations

Well infants
- blood glucose (exclude hypoglycaemia)
- full blood count (exclude anaemia)
- oesophageal pH monitoring (exclude reflux)
- electroencephalogram (EEG) (exclude seizures).

Unwell infants
- full infection screen (blood culture, lumbar puncture, urine culture, and chest radiograph)
- blood gases
- serum calcium, magnesium, and electrolytes
- cranial ultrasound scan
- abdominal radiograph (exclude NEC).

Management

The primary aim is to correct any underlying disorders, intermittently stimulate the infant during the events, and maintain monitoring. There is no evidence that well infants with mild apnoea (<10 per day) and quick responses to tactile stimulation need any more specific therapy. Therapy is summarised thus:

- Give gentle stimulation if not self-resolving.
- Monitor for hypoxaemia and administer supplemental oxygen if necessary.
- Use bag and mask if response to supplemental facial oxygen is poor.
- Transfuse if anaemic (keep $Hb \geq 12\,g/dl$).
- Administer methylxanthines—IV aminophylline (loading dose 6 mg/kg, maintenance 5 mg/kg per day) or oral theophylline (loading dose 5 mg/kg per day in three divided doses and then up to 8 mg/kg daily—therapeutic range 28–84 mmol/l (5–15 mg/l). Alternatively, caffeine (which is less toxic) may be given orally (loading dose 10 mg/kg and a once-daily maintenance of 2.5 mg/kg equivalent to 20 mg caffeine citrate/kg and 5 mg caffeine citrate/kg loading dose and maintenance, respectively. Caffeine and theophylline are equally effective.
- If methylxanthines fail, add doxapram, starting at 0.5 mg/kg per h and increasing to 2.5 mg/kg per h intravenously or orally. Load with 2.5–3.0 mg/kg IV over 15–30 min followed by maintenance therapy.

- If drug therapy fails, try nasal CPAP (4–6 cmH$_2$O).
- If CPAP fails, intubate and ventilate at low pressures and rates.

Prognosis

In otherwise uncomplicated preterm infants, there is no evidence that apnoea causes long-term neurological impairment when other complicating factors are controlled for.

Further reading

Henderson-Smart DJ. Apnea of prematurity. In: RC Beckerman, RT Brouillette, CE Hunt (eds). *Respiratory Control Disorders in Infants and Children.* Baltimore, MD: Williams & Wilkins, 1992: 161–77.

Henderson-Smart DJ. Recurrent apnoea. In: VYH Yu (ed.). *Baillère's Clinical Paediatrics, Pulmonary Problems in the Perinatal Period and their Sequelae.* London: Baillière Tindall, 1995: 203–22.

Polin RA, Fox WW, Abman SH (eds). *Fetal and Neonatal Physiology*, 3rd edn. Philadelphia: WB Saunders, 2004.

Spitzer AR (ed.). *Intensive Care of the Fetus and Neonate.* St Louis: CV Mosby, 1996.

Taeusch HW, Ballard R, Gleason CA. *Avery's Diseases of the Newborn*, 8th edn. Philadelphia: WB Saunders, 2005.

Related topics of interest

- acute collapse
- mechanical ventilation
- respiratory distress
- resuscitation
- seizures
- shock.

Assessment of gestational age

Antenatal

The measurement most frequently used to assess foetal gestation is the biparietal diameter at around 16 weeks' gestation. The 95% confidence interval of such a measurement is 0.8 weeks. If a scan is done between six and ten weeks, measurement of the crown–rump length is at least as accurate, but thereafter curling of the foetus may make this a difficult measurement. A combination of these measurements, combined if necessary with foetal femur length, is used for assessment at different gestations.

The accuracy of gestational assessment by scanning drops off dramatically as pregnancy progresses because of biological variation in growth. Later scans are useful for following an individual's growth, but a late first scan contributes little to gestational assessment. Ultrasonographic biometry in early pregnancy is a more accurate assessment of gestation and the expected date of delivery than maternal dates, even when the mother is certain!

Postnatal

In 1970, Dubowitz developed a scoring system for the assessment of gestational age in infants less than five days old based upon morphological and neurological characteristics. It is limited by the fact that only six babies of <30 weeks' gestation were included, and that, at its best, the confidence interval of the score was ±14 days. Thus, even in the best hands, an assessment of a baby's gestation as (say) 32 weeks means that the assessor is 95% sure that the true gestation is between 30 and 34 weeks. The confidence limits are even wider (>2.5 weeks) at lower gestations (or birth weight of <1500 g), the very ones that concern us most nowadays. Furthermore, the handling of sick preterm babies for this assessment is a problem. Parkin recognised this and developed a simplified score based only on morphological criteria that could be assessed with very minimal handling, but the confidence limit of his score was ±18 days. Further doubt was cast when experienced Norwegian paediatricians reported confidence limits of ±5 and ±6 weeks for the two scores, respectively. The Ballard score is an abbreviated version of the Dubowitz scoring system and is therefore subject to the same limitations. Notwithstanding the above limitations, a new expanded Ballard scoring system has been developed for very low-birth-weight and extremely low-birth-weight infants. The updated Ballard included 61 infants less than 26 weeks' and 89 between 26 and 31 weeks' gestation. This system provides a means of gestational assessment for all infants of gestational ages greater than 20 weeks. For the most immature infants, the assessment is more accurate when performed during the first 12 h of life. Other ways of estimating gestational age include nerve-conduction studies and examination of the anterior vascular capsule of the lens.

Nowadays, with accurate dating by antenatal ultrasound, there is neither need nor justification for a detailed postnatal assessment of gestation. However, the above methods of assessing gestational age may be extremely useful in the minority of pregnancies where the mother deliberately conceals her pregnancy, is unable (due to language or communication difficulties) or unwilling to divulge the requisite information, or is particularly unreliable (such as drug-abusing mother in unfavourable social circumstances). Thus, familiarity with at least one of the above assessment systems is advantageous.

Further reading

Ballard JL, Khoury JC, Wedig K et al. New Ballard score expanded to include extremely premature infants. *Journal of Pediatrics* (1991) **119:**417–23.

Dubowitz LMS. *The Neurological Assessment of the Preterm and Full-term Infant*, 2nd edn. Clinics in Developmental Medicine No. 148. Cambridge: Cambridge University Press, 1998.

Dubowitz LMS, Dubowitz V, Goldberg C. Clinical assessment of gestational age in the newborn infant. *Journal of Pediatrics* (1970) **77:**1–10.

Hitter H, Gorman W, Rudolph A. Examination of the anterior vascular capsule of the lens. II. Assessment of gestational age in infants small for gestational age. *Journal of Pediatric Ophthalmology and Strabismus* (1981) **18:**52–4.

Mongelli M, Wilcox M, Gardosi J. Estimating the date of confinement: ultrasonographic biometry versus certain menstrual dates. *American Journal of Obstetrics and Gynecology* (1996) **174:**278–81.

Parkin JM, Hey EN, Clowes JS. Rapid assessment of gestational age at birth. *Archives of Disease in Childhood* (1976) **51:**259–63.

Pearce MJ, de Chazal R. Establishing gestational age. In: K Dewbury, H Meire, D Cosgrove (eds). *Ultrasound in Obstetrics and Gynaecology*. Edinburgh: Churchill Livingstone, 1993: 211–21.

Vogt H, Haneberg B, Finne PH et al. Clinical assessment of gestational age in the newborn infant—an evaluation of two methods. *Acta Paediatrica Scandinavica* (1981) **70:**669–72.

Related topics of interest

- intrauterine growth restriction
- maternal drug abuse
- neurological evaluation
- postnatal examination.

Birth injuries

The continuing advances in antenatal and perinatal care have led to a progressive fall in foetal deaths due to trauma during delivery. Birth injuries, however, still cause a significant neonatal morbidity of which the neonatal staff should be aware. Difficult delivery by any method is a prime risk factor, but so is a very rapid delivery. An increased risk is also attached to preterm delivery, caesarean delivery, and multiple pregnancy.

Head and neck

Facial and superficial injuries

Facial bruising, cyanosis, and subconjunctival and petechial haemorrhages, which all resolve soon after birth, are common with face and brow presentations, as well as when the cord is wound tightly around the neck. Similarly, the use of forceps commonly leaves superficial bruising on the face that rapidly resolves. Scalp or facial cuts from scalpel injuries may follow caesarean births, and significant facial injuries may require an expert opinion.

The presenting part of the scalp often gives the skull an elongated and pointed appearance (caput succedaneum), which gradually settles. Prolonged traction during vacuum extraction may cause considerable injury to the foetal scalp, with haemorrhage, skin necrosis, and infection leading to permanent scars.

Scalp electrodes may also produce lacerations, which may become infected. Subperiosteal haemorrhages produce haematomas (cephalhaematomas) that are limited by the suture lines (parietal and occipital bones, mainly). The fluctulant swelling eventually calcifies and resolves. Significant cephalhaematomas may be associated with anaemia, underlying skull fracture, and the attendant hyperbilirubinaemia. Apart from some local hygiene and perhaps analgesia when the integrity of the skin has been breached, no treatment is usually required for the above injuries.

Vacuum extraction may result in a more serious often unrecognised subaponeurotic haemorrhage (bleeding beneath the epicranial aponeurosis), leading to significant anaemia and even shock. The immediate management involves volume replacement with blood (or colloid if blood is unavailable).

Intracranial injuries

Significant intracranial haemorrhage and injury may also result from perinatal trauma, most commonly as subarachnoid or subdural haemorrhages and less commonly as periventricular/intraventricular (PVH/IVH), intracerebral, and intracerebellar haemorrhages. PVH/IVH primarily occurs in preterm infants. Haemorrhage within the subarachnoid space arises from small blood vessels (mainly venous) within the subarachnoid space. Subarachnoid haemorrhages are commonly silent but may be accompanied by seizures and, rarely, rapid neurological deterioration. Diagnosis is by lumbar puncture (uniformly blood-stained CSF) and CT scan (better able to exclude other types of haemorrhages, especially in the posterior fossa). Prognosis is usually good.

Subdural haemorrhages may occur after excessive moulding forces on the head that produce dural tears and rupture of the closely applied vessels (mostly seen with difficult delivery of the head, in breech deliveries, and in association with severe birth asphyxia). Symptoms include irritability, seizures, apnoea, altered consciousness, bulging fontanelle, brainstem compression, and cranial nerve dysfunction (for example, third nerve palsy with unilateral fixed dilated pupils), associated with a rapid fall in haemoglobin. Diagnosis is by ultrasound scan (large subdurals produce midline shift) or CT scan (investigation of choice). One should perform coagulation studies, correct any defects, and administer vitamin K. Large subdurals over the surface of the brain with midline shifts or posterior fossa collections with major neurological signs should be decompressed (craniotomy and aspiration of clot or subdural tap). In the absence of concomitant birth asphyxia, small subdural haemorrhages are associated with a good outcome, but large, especially infratentorial haemorrhages may be fatal.

Neurological complication

Facial nerve palsy
The use of forceps may result in excessive pressure being applied on the facial nerve as it is against the mandible, resulting in a temporal, usually unilateral, weakness of the facial nerve. The eye cannot be shut on the affected side. The mouth is pulled forward to the opposite side when the infant cries. Complete resolution is common during the first weeks of life. There may be transient feeding difficulties and artificial tears required until recovery occurs. Distinguish from prenatal nerve injury, from which there may be little or no recovery.

Cervical spine and cord injuries

Injuries to the cervical spine and spinal cord
The spinal cord is especially prone to injury, as it can stretch only 0.5–1 cm as compared to the spine, which can stretch for up to 5 cm. Therefore, cervical bony disruption is always associated with severe spinal cord transectional injury. Injuries commonly occur at the C1–2 level (cephalic delivery) or C6–7/C8–T1 levels (breech delivery). The hyperextended foetus ('flying foetus') has a high risk of cord injury due to its unusual posture if delivered vaginally. The infant is initially hypotonic, hypoventilates and may have absent reflexes. Breathing may be diaphragmatic (unless the phrenic nerve is also paralysed), and paraparesis or quadriparesis is common in survivors. Magnetic resonance imaging (MRI) scans are the investigation of choice.

Injuries to the brachial plexus
If the spinal cord escapes injury, its nerve roots may still sustain injury, especially in the brachial plexus, with a prevalence of approximately one in 2300 births. Excessive pulling on the upper limbs or the head, shoulder dystocia, excessive flexion of the neck during both vertex and breech deliveries may all result in injury to the brachial plexus. Injury to the cervical sympathetic nerves produces myosis, ptosis, and enophthalmos (Horner's syndrome), and unilateral diaphragmatic paralysis follows damage to the ipsilateral phrenic nerve.

Erb's palsy

This is the commonest manifestation of brachial plexus injury and results from traumatic stretching of C5 and C6 nerve roots during delivery (as in traction on head during a shoulder dystocia). The affected arm is adducted and internally rotated with the elbow extended. The forearm is pronated and the wrist flexed (waiter's tip position). The biceps jerk is absent and the Moro reflex is asymmetric. Diaphragmatic paralysis, fractured clavicle, and cervical spine injury must be excluded. Spontaneous recovery is usual. Physiotherapy prevents joint contractures. In selected cases, surgery to the plexus may aid recovery.

Klumpke's paralysis

This follows lower brachial plexus (C8 and T1) injury and affects small muscles of the hand, wrist, and finger flexors (clawhand) and sympathetics (Horner's syndrome). The Moro reflex is reduced on the affected side. Exclude fractures of spine, clavicle, proximal humerus, and arm (radiography of the whole limb, shoulder, and spine is needed). Preserve full range of passive motion with physiotherapy until spontaneous recovery occurs (6–18 months). However, fewer than one in five patients have full neurological recovery, though functional outcome is good.

Abdominal injury

This may occur in the presence of abdominal distension, particularly in association with massive hepatosplenomegaly, malpresentation (especially breech), and rough handling during manipulation. Intra-abdominal haemorrhage may result with attendant shock. Subcapsular haemorrhage may remain 'latent' for a few days until rupture of the capsule, which is heralded by shock. Manage as for haemorrhagic shock and treat any underlying coagulopathy. Request a surgical review.

Perineal injury

Breech delivery is associated with vulval or scrotal bruising and haematomata. In males testicular viability may be threatened by marked scrotal oedema and consequent impaired testicular perfusion. Treatment is symptomatic and pain relief. Exclude congenital torsion of the testes, which requires immediate surgery.

Injury to the limbs

Long bones may sustain mid-shaft fractures (most commonly clavicular) epiphyseal avulsions (mainly humerus and femur) during difficult deliveries. While long-bone mid-shaft fractures are generally recognised immediately when they occur (by the obstetrician), epiphyseal separations often go undetected until the inflammatory phase (healing phase) commences. Risk factors include large infants (such as infants of diabetic mothers), difficult instrumental deliveries, congenital disorder (such as osteogenesis imperfecta), and being the first born.

The affected limb is swollen and tender, and shows minimal movement because of pain (pseudoparalysis). Epiphyseal separation may mimic septic arthritis/

osteomyelitis. The radial nerve may be injured if the humerus is fractured, producing wrist drop. Confirm fractures with appropriate radiographs. Mid-shaft fractures require only simple splinting (seek orthopaedic review), but no treatment (save analgesia) is required for fractured clavicles (often only recognised after the callus has formed). If septic arthritis cannot be ruled out easily, treat as such with intravenous antibiotics until the picture becomes clearer.

Cutaneous bruising and soft-tissue injury

Malpresentations (commonly breech) may result in extensive bruising of the presenting part due to the additional manipulations during the delivery. Preterm infants bruise easily and may develop significant haemorrhage into their muscles if handled roughly during manipulation. This also applies to term infants with coagulation defects. Hypovolaemia, anaemia, and hyperbilirubinaemia may result. Management is symptomatic (blood transfusion or phototherapy).

Further reading

Cyr RM, Usher RH, McLean FH. Changing patterns of birth asphyxia and trauma over 20 years. *American Journal of Obstetrics and Gynecology* (1984) **148:**490–8.

Evans-Jones G, Kay SPJ, Weindling AM et al. Congenital brachial palsy: incidence, cause, and outcome in the United Kingdom and Republic of Ireland. *Archives of Disease in Childhood, Fetal and Neonatal Edition* (2003) **88:**F185–9.

Falco NA, Eriksson E. Facial nerve palsy in the newborn: incidence and outcome. *Plastic and Reconstructive Surgery* (1990) **85:**1.

Geirsson RT. Birth trauma and brain damage. *Baillière's Clinical Obstetrics and Gynaecology* (1988) **2:**195.

Levene M, Chervenak FA, Whittle M (eds). *Fetal and Neonatal Neurology and Neurosurgery,* 3rd edn. Edinburgh: Churchill Livingstone, 2001.

MacKinnon JA, Perlman M, Kirpalani H et al. Spinal cord injury at birth: diagnostic and prognostic data in twenty-two patients. *Journal of Pediatrics* (1993) **122:**431–7.

Medlock MD, Hanigan WC. Neurologic birth trauma: intracranial, spinal cord, and brachial plexus injury. *Clinics in Perinatology* (1997) **24:**845–57.

Rossitch E Jr, Oakes WJ. Perinatal spinal cord injury: clinical, radiographic and pathological features. *Pediatric Neurosurgery* (1992) **18:**149–52.

Related topics of interest

- childbirth complications and foetal outcome
- hypoxic-ischaemic encephalopathy
- orthopaedic problems
- postnatal examination.

Bleeding disorders

Bleeding disorders during the neonatal period are quite common, particularly in preterm infants. Normal haemostasis requires vascular integrity, normal platelet function, and a functional coagulation system (clotting factors or procoagulants, procoagulant inhibitors, and fibrinolysis). In otherwise healthy infants, the commonest causes of bleeding are thrombocytopenia secondary to transplacental passage of maternal platelet antibodies, vitamin K deficiency, and, less commonly, congenital coagulation factor deficiencies.

Clinical features

- Infants with isolated platelet disorders normally appear well except for progressive petechiae, bruising, or mucosal bleeding.
- Vitamin K deficiency haemorrhagic disease or inherited coagulation defects occur in seemingly healthy infants with large bruises or localised bleeding (such as umbilical cord or large cephalhaematoma).
- Bleeding secondary to disseminated intravascular coagulation (DIC) or liver disease generally occurs in sick infants with multiple bleeding sites.
- Severe congenital coagulation factor deficiencies present with bleeding from the mucous membranes, umbilicus, and peripheral blood-sampling sites; bleeding following circumcision; and bleeding into the scalp forming large cephalhaematomas. A minority present with intraventricular haemorrhage (IVH) as the first manifestation.

Investigating the bleeding infant

One should start with a careful history of family bleeding problems, outcome of previous pregnancies, maternal illnesses (especially infections), maternal and neonatal drug administration, and ascertainment of vitamin K administration.

Laboratory investigations should include:

- full blood count (FBC) and film (screen platelet numbers and presence of fragmented red cells)
- coagulation screen
  —prothrombin time (PT)
  —partial thromboplastin time (PTT)—very heparin sensitive
  —thrombin time (TT)
  —reptilase time (RT)—fibrin-degradation products (FDPs), but not heparin, affect RT
  —Normal RT with prolonged PTT and TT suggest heparin contamination, while prolonged RT, PTT, and TT suggest DIC
  —plasma fibrinogen concentration (normal 1.56–4 g/l)
  —bleeding time (BT) rarely needed.

Abnormalities in the above tests usually guide the selection of additional tests such as specific factor or procoagulant assays. For a male child in whom haemophilia A or

B is suspected, specific factor assays must be performed regardless of the coagulation screen (PTT) results.

General management

Appropriate management depends on the correct identification of the haemostatic defect. Commonly FFP (10–20 ml/kg), platelet concentrates (10–20 ml/kg), and cryoprecipitate (one bag, which contains ~250 mg fibrinogen and 80–120 units of factor VIII) are used, and, where a specific defect is apparent, the specific factor concentrates are administered.

Thrombocytopenia

Defined as a platelet count of $<150000 \times 10^9/l$, thrombocytopenia is very common in newborns and may be found in 1–5% of newborns at birth, 22–35% of all infants admitted to the NICUs, and up to 50% of those admitted to NICUs who require intensive care. Severe thrombocytopenia (platelets $<50 \times 10^9/l$) occurs in 8% of preterm and 6% of all infants admitted to NICUs. It is most commonly found in small for gestational age (SGA) infants. Thrombocytopenic bleeding is uncommon if the count is $\geq 40 \times 10^9/l$. Bleeding may occur due to severe thrombocytopenia or impaired platelet function.

A most useful and pragmatic way of classifying thrombocytopenias is to divide them into early and late onset.

Early-onset thrombocytopenia (<72 h)

This is most frequently seen in preterm infants, and evolves slowly, with a platelet nadir at days 3–5, which resolves by 7–10 days. Severe thrombocytopenia (platelets $<50 \times 10^9/l$) is less common, but is usually due to severe sepsis (as in group B streptococcus infection [GBS]), and perinatal asphyxia. The most common cause is an unfavourable prenatal environment, with other causes as follows:

- placental insufficiency (as in IUGR or PET)
- perinatal infection (as in GBS)
- perinatal asphyxia
- alloimmune
- autoimmune
- DIC
- congenital infection (such as TORCH)
- thrombosis (as of the renal vein)
- inherited metabolic disease (such as propionic and methylmalonic acidaemia)
- congenital (for example, congenital amegakaryotic thrombocytopenia or thrombocytopenia with absent radii)
- Kasabach–Merritt syndrome
- bone marrow replacement (as in congenital leukaemia).

Late-onset thrombocytopenia (>72 h)

This is invariably caused by sepsis or NEC, and rapidly unfolds over 24–48 h, with a slow recovery over 4–5 days. In order of clinical relevance, the causes include:

- late-onset sepsis
- NEC
- autoimmune
- DIC
- congenital infection (for example, TORCH)
- inherited metabolic diasease (as in propionic and methylmalonic acidaemia)
- congenital (as in congenital amegakaryotic thrombocytopenia or thrombocytopenia with absent radii)
- Kasabach–Merritt syndrome.

Aetiology of thrombocytopenia

Impaired platelet production

Contrary to previously held belief, it is now apparent that the most important cause of neonatal thrombocytopenia is impaired platelet production (not consumption), due to impaired megakaryocytopoiesis. In 75% of cases, the thrombocytopenia is apparent at birth or within 72 h of life. It is more common in preterm infants. In order of clinical importance, the causes include:

- placental insufficiency (as in IUGR and PET)
- foetal hypoxia
- perinatal asphyxia
- amegakaryocytic thrombocytopenia (as in Wiskott–Aldrich syndrome)
- aplastic anaemia (as in Fanconi's anaemia and TAR syndrome)
- infiltrative disorders (such as congenital neuroblastoma) and bone marrow replacement (as in congenital leukemia).

Increased peripheral consumption and sequestration of platelets (25–35%)

- DIC or consumption coagulopathy. DIC is confirmed by marked thrombocytopenia, prolonged PT, PTT, marked hypofibrinogenaemia (<1 g/l), FDPs, and peripheral blood film schistocytes. Treatment starts with removing trigger factors, and then providing supportive therapy (FFP, platelet concentrate, or cryoprecipitate), exchange transfusion, and rarely, heparinisation.
- NEC
- sepsis
- giant haemangioma (Kasabach–Merritt syndrome). Local consumption of platelets and coagulation factors occurs, resulting in a bleeding tendency. Steroids are beneficial
- exchange transfusion
- polycythaemia
- thrombosis
- inherited metabolic disease.

Decreased platelet survival

- Neonatal alloimmune thrombocytopenia (NAITP). This is the commonest cause of severe thrombocytopenia in the first few days of life, resulting in 400–600 cases each year in the UK. Maternal IgG alloantibodies are directed against paternally derived antigens on the baby's platelets, which are absent from the mother's platelets (just as in haemolytic disease of the newborn). The human platelet antigen (HPA)-1a (Pl^{A1}) (present on platelets of 98% of the general population) is implicated in 80% of cases, and in 10–15%, the HPA-5b alloantigen is responsible. Severe NAITP may also occur with anti-HPA-3a and maternal HLA antibodies, either alone or in combination with HPA-1a antibodies. Note, however, that in up to 30% of cases no antibody may be found. Incidence is one in 1500 live births. NAITP commonly presents as isolated thrombocytopenia ($<10 \times 10^9$/l) in an otherwise well infant with petechiae, gastrointestinal haemorrhage, or serious intracranial haemorrhage. Mother's platelet count is normal. Transfuse-washed (to remove antibody) and irradiated maternal platelets or matched platelets (HPA1-negative irradiated CMV-negative) from unrelated donor. Random donor platelets will give temporary respite in the bleeding infant. Aim to keep a platelet count of $>30 \times 10^9$/l until haemorrhage stops. In all cases of suspected NAITP, when there is serious haemorrhage, or when there is severe thrombocytopenia (platelet count of $<30 \times 10^9$/l), transfuse with HPA-compatible platelets (HPA-1a and HPA-5b negative) until the diagnosis is established. If HPA-compatible platelets are not available, steroids (prednisolone 2 mg/kg per day) or IV immunoglobulin (IVIG) (1 g/kg per day on two consecutive days or 0.5 g/kg per day for four days) may also be beneficial, though the response to IVIG may be delayed for 24–48 h. NAITP usually resolves in two weeks.

- Autoimmune neonatal thrombocytopenia. This results from the transplacental passage of IgG platelet antibodies from mothers with idiopathic thrombocytopenia (ITP), systemic lupus erythematosus (SLE), or hyperthyroidism. Antibody is directed against maternal and neonatal platelets. It is less severe than NAITP. The maternal platelet count predicts the neonatal platelet count. Cord platelet count is rarely $<50 \times 10^9$/l, but the lowest platelet count occurs several days after birth (days 3–4) and rises spontaneously by day seven. Obtain a platelet count on cord blood, and daily thereafter, for the next four days. If platelet count is $<30 \times 10^9$/l, treat with IVIG (1 g/kg per day on two consecutive days or 0.5 g/kg per day for four days) and, if bleeding, transfuse irradiated platelets (10–20 ml/kg). Prednisolone (2 mg/kg per day) is also beneficial.
- Drug induced (as by quinine, hydralazine, tolbutamide, and thiazides).
- Hypersplenism—usually mild with platelet counts of $50–100 \times 10^9$/l.

Platelet function disorders
- acquired—mainly drugs (such as indometacin)
- congenital (as in Bernard–Soulier syndrome and Glanzmann's disease).

Congenital coagulation factor deficiencies

These are rare and the only severe deficiencies present in the neonatal period. The majority are X-linked disorders. Examples include:

- haemophilia A (factor VIII deficiency) with an incidence of 1:20000
- Christmas disease (factor IX deficiency)
- factor VIII-related antigen and von Willebrand's disease
- fibrinogen deficiency (afibrinogenaemia or hypofibrinogenaemia)
- factor XIII deficiency.

Vitamin K deficiency

Vitamin K deficiency bleeding (VKDB) (previously known as haemorrhagic disease of the newborn) classically occurs within the first week of life (early VKDB), but a late form (late VKDB), can develop at 2–12 weeks and as late as 26 weeks. Early VKDB typically presents on days 2–4 of life as haematemesis, melaena, bleeding from cord, bruising, or scalp haemorrhage. Late VKDB often presents as a sudden intracranial haemorrhage (ICH) after minor herald bleeding of the umbilicus or mucous membranes. Death and handicap can result from ICH. Late VKDB typically occurs in exclusively breast-fed infants who have received no or inadequate vitamin K prophylaxis, or infants with intestinal malabsorption (as in cholestatic jaundice). In Europe, the rate of late VKDB ranges from 4.4 to 7.2 per 100 000 births.

- VKDB is caused by a deficiency of vitamin K-dependent clotting factors (factors II, VII, IX, and X).
- In VKDB, the prothrombin time (PT) is prolonged.
- Emergency treatment in a bleeding baby is fresh-frozen plasma (FFP) and 1 mg of vitamin K IV.
- Vitamin K as phytomenadione (Konakion) 1 mg i.m. at birth prevents both early and late VKDB.
- Konakion MM is licensed for oral administration—the recommended dose is 2 mg orally at birth, a further 2 mg 4–7 days later for all babies, and a final 2 mg dose at one month for exclusively breast-fed babies. A single oral dose at birth does not protect all breast-fed babies against late VKDB. Repeated therapeutic doses of oral vitamin K are safe, but babies with malabsorption, diarrhoea, and vomiting, or babies whose mothers forget later doses may not be protected.
- Studies by Golding et al in the UK in the early 1990s suggested that i.m. vitamin K (compared to oral vitamin K) was associated with a twofold increase in childhood cancer. The UK National Cancer Registry challenged this. A similar Swedish study found no such association. The Vitamin K Ad Hoc Task Force of the American Academy of Pediatrics reviewed these and other reports and concluded that there had been no rise in childhood leukaemia or cancer since i.m. vitamin K was introduced there. However, further UK studies have not been able to exclude completely a small risk of an increased incidence of leukaemia, and national guidelines have not been established. Golding's observations were widely publicised by the press, and i.m. vitamin K became very unpopular, leading to a resurgence of late VKDB (1.2–1.8 cases of oral prophylaxis failure per 100 000 live births) even when multiple oral doses of vitamin K prophylaxis had been used. A single i.m. dose of vitamin K virtually prevents late VKDB with the rare exception of those with severe malabsorption syndromes. However, oral vitamin K appears to be as effective as i.m. vitamin K in the prevention of early VKDB.
- In the UK, it is estimated that if vitamin K were not given to other than high-risk infants (that is, preterm infants, infants with a complicated delivery, or infants who are ill, or who have liver disease or difficulty absorbing feeds, especially if breast-fed), 60–80 infants would suffer a bleed (15–20 having ICH), 10–20 would be brain damaged, and 4–6 would die annually.

Thrombosis

Thrombotic complications are increasingly being recognised in neonates partly due to the ubiquitous use of intravascular devices as well as the inherent genetic propensity to thrombosis in some infants. The genetic predisposition to thrombosis is known as thrombophilia, of which there are several types. Control of coagulation depends on a fine balance of procoagulants and anticoagulants. A deficiency of natural anticoagulants (such as antithrombin, protein C, and protein S) or an excess of procoagulants (such as factor VIII and lipoprotein A) may result in a tendency to thrombosis. In addition, mutations in natural anticoagulants (such as factor V Leiden and factor II Leiden) may also predispose to thrombosis.

Clinical features

Venous thrombosis
- congestion and cyanosis of affected limb or anatomical region (such as a leg)
- increased ventilatory support (pulmonary emboli)
- abdominal mass and haematuria (renal vein thrombosis)
- collateral vessel development (abdominal collaterals in inferior vena cava obstruction)
- purpura fulminans (protein C deficiency).

Arterial thrombosis
- PPPPPP (pain, pallor, paraesthesia, pulselessness, paralysis, and prostration)
- hypertension (renal artery thrombosis)
- seizures (intracranial thrombosis).

Diagnosis
- angiography (venography or arteriography)
- Doppler ultrasound
- MR angiography
- abdominal ultrasound with Doppler (renal artery or vein thrombosis).

Management
- Thrombolytic therapy for venous thrombosis has an uncertain role especially in newborns.
- Central venous lines which become occluded may be cleared by urokinase or tissue plasminogen activator flushes.
- Arterial thrombosis may be managed by whole-body anticoagulation (where risk of ICH is acceptable). Tissue plasminogen activator may be useful in this setting; 0.5 mg/kg infused over 10 min followed by 0.5 mg/kg per h until resolution of symptoms.
- Large discrete arterial thrombi (such as aorto-iliac thrombi) may require surgical embolectomy to prevent serious sequelae).
- Should it become apparent that a limb canot be salvaged, give sufficient time for the nonviable and viable tissues to be more clearly demarcated before proceeding to amputation.

Prevention

- Patency of central lines should be regularly monitored, with early intervention when signs of occlusion become evident.
- Arterial line infusions should always be heparinised.
- Never cannulate the radial and ulnar arteries on the same limb (risk of serious hand necrosis).
- Arterial lines are especially risky, particularly in extremely low-birth-weight (ELBW) and IUGR infants.
- Remove arterial catherters that produce signs of peripheral ischaemia or emboli (blue tips to fingers or toes, marked pallor, or absent pulses) or organ compromise (NEC).
- Limb cyanosis or pallor immediately after placement of an arterial line may be due to arterial spam and may be reversible. In sick ELBW infants, where such lines may be vital, it is acceptable to defer line removal while observing the regional perfusion for 30 min. If the pallor does not resolve, remove the line. If the pallor persists beyond 1 h, use a vasodilator (infuse a bolus of tolazoline (0.5 mg/kg) or apply nitroglycerine ointment to the area). If this fails, urgently assess arterial patency (see above), and proceed to thrombolysis or surgical exploration (if indicated), as there is a high risk of regional necrosis and gangrene.

Further reading

American Academy of Pediatrics. Controversies concerning vitamin K and the newborn. *Pediatrics* (2003) **112:**191–2.

Christensen R (ed.). Neonatal hematology. *Clinics in Perinatology* (2000); **27:**3.

Mammen EF. Pediatric thrombosis and hemostasis. *Seminars in Thrombosis and Hemostasis* (2003) **29:**325–8.

McNinch A, Draper G. Vitamin K for neonates: the controversy. *British Medical Journal* (1994) **308:**867–8.

Nathan DG, Orkin SH, Look T et al (eds). *Nathan and Oski's Hematology of Infancy and Childhood*, 6th edn. Philadelphia: WB Saunders, 2003.

Roberts I, Murray NA. Neonatal thrombocytopenia: causes and management. *Archives of Disease in Childhood Fetal and Neonatal Edition* (2003) **88:**F359–64.

Smith OP, Hann IM. *Essential Paediatric Haematology*. London: Martin Dunitz, 2002.

Von Kries R. Neonatal vitamin K prophylaxis: the Gordian knot still awaits untying. *British Medical Journal* (1998) **316:**161–2.

Wong AF, McCulloch LM, Sola A. Treatment of peripheral tissue ischaemia with topical nitroglycerine ointment in neonates. *Journal of Pediatrics* (1992) **121:**980–3.

Related topics of interest

- acute collapse
- liver disorders
- pulmonary haemorrhage
- germinal matrix-intraventricular haemorrhage.

Blood-glucose homeostasis

Perinatal metabolic adaptation

During foetal life, glucose is the principal energy substrate and provides 50% of the total energy needs. The foetal glucose consumption is 5 mg/kg per min. At birth, the newborn switches from a state of net glucose uptake and glycogen synthesis to one of independent glucose production. The ability of an infant to maintain normoglycaemia then depends on the adequacy of glycogen stores, glycogenolysis, gluconeogenesis, and the production of alternative metabolic substrates (such as free fatty acids, lactate, and ketone bodies). This process by which the body mobilises glucose and other fluids is called counterregulation. The main counterregulatory hormones are glucagon and adrenaline. However, the brain does not depend solely on glucose for its energy supply but also on a number of other alternative metabolic fuels, including lactate, fatty acids, and ketone bodies. The blood glucose concentration is therefore only one component of the infant's metabolic milieu and cannot be interpreted in isolation. Blood glucose homeostasis is thus controlled by the opposing actions of insulin and counterregulation (mainly glucagon), and its failure produces hypo- or hyperglycaemia.

Hypoglycaemia

Definition

A normal range for blood glucose in healthy term newborns has not been adequately described. Consequently, there is no universally acceptable definition of hypoglycaemia. Values are influenced by gestation, birth weight, postnatal age and feeding practice. Current evidence suggests that a blood glucose level persistently of <2.6 mmol/l is associated with neurodevelopmental impairment. However, this limit is derived from preterm infants.

Hypoglycaemia may be described as symptomatic (associated with clinical signs of apnoea, cyanosis, jitteriness, lethargy, abnormal cry, or convulsions) or asymptomatic (without clinical signs). Symptomatic hypoglycaemia in term or preterm infants is associated with adverse neurodevelopmental sequelae. Preterm infants may be more (not less!) susceptible to the detrimental effects of hypoglycaemia. Symptomatic hypoglycaemia should be treated rapidly whatever the measured blood glucose level, as there is no definitive threshold for an 'unsafe' blood glucose level.

Incidence

Incidence varies with the definition. A review of literature suggests incidences of 0–8% in term infants (when hypoglycaemia was defined as blood glucose of <1.6 mmol/l in infants <48 h old) and 3–15% in preterm infants (when hypoglycaemia was defined as blood glucose of <1.1 mmol/l).

Conditions predisposing to hypoglycaemia

- sepsis
- asphyxia

- cold stress
- erythroblastosis fetalis
- congenital heart disease (CHD)
- infants of diabetic mothers (IDMs) (transient hyperinsulinism)
- large-for-gestation term infants, birth weight over 90th percentile (hyperinsulinism)
- prematurity (reduced glycogen and fat stores, elevated insulin:glucose ratio, and impaired counterregulation)
- infants small for gestational age (SGA) (reduced fat and glycogen stores, impaired counterregulation, and hyperinsulinism)
- intravenous administration of >10g glucose/h during labour
- prolonged oral and short-term intravenous administration of beta-agonists to suppress preterm labour.

Screening for hypoglycaemia
- There is no need to screen healthy term infants.
- Reagent strip methods (such as Dextrostix [Ames] or BM Stix [Boehringer]) are prone to errors at low glucose levels and are unsuitable for diagnosing neonatal hypoglycaemia. Therapy should not be instituted on the basis of these tests alone— they should always be confirmed with blood glucose measurement.
- Glucose electrode-based analysers are accurate even at low glucose levels.

Causes of refractory hypoglycaemia
Hyperinsulinism
- islet cell adenoma
- Beckwith–Wiedemann syndrome
- nesidioblastosis (B-cell dysregulation syndrome).

Endocrine deficiency
- hypopituitarism
- cortisol deficiency
- glucagon deficiency
- growth hormone deficiency.

Inherited metabolic diseases
- disorders of carbohydrate metabolism (as in galactosaemia and glycogen storage disease type I)
- disorders of fatty acid metabolism (such as medium chain acyl-CoA dehydrogenase deficiency)
- disorders of amino acid metabolism (such as propionic acidaemia and methylmalonic acidaemia).

Investigations for refractory hypoglycaemia
During an episode of hypoglycaemia, the following assays should be performed :

- blood glucose
- cortisol
- growth hormone
- insulin (C-peptide and proinsulin).

It may be necessary also to assay β-hydroxybutyrate, amino acids, glycerol, pyruvate, ketones, free fatty acids, and lactate.

Prevention of hypoglycaemia
- Avoid preventable risk factors (such as cold stress).
- Early (<3–4h) enteral feeding in healthy term or preterm infants should be given priority.
- At-risk well newborns unable to feed orally should be fed by gavage within 1–3h of birth.
- For at-risk newborns, breast milk is nutritionally most appropriate and the safest food (unless mother has HIV infection).
- If enteral feeds are contraindicated (as in extreme prematurity cardiorespiratory distress and birth asphyxia), give 10% dextrose intravenously at a rate approximating the endogenous rate of hepatic glucose production (that is, 3–5mg/kg per min for term AGA infants, 4–6mg/kg per min for preterm AGA infants, and 6–8mg/kg per min for SGA infants). Note that 60ml/kg per day of 10% dextrose = 4.2mg glucose/kg per min. Amount of glucose administered in mg/kg per min = concentration of glucose infusion (%) × rate of infusion (ml/h) ÷ weight of baby (kg) ÷ 6.
- Check capillary glucose every 3–4h for the first 24h in the at-risk groups.

Treatment
Asymptomatic hypoglycaemia
- Send sample for true blood glucose, if possible.
- Feed the infant (breast, bottle, or gavage).
- Correct any precipitating factors (such as hypothermia).
- Repeat reagent strip test (BM Stix or Dextrostix) within 1h.
- If accurate, ward-based glucose electrode measurement or laboratory glucose measurement is <1.5mmol/l, treat as for symptomatic hypoglycaemia.
- Continue at least 3-hourly capillary glucose measurements until result is consistently ≥3mmol/l (12–24h).

Symptomatic hypoglycaemia
- This is an emergency. Measure blood glucose immediately but do not wait for result!
- Commence intravenous 10% glucose infusion giving a 3ml/kg 10% dextrose priming bolus followed by an infusion of 8mg/kg per min. Do not give intermittent glucose boluses alone!
- If venous access is difficult, give glucagon 0.1 mg/kg i.m. or hypostop (a 40% dextrose gel) 0.5 ml/kg massaged into buccal mucosa.
- Adjust the rate of infusion until plasma glucose is corrected and stabilised.
- If fluid overload is likely, change to 15% dextrose or a greater concentration (via central line).
- Gradually reduce glucose infusion while increasing volume of enteral feeds.

Refractory hypoglycaemia
A glucose requirement of >12mg/kg per min suggests transient or permanent hyperinsulinism. The following may help.

- hydrocortisone 5 mg/kg IV/i.m. every 12 h
- glucagon 200 µg IV intermittently or as a continuous infusion (10 µg/kg per h)
- diazoxide 10 mg/kg per day at 8-hourly intervals (maximum 25 mg/kg per day) concurrently with chlorothiazide (to prevent fluid retention) and potentiate the action of diazoxide. Diazoxide inhibits pancreatic insulin secretion, increases gluconeogenesis, and reduces peripheral glucose utilisation
- somatostatin or octreotide (the long-acting analogue at 5 µ/kg 6-hourly).

If the above medical measures are unsuccessful, refer to a specialist centre for more detailed investigations (pancreatic ultrasonography and coeliac angiogram) and possible surgery (partial or total pancreatectomy).

Hyperglycaemia

Definition
Hyperglycaemia is defined as a blood glucose level of >8 mmol/l.

Causes
- stress (as in asphyxia)
- drug therapy (dexamethasone and aminophylline)
- excess glucose administration in total parental nutrition
- intolerance to a 'normal' glucose load, especially in very low-birth-weight (VLBW) infants
- permanent (PNDM) or transient neonatal diabetes mellitus (TNDM).

Management of hyperglycaemia
- Reduce the amount of glucose being infused by reducing the volume or concentration of glucose.
- Exclude sepsis as a cause.
- Take steps to avoid an osmotic diuresis and electrolyte disturbance from glycosuria.
- Occasionally, insulin therapy is required (0.05–0.1 units/kg per h)—when there is danger of unrecognised serious hypoglycaemia.

Neonatal diabetes
PNDM and TNDM are extremely rare, with an incidence of one in 400000 in the UK. Commonly, it is the VLBW term infants that develop hyperglycaemia requiring insulin during the first six weeks of life, the condition resolving in 3–6 months. There is a predisposition to impaired glucose tolerance and type 2 diabetes in later life. Paternal uniparental isodisomy of chromosome 6 (inheritance of both number 6 chromosomes from the father) is implicated.

Further reading

Aynsley-Green A, Hussain K, Hall J et al. Practical management of hyperinsulinism in infancy. *Archives of Disease in Childhood Fetal and Neonatal Edition* (2000) **82**:F98–107.
Cornblath M, Hawdon JM, Williams AF et al. Controversies regarding definition of neonatal hypoglycemia: suggested operational thresholds. *Pediatrics* (2000) **105**:1141–5.

Cornblath M, Ichord R. Hypoglycemia in the neonate. *Seminars in Perinatology* (2000) **24:**136–49.

de Lonlay P, Touati G, Robert JJ et al. Persistent hyperinsulinaemic hypoglycaemia. *Seminars in Neonatology* (2002) **7:**95–100.

Halamek LP, Benaron DA, Stevenson DK. Neonatal hypoglycemia. I. Background and definition. *Clinics in Pediatrics* (1997) **36:**675–80.

Halamek LP, Stevenson DK. Neonatal hypoglycemia. II. Pathophysiology and therapy. *Clinics in Pediatrics* (1998) **37:**11–16.

Sarici SU, Alpay F, Dundaryz MR et al. Neonatal diabetes mellitus: patient report and review of literature. *Journal of Pediatric Endocrinology and Metabolism* (2001) **14:**451–4.

Yager JY. Hypoglycemic injury to the immature brain. *Clinics in Perinatology* (2002) **29:**651–74.

Related topics of interest

- intrauterine growth restriction
- infants of diabetic mothers
- inherited metabolic disease – investigation and management
- inherited metabolic disease – recognisable patterns
- nutrition
- fluid and electrolyte therapy.

Blood pressure

The normal blood pressure profile in newborns and in particular the extremely low-birth-weight (ELBW) (<1000 g) infants has not been completely described. While blood pressure can be measured directly and accurately, the appropriate level of mean blood pressure at which intervention is appropriate remains controversial. Even more controversial is how hypotension should be managed. Hypertension which is persistent is, by comparison, rare in neonates.

Blood pressure should be measured on a regular or continuous basis in all sick infants. Noninvasive Doppler or oscillometric devices may be used. Automatic oscillometric devices (such as Dinamap) tend to overestimate blood pressure in the sick ELBW infants and are unreliable in the presence of limb oedema. Indwelling arterial catheters give more reliable measurements.

Hypotension

Hypotension is one of the commonest cardiovascular problems encountered in the management of VLBW infants soon after birth and affects a significant proportion of all admissions to the neonatal intensive care unit (NICU). The definition of hypotension is disputed.

- The British Association of Perinatal Medicine and Royal College of Physicians defined hypotension as a mean systemic blood pressure less than an infant's gestational age in completed weeks.
- The major concern about hypotension is its association with IVH, periventricular leucomalacia (PVL), and poor neurodevelopmental outcome.

Clinical features
- tachycardia
- metabolic acidosis
- impaired renal function (pre-renal failure)
- decreased pulmonary blood flow (PBF) (impaired gas exchange)
- capillary refill time of >3s (best sites are on the forehead and midpoint of sternum)
- wide central-peripheral temperature gap (>2 °C), but this is less reliable during the first three days of life.

Causes
Cardiovascular disorders
- myocardial dysfunction
- marked tachycardia (as in supraventricular tachycardia [SVT])
- cardiac failure (as in patent ductus arteriosus [PDA])
- hypovolaemia (as in acute blood loss)
- immaturity of cardiovascular regulatory mechanisms.

Pulmonary disorders
- pulmonary air leaks (as in tension pneumothorax)
- excessive ventilation pressures (high thoracic pressure reduces venous return).

Gastrointestinal disorders
- perforation and peritonitis
- NEC (hypovolaemia)
- gross ascites or oedema (hypovolaemia)

Sepsis (vasoparalysis from endotoxin or excessive production of endogenous vasodilators such as nitric oxide)

Drug therapy (vasodilators)
- opiates
- tolazoline
- prostacyclin
- beta-blockers.
- magnesium sulphate

Artefact (air in intra-arterial catheter or transducer or erroneous measurements)

Management
- Replace blood volume with colloid or blood in the infant with an obvious recent acute blood loss (as in a cord accident or foetomaternal haemorrhage)—the infant is very pale.
- The hypotensive, hypothermic, pale, sick newborn infant may benefit from volume expansion (FFP, human albumin, or blood) at 10–20 ml per kg over 30 min. If blood pressure remains suboptimal, commence dopamine (10 μg/kg per min) and gradually increase to 20 μg/kg per min in 5 μg/kg per min increments.
- Add dobutamine (10 μg/kg per min) and increase to 20 μg/kg per min if BP remains suboptimal.
- Alternatively, or in addition, hydrocortisone may be added in VLBW infants (2.5 mg/kg IV 6-hourly for 48 h, then 1.25 mg/kg 6-hourly for 48 h, and finally 0.625 mg/kg 6-hourly for 48 h).
- For refractory hypotension, add an infusion of noradrenaline (0.05–1 μg/kg per min).
- Asphyxiated infants may respond better to inotropes as opposed to volume expansion with colloids.
- Perform cardiac echocardiography in infants with severe hypotension to ascertain myocardial function and rule out associated congenital heart disease or pericardial effusion.

Special notes
- The routine administration of colloid to preterm infants of <32 weeks' gestation is of no proven value.
- Dopamine is more effective than dobutamine in raising mean arterial blood pressure.
- At high dose, the α-adrenergic effects of dopamine produce decreased renal blood flow, decreased PBF (from pulmonary vasoconstriction), and increased myocardial oxygen consumption.

- Dobutamine, with a predominantly β-adrenergic effect, increases left ventricular output and is less likely to increase pulmonary vascular resistance (PVR) than dopamine.
- Normal saline (0.9% NaCl solution) is as effective as 5% albumin in treating hypotension in preterm infants (<34 weeks' gestation).
- Early hypotension (within the first few hours of life, <24h) is *not* usually due to hypovolaemia.
- Low blood pressure is a poor predictor of hypovolaemia in VLBW infants.
- The use of human albumin in critically ill patients is currently debatable, as it may increase mortality.

Hypertension

Hypertension in infants and children is defined as a systolic and/or diastolic pressure ≥95th centile for age and sex on ≥3 separate occasions. Infants must be at rest, and the cuff width should be at least 2/3 of upper arm length.

Clinical features
- tachypnoea
- lethargy
- impaired renal function
- congestive cardiac failure
- haematuria and proteinuria
- oedema (salt and water retention)
- seizures (hypertensive encephalopathy).

Causes of hypertension
Raised intracranial pressure
- IVH
- cerebral oedema (as in asphyxia).

Stress (pain or cold)

Sodium and fluid retention
- renal failure
- excess sodium administration
- adrenal disorders (such as congenital adrenal hyperplasia [CAH])

Drug therapy
- dexamethasone
- dopamine.

Renin-angiotensin mediated
- renal artery stenosis
- coarctation of the aorta
- obstructive uropathy
- cystic/dysplastic kidneys.

Renal artery occlusion accounts for >75% of neonatal hypertension, and renal artery stenosis accounts for approximately 20% of cases.

Management of hypertension
Treatment depends on the cause, but a renal cause will be found in over four out of five cases. Renal ultrasound scan, dimercaptosuccinic acid (DMSA), mercapto-acetyl-triglycerine-3 (MAG-3) renogram, and renal angiogram may all be required (see 'Renal and urinary tract disorders').

- To control hypertension acutely, use diazoxide 3–5 mg/kg IV or hydralazine 0.5–1 mg/kg IV followed by maintenance therapy with oral agents.
- Captopril is useful in severe hypertension (100–300 µg/kg per dose 8-hourly), but watch renal function.
- Mild hypertension may respond to diuretics (especially with fluid overload) or beta-blockers (such as propranolol 0.5–4 mg/kg per day given 6–8-hourly).
- Echocardiography will demonstrate coarctation of the aorta (upper limb BP > lower limb BP).
- Neonatal hypertension commonly has a treatable cause and a good prognosis.

Further reading

Bourchier D, Weston PF. Randomised trial of dopamine compared with hydrocortisone for the treatment of hypotensive very low birth weight infants. *Archives of Disease in Childhood Foetal and Neonatal Edition* (1997); **76:**F174–8.

Cunningham S. What is an adequate blood pressure in the newborn? In: TN Hansen, N McIntosh (eds). *Current Topics in Neonatology 3*, London: WB Saunders, 1999: 62–92.

Dasgupta SJ, Gill AB. Hypotension in the very low birthweight infant: the old, the new, and the uncertain. *Archives of Disease in Childhood Foetal and Neonatal Edition* (2003) **88:**F450–4.

Hope P. Pump up the volume? The routine early use of colloid in the very preterm infants. *Archives of Disease in Childhood Foetal and Neonatal Edition* (1998) **78:**F163–5.

Klarr JM, Faix RG, Pryce CJE et al. Randomised, blind trial of dopamine versus dobutamine for treatment of hypotension in preterm infants with respiratory distress syndrome. *Journal of Paediatrics* (1994) **125:**117–22.

National High Blood Pressure Education Program Working Group on High Blood Pressure in Children and Adolescents. The Fourth Report on the Diagnosis, Evaluation, and Treatment of High Blood Pressure in Children and Adolescents. *Pediatrics* (2004) **114:**555–76.

Seri I. Circulatory support of the sick preterm infant. *Seminars in Neonatology* (2001) **6:**85–95.

Seri I, Tan R, Evans J. Cardiovascular effects of hydrocortisone in preterm infants with pressor-resistant hypotension. *Pediatrics* (2001) **107:**1070–4.

Related topics of interest

- acute collapse
- respiratory distress syndrome
- resuscitation
- transfusion of blood and blood products.

Breast-feeding

It is now widely accepted that breast-feeding gives babies the best start in life. In the UK, 30% of mothers do not, or cannot, breast-feed. By the time babies are six weeks old, only 42% of all infants are being breast-fed, while only one in five mothers are breast-feeding after six months. The UK picture is typical of much of Europe, which has the lowest breast-feeding rates of any global region. By contrast, mothers in the developing world breast-feed on average for two years. Steps have been taken to reduce advertisements for infant formulas: (under the Infant Formula and Follow-on Formula Regulations, it is an offence for formula manufacturers in the UK to provide free or discounted products to pregnant women). The Baby-Friendly Hospital Initiative (BFHI), launched in 1991, is an effort by UNICEF and the World Health Organisation to ensure that all maternity units support breast-feeding. The WHO recently concluded that in the global context, six months of exclusive breast-feeding offers benefit over shorter periods.

Breast-feeding fulfils the following important functions:

- It provides infant nutrition.
- It provides digestive enzymes, such as milk lipases and amylase, that may assist digestion.
- It provides antimicrobial factors (such as lysozyme and interferon) and immunological protection (primarily secretory IgA) to the gut and respiratory tract.
- The antibodies produced in milk are directed against organisms to which the mother has been exposed via the gut and respiratory tract. Breast milk contains nucleotides, which may promote cell-mediated immunity, as well as large numbers of macrophages, polymorphonuclear leucocytes, and T and B cells, whose biological roles are still unclear.
- It provides a variety of hormones (such as erythropoietin) and growth factors (such as epidermal growth factor) that may influence neonatal metabolism and development.
- It provides health benefits for the mother, including a speedier return to the prepregnancy figure and a reduction of postpartum bleeding by increasing uterine contraction. It lowers the risk of premenopausal breast and ovarian cancer, reduces lifetime menstrual blood loss, reduces postmenopausal spinal and hip fractures, and may improve mother–infant bonding, self-esteem, and success with mothering.

Composition of human milk and cow's milk

The composition of human milk changes during each feed, diurnally and throughout lactation.

- The protein content of mature human milk is low (1 g/100 ml) compared to cow's milk (3.5 g/100 ml). Human milk is whey (60%) predominant while cow's milk is largely (80%) casein. The dominant protein in human whey is α-lactalbumin followed by lactoferrin. In cow's milk, the dominant protein is β-lactoglobulin, which is absent from human milk and may be antigenic when fed to human infants. Whey proteins have a high nutritive value for human infants and have a high essential amino-acid content. During early lactation, milk protein content is much higher than in mature milk.

- Human milk and cow's milk have similar fat contents, and most of the lipid is triglyceride (98%), the main difference being the pattern of fatty acids. Human milk has a higher proportion of unsaturated fatty acids than cow's milk and a greater concentration of essential fatty acids. The fat content of human milk rises sharply during a feed (from 2 g/100 ml to 4 g/100 ml), and in an individual the fat content increases during early lactation and then later declines.
- Carbohydrate, as lactose, is present in higher concentrations in human milk (7 g/100 ml) than in cow's milk (4.7 g/100 ml). Lactose enhances calcium absorption and may encourage the growth of lactobacilli (bifidobacteria), which protect against gastroenteritis.
- The major minerals (sodium, potassium, calcium, magnesium, phosphorus, and chloride) are present in higher concentration in cow's milk than in human milk, but, as with trace elements (copper, iodine, iron, manganese, and zinc), the bioavailability is more meaningful than the absolute amounts. Trace elements in human milk are more available. However, there are grounds for supplementing iron in breast-fed infants.
- The energy content of breast milk is 60 kcal/100 ml; for unmodified cow's milk it is 67 kcal/100 ml; for most modern cow's milk-based term infant formulas, it is 65–70 kcal/100 ml; and for special preterm infant formulas, it is 80–82 kcal/100 ml.
- In the developed nations, breast milk from well-nourished mothers has adequate amounts of all vitamins except D and K. To protect breast-fed infants against haemorrhagic disease, 1 mg vitamin K given intramuscularly is effective. Due to concerns about the potential carcinogenicity of intramuscular vitamin K, an oral preparation has been made available. It is recommended that at least three doses be given, though late haemorrhagic disease of the newborn has been reported in breast-fed infants who received three oral doses. It is recommended, however, to give vitamin D supplements (400 IU/day) to breast-fed infants living in inner-city areas and infants of dark-skinned racial groups, who may be unable to synthesise adequate vitamin D (cholecalciferol) in their skin from the available sunlight.

Breast versus bottle

Benefits of breast-feeding

- In the developing countries, the evidence that breast-feeding has a major influence on infant mortality and morbidity is strong. In the developed countries, an increased morbidity (but not mortality) due to infection in bottle-fed babies is supported by recent evidence. Infants who are breast-fed for at least 13 weeks have a lower incidence of gastroenteritis and respiratory tract infections than formula-fed infants, and the benefits persist up to the age of one year. The risk of ear infections and probably *Haemophilus influenzae* is also reduced.
- Previously breast-fed term infants have higher cognitive performance than bottle-fed infants. Similarly, preterm infants fed on their mother's milk have higher developmental scores at 18 months and higher IQ at 7.5–8 years of age than those fed other diets.

- Exclusive breast-feeding for more than four months has a preventive effect on the early development of allergic disease (asthma, atopic dermatitis, suspected allergic rhinitis, and multiple allergic diseases) up to two years of age.
- There is emerging evidence of other longer-term benefits of breast-feeding, including a lower incidence of childhood diabetes and malignancies (particularly lymphoma), and reduced systolic blood pressure at school age.
- Preterm infants fed on human milk have more rapid gastric emptying, tolerate enteral feeds sooner, and are at a substantially reduced risk (up to six times lower) of necrotising enterocolitis.
- Despite similar weight gain over the first three months of life, formula-fed infants become fatter than their breast-fed peers between four and 18 months. Breast-feeding exerts a small protective effect against later obesity in 12–18-year-olds.
- Breast feeds are convenient, sterile, and always available at the right temperature.

Benefits of bottle feeding
- *Convenience.* The mother does not have to do all the feeding and can leave the baby with other carers. However, breast-feeding mothers may also express their milk into a bottle to give themselves a break.
- *Comfort.* Some breast-feeding mothers develop sore nipples, engorgement, lumpy breasts (blocked milk ducts), and mastitis.
- *More sleep.* Formula is more difficult to digest, so infants sleep longer.
- *Less anxiety.* The mother can measure how much milk the baby is taking in, whereas breast-feeding mothers have to monitor their infant's weight gain.

Potential problems with breast-feeding
- Maternal medications may cause toxicity in the infant; therefore, the safety of any maternal drugs administered during pregnancy and breast-feeding should be ascertained.
- Addictive drugs (including alcohol) may be detrimental to the breast-fed infant's health.
- Some rare inborn errors of metabolism (such as alactasia, galactosaemia, and phenylketonuria [PKU]) in the infants may preclude breast-feeding.
- Pesticides (such as dioxins) are excreted in breast milk in 10–50 times the concentration in cow's milk or formulas. They are carcinogenic and toxic to the immune and nervous systems, liver, and skin. The long-term significance of these findings is unknown.
- CMV infections. CMV is commonly present in breast milk and is often transmitted to babies. Postnatal primary CMV infection is not usually associated with significant disease in term infants, as passively acquired CMV antibodies usually protect them. In contrast, very premature babies do not have this protection, as transfer of antibodies occurs principally after 28 weeks. Postnatally acquired CMV can cause serious disease in the very premature infants and long-term sequelae, including severe neurological impairment. However, freezing of breast milk at $-20\,^{\circ}$C for >72 h may reduce CMV viral titres by 99%.
- HIV infection. Babies stand a 10% risk of contracting HIV through breast milk. The risk of HIV transmission is higher in infants who are breast- and bottle-fed than in infants exclusively breast-fed.

- Hepatitis B and C (HBV and HCV) found in the breast milk of seropositive mothers are transmissible to the infant.

Collection and storage of human milk

Infants may be fed their own mother's breast milk (maternal expressed breast milk [MEBM]) or milk donated by other mothers (expressed donor milk [EDM]). Human milk composition also varies according to its source, the postconceptional and postnatal age of the donor, and the manner in which it is collected and stored. Mothers who deliver their infants prematurely produce a preterm milk which has a higher concentration of protein, sodium, iron, magnesium, copper, and zinc (for the first four weeks) than that produced by mothers who deliver at term. Indeed, the concentration of most breast-milk nutrients declines after the first 2–3 months of lactation. EDM may be obtained before (fore milk) or after the donor's own infant has breast-fed (hind milk). Fore milk has a lower fat and energy content than hind milk. Milk dripping spontaneously from the contralateral breast during feeding (drip breast milk) is similar to fore milk (energy content 50 kcal/100 ml vs 65 kcal/100 ml in MEBM).

In order to meet the nutrient needs of preterm, low-birth-weight infants, human milk may be fortified with additional energy, protein, minerals, and vitamins. Fortifiers have been demonstrated to improve short-term growth, nutrient retention, and bone mineralisation.

Expressing breast milk

For the following reasons, mothers may wish to express their breast milk:

- Breasts may feel full and uncomfortable.
- The baby may be too immature or sick to breast-feed.
- The mother may need to be away from the baby, as for a social function.
- The mother may be returning to work.

Methods of expressing breast milk

There are three methods of expressing breast milk:

- by hand
- a hand pump (manual or battery operated)
- an electric pump.

There should be careful hand washing before milk expression, and all containers and pump pieces must also be thoroughly cleaned and sterilised before use. Breast massage and simultaneous (both breasts simultaneously) pumping increase the volume of milk expressed. Frequent (minimum of 6–8 times in 24 h, including once during the night) and efficient milk removal is essential for continued production of milk.

Milk banking

Breast milk (labelled and dated) may be stored in a refrigerator at 2–4 °C for 3–5 days, for a week in the ice compartment of a refrigerator, or for up to three months in a freezer. Babies fed fresh breast milk gain weight better than those who receive it after freezing. Frozen breast milk should be thawed slowly in a refrigerator or at room temperature (not in a microwave) and, once thawed, used within 24 h or discarded, but *never* refrozen. Dedicated human milk banks require significant funding and organisation; effective donor screening for HIV, HBV, and HCV; effective pasteurisation; bacteriologic monitoring; nutrient quality control; and adequate manpower to ensure the smooth running of the facility. It should be noted that the above 'processing' of human milk has a deleterious effect on its biological (that is, antimicrobial activity) and biophysical properties (that is, reduction in fat, riboflavin, and vitamin A and C content).

Parent information and support groups

Association of Breastfeeding Mothers
PO Box 207
Bridgewater
Somerset TA6 7YT, UK
Tel: 0870 401 7711
www.abm.me.uk

The Breast-Feeding Network
PO Box 11126
Paisley PA2 8YB
UK
Tel: 0870 900 8787
www.breastfeedingnetwork.org.uk

La Leche League (Great Britain)
PO Box 29
West Bridgford
Nottingham NG2 7NP, UK
Tel: 0115 981 5599
www.laleche.org.uk

National Childbirth Trust
Alexandra House
Oldham Terrace
Acton
London W3 6NH, UK
Tel: 0870 770 3236
www.nctpregnancyandbabycare.com

Useful websites

www.breastfeeding.co.uk
The prime Internet resource for breast-feeding information.

www.babyfriendly.org.uk
A global programme of UNICEF and the WHO that works with the health services to help parents make informed choices about feeding and caring for their children.

Further reading

Fewtrell M, Lucas A. Feeding the full-term infant. In: JM Rennie, NRC Roberton (eds). *Textbook of Neonatology*, 3rd edn. Edinburgh: Churchill Livingstone, 1999: 325–38.
Fewtrell M, Lucas A. Feeding low birth weight infants. In: JM Rennie, NRC Roberton (eds). *Textbook of Neonatology*, 3rd edn. Edinburgh: Churchill Livingstone, 1999: 338–48.
Lang S. *Breastfeeding Special Care Babies*, 2nd edn. Edinburgh: Baillière Tindall, 2002.
Lawrence RA, Lawrence RM. *Breastfeeding—A Guide for the Medical Profession*, 5th edn. St Louis, MO: Mosby, 1999.
Mohrbacher N, Stock J. *The Breastfeeding Answer Book*, 3rd edn. Schaumburg: La Leche League International, 2003.
Newman J, Pitman T. *The Ultimate Breastfeeding Book of Answers*, Roseville, CA: Prima Publishing, 2000.
Nicoll A, Williams A. Breastfeeding. *Archives of Disease in Childhood* (2002) **87**:91–2.

Related topics of interest

- intrauterine growth restriction
- necrotising enterocolitis
- nutrition.

Cardiac arrhythmias

Milind Chaudhari

Normal rhythm

The heart rate of a healthy neonate shows considerable variations depending on the state of sleep or activity. The normal resting heart rate of the neonate varies between 110 and 150 beats/min with a mean heart rate of 120. Sinus arrhythmia occurs in most normal neonates. Benign supraventricular and ventricular ectopic beats are also common, and most subside spontaneously in the absence of structural heart defects. Persistently abnormal rhythms, as in bradycardia (<100 beats/min), tachycardia (>150 beats/min), or ectopic rhythms, need cardiac evaluation even in the absence of other cardiac symptoms.

Abnormal rhythms

Tachyarrhythmias

Sinus tachycardia

This is the result of a rate of sinus node discharge higher than normal for the age (>150 beats/min in neonates). Common causes are fever, pain, sepsis, blood loss, shock, hyperthyroidism, and drugs (such as catecholamines and caffeine). The ECG shows regular rhythm with normal P-wave axis, P-QRS-T wave sequence, and normal QRS duration. Therapy is aimed at treating the underlying cause.

Supraventricular tachycardia (SVT)

Paroxysmal SVT is characterised by rapid heart rates, usually 200–300 beats/min. Episodes usually begin and end abruptly, and the duration of tachycardia is variable. Short episodes of SVT are well tolerated in most neonates. Sustained SVT presents as pallor, irritability, poor feeding, and respiratory distress, and it can progress to heart failure with cardiovascular collapse within 24–48 h after onset. There is a 20% recurrence risk, which drops significantly after one year of age.

Wolff–Parkinson–White (WPW) syndrome is responsible for up to 40% of SVT in neonates. The majority of neonates with SVT have no structural cardiac abnormality. However, up to 25% have an associated heart defect. Ebstein's anomaly, corrected transposition of great arteries, tricuspid atresia, and cardiac rhabdomyoma are the more common associations. The diagnosis is confirmed by ECG, which shows heart rate >200/min, abnormal P wave morphology, and P wave axis with normal QRS duration. In the WPW syndrome, ECG during sinus rhythm shows a short P–R interval, the presence of a delta wave, and a wide QRS complex changing to inverted (retrograde) P-waves and narrow QRS complexes during tachycardia.

Management of SVT

SVT with cardiovascular collapse

This is managed with synchronised cardioversion: 0.5 J/kg. If the tachycardia persists, repeat cardioversion with double the dose, that is, 1.0 J/kg. If conversion to sinus rhythm is still not accomplished, reconsider the diagnosis of SVT in consultation with the cardiologist.

SVT without cardiovascular compromise
Vagal manoeuvres—for example, application of an ice bag to the face—can convert SVT to sinus rhythm. Adenosine is the drug of choice with an initial dose of 50 μg/kg as rapid IV bolus with constant ECG monitoring. If there is no response, give a second dose of 100 μg/kg after 1–2 min. A third dose of 150 μg/kg can be given after a further 1–2 min. Adenosine is a potent blocker of A-V nodal conduction with an extremely short half-life (<10 s) and can successfully terminate acute attacks of SVT in up to 90% of cases. Intravenous infusion of amiodarone or flecainide forms the second line of therapy for refractory episodes of SVT.

Long-term therapy
Maintenance treatment is required to prevent recurrent episodes of SVT, especially when the attacks are frequent, long-lasting, and difficult to control and also after an episode of SVT associated with cardiovascular compromise. Digoxin (for non-WPW SVT) or beta-blockers (propranolol or sotalol) are commonly used for this purpose. Most infants outgrow their SVT by the age of one year, when maintenance therapy can be discontinued.

Ventricular tachycardia (VT)
VT is uncommon in neonates and is characterised by tachycardia with wide and abnormal QRS complexes (>0.08 s), A-V dissociation, and secondary ST and T-wave changes. In neonates, VT is seen with cardiac tumours, myocardial diseases, prolonged QT syndrome, asphyxia, acidosis, hypokalaemia, or hyperkalaemia. VT associated with cardiovascular compromise needs synchronised cardioversion beginning with 2 J/kg followed by 4 J/kg if no response occurs. During cardioversion, the patient should ideally be intubated and ventilated with 100% oxygen with adequate sedation and analgesia. Underlying acid–base and electrolyte abnormalities should be promptly corrected. Cardiac evaluation and maintenance therapy should be planned in close consultation with the paediatric cardiologist. Beta-blockers are commonly used in patients with prolonged QT syndrome for prevention of VT.

Bradyarrhythmias
Sinus bradycardia
This is defined as a heart rate of <100 beats/min with a normal P-wave preceding each QRS complex. Persistent sinus bradycardia in neonates is seen with hypoxia, hypothermia, acidosis, hypothyroidism, hyperkalaemia, raised intracranial pressure, and obstructive jaundice. Therapy should be aimed at the precipitating cause.

Complete heart block (CHB)
CHB is characterised by independent beating of atria and ventricles. ECG reveals regular P waves (constant P-P interval) and regular QRS complexes (constant R-R interval), but with complete A-V dissociation and slow ventricular rate. Congenital CHB occurs in one in 25 000 live births. Up to 30% of cases can be associated with structural heart disease, as in atrioventricular septal defects or corrected transposition of great arteries. There is a strong association of connective tissue disorders (SLE) in

mothers of neonates with congenital CHB. Most mothers are asymptomatic at the time of delivery, but about two-thirds will develop evidence of connective tissue disorder later. The majority of the patients with congenital CHB are asymptomatic at birth. Symptoms of heart failure develop with persistent bradycardia. Occasionally, in its most severe form, congenital CHB presents as hydrops fetalis, necessitating early delivery. Symptomatic neonates require isoprenaline infusion followed by pacemaker implantation. Prognosis is good for isolated CHB. However, it is unfavourable in infants with persistent bradycardia (<50/min), associated structural heart defects, or prolonged Q-T interval on ECG.

Further reading

Allen HD, Gutgesell HP, Clark EB et al. *Moss and Adams' Heart Disease in Infants, Children, and Adolescents*, 6th edn. Philadelphia: Lippincott, Williams & Wilkins, 2000.

Burton DA, Cabalka AK. Cardiac evaluation of infants. *Pediatric Clinics of North America* (1994) **41:**991–1011.

Gilette PC, Garson A. *Clinical Pediatric Arrhythmias: Electrophysiology and Pacing*, 2nd edn. Philadelphia: WB Saunders, 1998.

Park MK. *Pediatric Cardiology for Practitioners*, 3rd edn. Chicago: Year Book Medical Publishers, 1996.

Park MK, Guntheroth WG. *How to Read Pediatric ECGs*, 2nd edn. Chicago: Year Book Medical Publishers, 1987.

Silove ED. Assessment and management of congenital heart disease in the newborn by the district paediatrician. *Archives of Disease in Childhood* (1994) **70:**F71–4.

Related topics of interest

- acute collapse
- congenital heart disease—congestive heart failure
- congenital heart disease—cyanotic defects
- heart murmurs in neonates.

Cerebral palsy

'Cerebral palsy' (CP) is an umbrella term that covers a group of nonprogressive but often changing disorders where there is primarily a disorder of voluntary movement and coordination. It is caused by damage to the developing brain sometime during pregnancy or delivery, or shortly after birth.

However, CP is difficult to define, has a varied aetiology and can be difficult to diagnose, especially in young children. Furthermore, although CP results from permanent nonprogressive damage to the immature brain, its clinical picture often changes as the child grows older; in some cases, all signs of CP completely resolve. Consequently, to avoid labelling other conditions as CP, the age of ascertainment of CP is set at five years. Finally, although CP remains the most common cause of physical disability in childhood, its severity varies greatly from barely detectable clumsiness to profound and multiple impairments.

Epidemiology and trends in CP

- In spite of the difficulties in defining and classifying CP, the rates of CP around the world are comparable at 1.2–3.0 per 1000 live births (UK 2.0–2.5 per 1000 live births).
- Rates of CP among normal birth-weight groups have remained relatively constant over time (~1 per 1000 live births). Rates among low-birth-weight (LBW, 1500–2499 g) and very low birth weight (VLBW, 1000–1499 g) infants have increased threefold during the late 1970s and 1980s, respectively. Rates among the extremely low-birth-weight (ELBW, <1000 g) infants are also reported to be increasing, though in the late 1980s rates appeared to have stabilised with no further increases. Although LBW infants comprise 5–7% of all live births in the developed nations, they constitute approximately 50% of all cases of CP.

Aetiology
- There are many causal pathways leading to the development of CP, and the mechanisms and timing of events leading to CP in preterm infants are different from those in term infants.
- Current evidence suggests that the majority of cases of CP have a prenatal origin (environmental and genetic factors in particular), with intrapartum asphyxia now thought to be responsible for as little as 10% of all CP cases.

Key risk factors
Risk factors are events that have a statistical association with but do not necessarily cause CP. They may contribute to a chain of events that ultimately leads to CP.

Birth weight and gestation
Rates of CP increase with declining birth weight and gestation. Preterm infants have a risk of developing CP that is 50–70 times that of term infants. One Swede reported specific rates of CP of one per 1000 live births among term infants, eight per 1000 live births among infants of 32–36 weeks' gestation, and 60 per 1000 live births among infants born between 28 and 32 weeks' gestation.

Foetal growth

IUGR is associated with an increased risk (more than seven times in term infants and more than five times in preterm infants) of developing CP. Large-for-gestational-age (LGA) infants also have an increased risk of CP.

Sex

There is an excess of boys with CP, with a sex ratio of 1.3:1 for all birth weights.

Multiple pregnancies

Multiple births are at higher risk of morbidity and mortality. The relative risk of CP (compared to singletons) has been calculated as 4.5 for twins and 18.2 for triplets. The risk is especially high when one twin or triplet dies in utero.

Congenital malformations

Cerebral malfunctions are strongly associated with CP. Data collected in Western Australia on CP showed that 29% of children with moderate or severe CP had a congenital malformation compared to 4.9% for the control group and normal population.

Genetic defects

Rates of foetal and neonatal loss are higher in families with all types of CP. Genetic factors have been recognised in a few families, but inheritance appears to be multifactorial.

Maternal infections

Maternal infections may have an important role in the development of CP. Bacterial and mycoplasmal infections may contribute to CP through two routes. First, they are associated with preterm labour—itself a risk factor for CP. Secondly, it is thought that inflammatory cytokines released from the site of the infection reach and damage specific parts of the brain. A recent study from California showed an association between CP and infection in term infants weighing over 2500 g. Chorioamnionitis had an increased risk of 4.2- to 12-fold of CP, and up to 31-fold for quadriplegia. Additional reports from France and the USA have also reported an association of chorioamnionitis and prolonged rupture of membranes with periventricular leucomalacia (PVL). Cystic PVL, which can develop in association with placental infection, is strongly correlated with CP. Indeed, one report suggested that 44% of CP was 'postinfection'.

Birth asphyxia

Up to the 1980s, birth asphyxia was thought to be a major cause of CP. Recent studies however, suggest that only 3–14% of all cases of CP may be attributable to birth asphyxia.

Postnatal dexamethasone

A number of studies have shown an association between postnatal dexamethasone (usually given for CLD) and the development of CP. A multicentre, randomised trial is now under way and may provide a definitive answer. Antenatal steroids, however, have no statistical association with CP, and remain an essential treatment when preterm labour is anticipated.

Classification

Historically, the description and classification of CP into subtypes have been the subject of much debate. However, one of the best-known classifications was by the Swede Hagberg (the 'Swedish classification'). This divides CP into three main syndromes—spastic, ataxic, and dyskinetic. The distribution of subtypes differs between preterm infants (dominated by spastic diplegia) and term infants with CP (dominated by spastic hemiplegia).

Spastic CP (75–80% of all CP)

Spasticity or hypertonia refers to increased tone evident through observation, examination, or both. There is a high risk of developing contractures, which may further limit mobility. Concerted physiotherapy is required to prevent contractures. Spastic CP is further divided into hemiplegia, diplegia, and quadriplegia.

Hemiplegia (~30% of all CP)

- One side of the body (more commonly the right) is more affected than the other.
- Prenatal causes are present in approximately 75%.
- Accounts for approximately 20% of all CP in preterm infants but about 50% of all CP in term infants.
- The majority of children with hemiplegia achieve walking and normal intelligence. Where learning disability is present, it is mild (IQ $\geq$ 70) with problems of impaired concentration, perception, and spatial awareness. The most commonly associated problems are seizures, mild visual impairment, and behavioural problems.

Diplegia

- The legs are more severely affected than the arms.
- When lower limbs only are affected, the term 'paraplegia' is used (always consider the possibility of a spinal cord lesion in this case).
- Fifty per cent are preterm infants, classically associated with PVL.
- Reported associations include abnormal labour or delivery, or both (50%), antepartum haemorrhage (APH) (40%), and PET (25%).
- A third have learning disability (moderate to severe: IQ < 70), and mild visual problems are common, but seizures are not.
- More children will achieve walking but may need to use aids (crutches or walkers).

Quadriplegia (tetraplegia or bilateral hemiplegia)

- This is a profound disabling disorder produced by bilateral lesions of the cerebral cortex in which all four limbs are involved. Speech and feeding are very difficult.
- Aetiological factors are prenatal in 30%, perinatal in 16%, and postnatal in 18%.
- Intelligence is greatly reduced, and most patients have intractable epilepsy and visual impairment.
- Oesophageal reflux and aspirations are common, as is growth failure.
- Death by aspiration or during status epilepticus is common, with 50% dying before the age of 16 years.

Ataxic CP (7% of all CP)

Ataxia implies incoordination of postural control, gait, and the skilled movements of hand manipulation and speech. Movements are disordered and characteristically short and jerky. In pure ataxia, muscle tone is reduced or normal. Prenatal factors are dominant but the pathogenetic mechanisms are unclear. Ataxic CP has a subtype, ataxic diplegia.

Ataxic diplegia
There is tremor and ataxia with spasticity of the legs. Some achieve independent walking in the later years. The commonest associated impairments include visual problems, problems of articulation of speech, and learning disability (mild to moderate).

Dyskinetic CP (9% of all CP)
Dyskinesia comprises slow writhing movements with variable muscle tone. Dyskinetic CP is largely (80%) due to perinatal brain damage following jaundice, asphyxia, and prematurity. While this represents under 10% of CP in the UK, in countries where G6PD deficiency is common, it may represent up to a third. Generally, jaundice causes a pure choreoathetoid form of CP, asphyxia a choreoathetoid form associated with spasticity, and prematurity rigidity without choreoathetosis. The majority of children with dyskinetic CP are unable to walk due to incoordination and involuntary movements, and lack of head, neck, and trunk control. Communication and feeding are also difficult. Dyskinetic CP is further divided into athetosis and dystonia.

Athetosis
There is generalised incoordination, and movements are hyperkinetic.

Dystonia (tonus changing)
This is a more severe form of dyskinesia with reliance on primitive reflexes, usually affecting all four limbs.

Severity of CP
Pooled data from four UK CP registries show that:

- One in three children with CP is unable to walk.
- One in four has no useful function of arms or hands.
- One in four has a severe learning disability.
- One in ten has no useful vision.
- One in 200 has no useful hearing.

Life expectancy
- The majority of people with CP have the same life expectancy as the rest of the population. However, only 40% of those with three severe impairments will survive 30 years.
- Differential survival is reported among subgroups of children, with CP mortality being higher among those more severely affected (those with severe learning disability, epilepsy, and inability to walk), and the highest mortality rates being in those with spastic quadriplegia.
- Boys with CP have poorer survival rates than girls and full-term infants with CP also have poorer survival rates than preterm infants.

Disorders commonly associated with CP

Epilepsy
Between 20% and 50% of children with CP suffer from epilepsy, the majority having bilateral hemiplegia, and 50% of those with hemiplegia have fits.

Visual disorders
Squints (which may be paralytic) are very common in CP. Optic atrophy, cortical blindness, and visuospatial and visuomotor problems (as in fastening buttons or tying shoe laces) are also common.

Communication problems
The child may suffer from a pseudobulbar, hypokinetic, hyperkinetic, or ataxic bulbar palsy. Speech therapists may be required from an early age to encourage proper lip closure and bite, and improve feeding. Later the child may need formal speech therapy and/or an alternative communication system (such as sign language). Speech therapists may help children with severe drooling.

Behaviour disorders
During the first months of life, the infant is irritable and slow to feed, and often shows a reverse sleep pattern, being difficult to get off to sleep and resistant to hypnotic drugs. The older child shows poor concentration and a decreased threshold for fight and flight.

Educational problems
The majority of children with moderate or severe CP are of subnormal intelligence (25–33% have an IQ of <55) and therefore need to be educated in special schools. However, as many handicapped children as possible should be educated in normal schools.

Independence
To achieve personal and social independence, such children may need the help of an occupational therapist along with modified clothing and special physical adaptations (such as rails and ramps).

Treatment and therapy in CP
The basic tenet of any therapy in CP is to improve function and prevent deformity.

Physiotherapy
Various techniques can be applied to reduce muscle tone. Such techniques should be used with knowledge of the appliances in the management of postoperative cases, serial plastering, splinting, and the prevention of positional deformity.

Orthotics
Stretching a muscle over a prolonged period (as with night splints) encourages increase in muscle length. Jackets prevent positional deformities and try to prevent scoliosis during the pubertal growth spurt.

Independent mobility
Mobility will depend on the type of CP and the age at which certain milestones are achieved. Generally, of children who sit independently by two years of age, most (97%) can be expected to walk independently; if sitting is achieved by three years of

age, 50% will walk with or without support; by four years of age, very few (3%) will ever walk, and if there is still a persistent asymmetric tonic reflex, probably none of those with this reflex will ever walk.

Drugs

Drugs can be useful in reducing the marked extensor spasms and spasticity. Benzodiazepine (nitrazepam) in regular small doses and baclofen, which may be given orally or intrathecally, have been used successfully. Botulinum toxin injections abolish voluntary and involuntary movements, dystonia, spasticity, and reflex excitability. The effect lasts several months.

Surgery

Orthopaedic surgery is used to improve ambulation, improve seating, help nursing, and treat pain or discomfort. Deformity that may lead to irreversible loss of function may be treated or prevented (as in scoliosis or hip dislocation). Orthopaedic surgery is most commonly used for fixed contractures producing deformities. In selective dorsal rhizotomy, there are multiple divisions of dorsal sensory afferent rootlets in an attempt to relieve spasticity and avert the future need for multiple orthopaedic procedures.

Needs and services of children with CP

Health authorities in the UK have a duty to establish and maintain a register of children with disability for the purpose of providing services and evaluating the extent to which needs are met. The guiding principles include working in partnership with children and their families on matters relating to their care and welfare, supporting the family, and improving coordination between the various agencies involved in the child's care.

Website resources

www.scope.org.uk
A UK-based organisation concerned with the needs of people with cerebral palsy.

www.fhs.mcmaster.ca/canchild
CanChild center for Chidhood Disability Research.

www.ucpa.org
United Cerebral Palsy Association.

www.aacpdm.org
American Academy for Cerebral Palsy and Developmental Medicine. The preeminent multiprofessional childhood disability organisation in the world.

www.eacd.org
European Academy of Childhood Disability.

Further reading

Bakketeig LS. Only a minor part of cerebral palsy cases begin in labour. *British Medical Journal* (2000) **319**:1016–17.

MacLennan A, for the International Cerebral Palsy Task Force. A template for defining a causal relation between acute intrapartum events and cerebral palsy: International Consensus Statement. *British Medical Journal* (1999) **319:**1054–9.

Parkes J, Donnelly M, Hill N. *Focusing on Cerebral Palsy. Reviewing and Communicating Needs for Services.* London: Scope, 2001.

Rosenbaum P. Cerebral palsy: what parents and doctors want to know. *British Medical Journal* (2003) **326:**970–4.

Stanley F, Blair E, Alberman E. Cerebral palsies: epidemiology and causal pathways. *Clinics in Development Medicine*, No. 151. London: MacKeith Press, 2000.

Wheater M, Rennie JM. Perinatal infection is an important risk factor for cerebral palsy in very-low-birth weight infants. *Developmental Medicine and Child Neurology* (2000) **42:**364–7.

Related topics of interest

- extreme prematurity
- germinal matrix-intraventricular haemorrhage
- hypoxic-ischaemic encephalopathy
- periventricular leucomalacia.

Childbirth complications and foetal outcome

Labour is the whole process whereby the products of conceptions are expelled from the mother. Modern management of labour has greatly reduced the maternal and foetal morbidity and mortality previously associated with childbirth by applying careful monitoring techniques aimed at anticipating the complications and potential risks of both predictable and unpredictable acute emergencies. These include malpresentation, malposition, cord accidents, dystocia, and trauma.

Dystocia

Dystocia signifies difficult labour. A difficult labour is one where the hazards significantly exceed those of minimal-risk labours. There should be an assessment of the adequacy of the passages in relation to the size of the foetus. Pelvic anomalies or an unusually large baby both have the potential to cause difficult deliveries.

Maternal risks
- trauma (uterine, pelvic, and perineal)
- excessive blood loss.

Foetal risks
- fractured clavicle(s) or limb(s)
- Erb's palsy
- injury to the cervical spine
- severe birth asphyxia (seizures and impaired neurodevelopmental outcome)
- intracranial haemorrhage
- death.

Malpresentation

Malpresentation includes breech, transverse or oblique lie with shoulder, face, brow, compound, and cord presentation. Abnormal presentations occur in about 4% of singleton deliveries, the vast majority (3%) being breech. They account for significant mortality in both mother and foetus.

Maternal risks
- prolonged labour
- rupture uterus
- increased risk of infection
- trauma to vagina, cervix, perineum, and uterus
- risks of emergency anaesthesia and caesarean section
- obstructed labour (vesicovaginal and rectovaginal fistula in developing nations)
- venous thrombosis and fatal pulmonary embolism in puerperium.

Foetal risks
- foetal death
- meconium aspiration
- traumatic instrumental delivery
- cord prolapse and severe asphyxia
- injuries to spine or abdominal contents
- prolonged rupture of membranes and infection.

Breech presentation and labour

Some 30–40% of singletons present by breech at 20–25 weeks and 15% at 32 weeks, but by 34 weeks most have undergone spontaneous version to a cephalic presentation. Subsequent reversion to breech is rare, occurring in 4%. Conditions predisposing to breech include multiple pregnancy, oligohydramnios or polyhydramnios, abnormal uterine shape, hydrocephaly, intrauterine foetal death, or, rarely, pelvic tumours.

There are three types of breech presentation:

- extended or frank breech
- flexed or complete breech
- footling or incomplete breech.

Frank breech occurs in 60–70% of cases and has a low incidence of cord prolapse due to snug fitting presenting part which engages early. Flexed breech has a four times higher incidence of cord prolapse than frank breech, and the incidence is higher still in footling breech presentation. Breech presentation is the commonest association with prolapse of the cord, occurring in 40–50% of cases.

Maternal risks
- sepsis
- trauma to the vagina, cervix, and perineum
- ruptured uterus from external cephalic version
- risks of emergency anaesthesia and caesarean section.

Foetal risks
- prematurity
- cord tears and prolapse
- placental abruption and asphyxia
- fractures of long bones and the skull
- brachial plexus injury and cord transection
- occipital injury and intracranial haemorrhage
- foetal distress and death (following external cephalic version)
- lower Apgar scores (three times as common as with cephalic presentation)
- perinatal mortality may be four times higher than that of vertex presentation
- increased risk of congenital abnormality (6.3% incidence vs 2.4% in nonbreech cases).

Malposition

Malposition of the foetal head is present when it engages the pelvis in the occipitopos-terior position. This occurs in 10% of cephalic presentations and causes difficulties in approximately 10%. The diagnosis is suggested by severe backache in labour with early rupture of membranes. The head presents a larger diameter in the maternal pelvis and may become arrested in the occipitoposterior position deep in the pelvis.

Maternal risks
- prolonged labour
- perineal trauma and bruising
- instrumental delivery or caesarean section
- puerperal complications of instrumental or caesarean deliveries.

Foetal risks
- foetal distress
- birth asphyxia
- trauma and facial bruising
- feeding difficulties (following facial trauma).

Cord presentation and prolapse

This has an incidence of one in 200–300. While the membranes are intact, the condition is labelled cord presentation, but it becomes cord prolapse when the sac ruptures.

Aetiology
- multiparity (head not engaged until labour starts)
- malpresentation, especially breech presentation
- prematurity (small foetus and relatively copious liquor)
- cord abnormality (long cord or low placental insertion)
- operative manoeuvres (forewater amniotomy or manual rotation).

Management
Immediate delivery is ideal if the foetus is alive and sufficiently mature. Cord presen-tation must be treated with the same urgency as cord prolapse. A corrected mortality of 10–17% has been reported, but the rate was only 5.5% if delivery was effected within 10 min.

Foetal risks
- death
- severe asphyxia.

Useful website

www.safehands.org
A charity concerned with helping health professionals prevent deaths and suffering in pregnancy and childbirth.

Further reading

Chamberlain G, Steer P. *Turnbull's Obstetrics*, 3rd edn. Edinburgh: Churchill Livingstone, 2001.

Geirsson RT. Birth trauma and brain damage. *Baillières Clinical Obstetrics and Gynaecology* (1988) **2:**195.

James D, Steer PJ, Weiner CP et al. *High Risk Pregnancy*, 2nd edn. Philadelphia: WB Saunders, 1999.

Medlock MD, Hanigan WC. Neurologic birth trauma: intracranial, spinal cord and brachial plexus injury. *Clinics in Perinatology* (1997) **24:**845–57.

Related topics of interest

- birth injuries
- hypoxic-ischaemic encephalopathy
- pregnancy complications and foetal health
- resuscitation.

Chromosomal abnormalities

Despite their relative infrequency, chromosomal abnormalities constitute a significant workload in the care of newborns. Autosomal chromosomal abnormalities are present in up to four of every 1000 births, and sex chromosome abnormalities occur in up to three births per 1000. Of the autosomal abnormalities, approximately 1.5 in every 1000 are trisomies (mainly trisomy 21), balanced translocations largely accounting for the remainder. Up to 50% of miscarriages, however, may have associated chromosomal abnormalities.

Trisomies

Trisomy 8
This is quite uncommon, most abnormalities being mosaic for trisomy 8/normal karyotype.

Clinical features
Facial
Coarse features with broad nasal root, thick lips, prominent forehead, and protuberant ears.

Limbs
Deep grooves on the soles and palms, mild captodactyly, and limited elbow extension.

Trisomy 9
This is a relatively uncommon chromosome abnormality. Neonatal mortality is high, and most survivors are severely mentally retarded. Cytogenetic analysis delineates two groups: mosaic and nonmosaic complete trisomy 9. Outcome is dismal for infants with complete trisomy 9. Mosaicism for trisomy 9 is predictive of longer survival, but the degree of mosaicism does not predict survival or degree of impairment. Other chromosome variations are found with increased frequency in patients or their parents.

Clinical features
Prenatal
Intrauterine growth restriction.

Facial
Large bulbous nose (in over 50%), widely spaced and deep-set eyes, epicanthic folds, antimongoloid slant of the eyes, microphthalmia, down-turned mouth, micrognathia, protruding ears with abnormal antihelix, hypoplastic phalanges, extra neck skin folds, microcephaly, and large fontanels.

Other
Mental retardation, skeletal anomalies, congenital heart defects, genital anomalies, and intracranial and renal cysts.

Trisomy 13 (Patau's syndrome)

This is even rarer with an incidence of one in 7000 and poor prognosis, most infants dying during the first year of life. The recurrence risk of another chromosomal anomaly is 1%, but this is lower for trisomy 13.

Clinical features
Facial
Small triangular head with sloping forehead, small eyes with frequent colobomata of the iris, and cleft lip and palate.

Limbs
Polydactyly, overlapping fingers, and rocker bottom feet.

Cardiovascular
Congenital heart defects in 80%.

Urogenital
Renal abnormalities.

Gastrointestinal
Gut malrotation.

Trisomy 18 (Edwards' syndrome)

This is relatively rare with an incidence of one in 5000 and poor prognosis, only one in ten surviving the first year of life. The incidence increases with the maternal age. The recurrence risk is 1%.

Clinical features
Prenatal
Intrauterine growth restriction.

Facial
Small chin and mouth, long head, low set and malformed ears, wide epicanthic folds, and ptosis.

Limbs
Second finger overlaps third and fifth and may overlap fourth. Rocker bottom feet, hypoplastic nails, and flexion deformities are common.

Urogenital
Cryptorchidism and renal defects.

Cardiovascular
Atrial septal defects or patent ductus arteriosus.

Neurodevelopmental
Severe mental retardation.

Trisomy 21 (Down's syndrome)

This is the commonest autosomal anomaly with an overall incidence of one in 600–700 births. The incidence varies with maternal age from approximately one in 1200 births at age 20 years to one in 100 births at age 40 years, but with a rapid rise thereafter to one in 40 births at age 45 years. Up to 95% are due to an extra chromosome 21 caused by nondysjunction during oogenesis in the mother. In 2.5%, there are chromosomal translocations, mostly 14/21 translocations and the remainder mosaics.

Clinical features

Facial

Upward slanting eyes, prominent epicanthic folds, protruding tongue, nasal bridge, Brushfield's spots, short neck, and flat occiput.

Limbs

Short broad hands, short incurved little fingers, single palmar creases, gap between first and second toes, and increased risk of congenital hip dislocation.

Cardiovascular

Atrial and ventricular septal defects and atrioventricular canal defects are the commonest. Cardiac defects are present in 40% of cases.

Gastrointestinal

Gut stenoses and atresias (especially duodenal) are more common, including Hirschsprung's disease.

Neuromuscular

Hypotonia, feeding difficulties, and motor delay.

Management

Inform parents of the diagnosis at the earliest opportunity. Confirm the diagnosis with chromosomal analysis. Give parents information on prognosis and general management. Parents may wish to establish links with the local Down's Syndrome Association. Genetic counselling on risks to future children and prenatal diagnosis are essential. The chance of having an affected child is significantly influenced by the maternal age, being one in 2300 at age 18 years but one in 100 at 40 years. After one trisomic child (mother under 40 years), the recurrence rate is 1%, but it is 10% if the mother is a 14/21 translocation carrier (2% if the father is the translocation carrier) and 100% if either parent is a balanced Robertsonian 21/21 translocation carrier.

Trisomy 22

Clinical features

Facial

Preauricular skin tags, beaked nose, anteverted nostrils, antimongoloid slant to the eyes, cleft palate, and short neck.

Limbs

Broad thumbs.

Cardiovascular
Congenital defects in 50%.

Cat's-eye syndrome
Cat's-eye syndrome (commonly associated with anal atresia and colobomata) is a partial trisomy of the long arm of chromosome 22.

Chromosomal deletion syndromes

Deletion of short arm of 4 (4p-) (Wolff–Hirschhorn syndrome)
This syndrome has a dismal prognosis with half the affected infants dying before six months of age. Severe growth restriction is characteristic.

Clinical features
Facial
Fish mouth, cleft lip and palate, colobomata of the iris, low-set simple ears, and preauricular pits and tags are common. Hypertelorism, a prominent glabella, and absence of an angle between the broad nasal bridge and forehead commonly co-exist, giving the face a 'Greek warrior helmet' appearance.

Neurodevelopmental
Grand mal epilepsy and neurodevelopmental delay.

Deletion of short arm of 5 (5p-) (cri-du-chat syndrome)
In addition to the characteristic cry, other features are usually apparent.

Clinical features
Facial
Characteristic small head with small round face, widely spaced eyes, antimongoloid slant to the eyes, marked epicanthic folds, low set ears, and cleft lip and palate.

Other
Renal and cardiac abnormalities.

Deletion of the long arm of 18 (18q-)
This commonly gives a distinct syndrome which can be diagnosed on clinical grounds.

Clinical features
Facial
Characteristic mild facial flattening with prominent protruding jaw and down-turned and 'carp-like' mouth. Hypertelorism, nystagmus, epicanthic folds with pale discs, and prominent ears with the narrow external canal associated with deafness.

Limbs
Fingers are tapered and thumbs are proximally implanted with dimples over extensor surfaces of joints.

Deletion of the long arm of 22 (22q11) (DiGeorge syndrome)

This disorder, also known as the velocardiofacial syndrome or Shprintzen syndrome, is one of the most common human genetic disorders with at least 185 reported anomalies. It is inherited in an autosomal dominant fashion (93% of probands have de novo mutations and 7% inherit from one parent). The 22q11.2 deletion syndrome is diagnosed in individuals with a submicroscopic deletion of chromosome 22 detected by fluorescence in situ hybridisation FISH with DNA probes from the DiGeorge chromosomal region (DGCR). Less than 5% of affected individuals have a negative FISH test, having variant DGCR deletions or other deletions. Microdeletions of chromosome 22q11.2 have also been detected in patients with the conotruncal anomaly face syndrome (CTAF), some cases of 'Opitz' G/BBB syndrome, and Caylor cardiofacial syndrome.

Clinical features
Cardiovascular
Congenital heart defects are present in 74% of patients (especially tetralogy of Fallot, interrupted aortic arch, ventricular septal defect [VSD], and truncus arteriosus).

Palatal abnormalities
These are present in 70%, especially velopharyngeal incompetence, submucosal cleft palate, overt cleft palate, and bifid uvula.

Feeding difficulties
Some 30% have feeding difficulties, often severe, due to dysmotility in the pharyng-oesophageal area. Nasal regurgitation, gastrooesophageal reflux (GOR), constipation, and failure to thrive are common in infancy.

Immunological
Up to 77% of patients have an immunological deficiency; impaired T-cell production, impaired T-cell function, humoral defects, and IgA deficiency. However, T-cell production improves with time.

Parathyroid function
Some 30% of patients have hypocalcaemia, but calcium homeostasis typically improves with age.

Craniofacial
Auricular abnormalities, nasal abnormalities, hooded eyelids, malar flatness, suborbital congestion, open-mouthed expression, asymmetric face, retrognathia, microcephaly, hypotonia, flaccid facies, and abundant scalp hair may be present in most Caucasians but rare in others.

Eyes
Ptosis, epicanthia folds, posterior embryotoxon, tortuous retinal vessels, deep iris crypts, small optic nerves, strabismus, and amblyopia may be present.

Ear, nose, and throat
Auricular abnormalities, preauricular pits or tags, narrow external auditory meati,

prominent nasal root, chronic otitis media and chronic sinusitis, mild conductive and sensorineural hearing loss, laryngomalacia, and laryngeal webs have all been reported.

Endocrine/metabolic
Relatively small stature, growth hormone deficiency, hypoplasia of the pituitary gland, hypothyroidism, hypoparathyroidism, and pseudohypoparathyroidism have all been reported.

Neurodevelopmental
Hypotonia in infancy and learning difficulties are common. Seizures, strokes, periventricular cysts (mostly anterior horns), multicystic white-matter lesions of unknown significance, enlarged sylvian fissure, cerebellar hypoplasia/dysgenesis, and cerebellar ataxia are reported less frequently. Motor development is delayed, as is mental development, along with speech and language impairment and attention-deficit hyperactivity disorder (ADHD).

Genitourinary
Renal tract abnormalities (such as single kidneys, multicystic dysplastic kidneys, horseshoe kidneys, hydronephrosis, renal tubular acidosis, hypospadias, and cryptorchidism) may be found in 30%.

Autoimmune disease
Idiopathic thrombocytopenia, hyperthyroidism, hypothyroidism, vitiligo, coeliac disease, and haemolytic anaemia have been reported.

Musculoskeletal system
Cervical spine abnormalities, rib abnormalities, vertebral anomalies (such as butterfly and hemivertebrae), upper and lower limb abnormalities (such as polydactyly, syndactyly, talipes, and joint dislocations), scoliosis, and chronic leg pains have all been reported.

Turner's syndrome (45, XO)
With an incidence of approximately one in 5000 births, this syndrome has, by comparison, a favourable prognosis.

Clinical features
Prenatal
Nuchal swelling or hydrops.

Facial
Webbed neck (pterygium colli) and low trident posterior hairline.

Limbs
Lymphoedema of dorsum of hands and feet, increased carrying angle at the elbow, and convex deep-set nails.

Cardiovascular
Cardiac defects, especially coarctation of the aorta (20%).

Other

Widespread nipples and broad chest, renal anomalies, but good neurodevelopmental outlook.

Family support groups and information

www.cafamily.org.uk/
Contact a Family: National charity dedicated to helping families who care for children with any disability or special need.

www.downs-syndrome.org.uk
Down's Syndrome Association.

www.vcfsef.org
Velo-cardio-facial syndrome education foundation.

www.geneticalliance.org
Alliance of Genetic Support Groups.

Useful websites

www.ncbi.nlm.nih.gov/Omim/
On-line Mendelian Inheritance in Man (OMIN) is a fully referenced mine of information.

www.phgu.org.uk
Public Health Genetics Unit in Cambridge.

www.kumc.edu/gec
University of Kansas Medical Center – Genetics Education Center.

www.geneclinics.org
GeneTests website – a huge medical genetics information resource funded by the US National Institutes of Health.

Further reading

Arnold GL, Kirby RS, Stern TP et al. Trisomy 9: review and report of two new cases. *American Journal of Medical Genetics* (1995) **56:**252–7.
Baraister M, Winter RM. *Colour Atlas of Congenital Malformation Syndromes.* London: Mosby-Wolfe, 1996.
Gilbert P. *The A–Z Reference Book of Syndromes and Inherited Disorders,* 2nd edn. London: Chapman & Hall, 1996.
Hall JG (ed.). Medical Genetics I & II, *Pediatric Clinics of North America* (1992) **39:**(1 and 2).
Harper PS. *Practical Genetic Counselling,* 3rd edn. Oxford: Butterworth-Heinemann, 1991.
Jones KL. *Smith's Recognizable Patterns of Human Malformation,* 5th edn. Philadelphia: WB Saunders, 1997.

Related topics of interest

- congenital malformations and birth defects
- intrauterine growth restriction
- prenatal diagnosis.

Chronic lung disease

The introduction of mechanical ventilation to neonatal medicine in the 1960s ushered in a hitherto undescribed disorder, bronchopulmonary dysplasia (BPD). Classic BPD was originally described by Northway in 1966. Its diagnosis was based on progressive radiographic changes in preterm infants and who had prolonged ventilator and oxygen dependence as a consequence of their treatment for respiratory distress syndrome (RDS). Northway described four distinct radiographic stages of BPD: (1) RDS, (2) diffusely hazy, (3) diffusely bubbly, interstitial pattern, and (4) hyperaeration, focal hyperlucency, and alternating strands of opacification. Later, Bancalari's definition (1979) required a history of assisted ventilation, radiographic abnormalities, and oxygen dependence at 28 days, with continuing respiratory symptoms. Shennan (1988) noted that the need for supplemental oxygen beyond 36 weeks postconceptual age (PCA) in these infants was more predictive of later pulmonary morbidity. He recommended that oxygen dependence at 36 weeks PCA, instead of 28 days after birth, be used to define BPD. The advances in neonatal care have decreased the incidence of BPD only in the larger, more mature preterm infants, and not in VLBW infants, although the disease is now less severe than in the past. As many infants now do not have the radiographic changes of classic BPD, the term 'chronic lung disease' (CLD) is now preferred. The term is also used to denote persistent pulmonary insufficiency and oxygen requirement beyond 36 weeks' PCA regardless of the cause or need for mechanical ventilation. The risk of CLD is directly proportional to the severity of the initial lung disease, duration of ventilation, and oxygen administration, and is inversely related to birth weight and gestational age (the most immature infants have the highest risk). For VLBW infants who require ventilation support, 60% are oxygen dependent at 28 days, and 30% remain oxygen dependent at 36 weeks PCA.

Pathogenesis

The pathogenesis of CLD is complex and multifactorial.

- Pulmonary oxygen toxicity is a major contributor, as high concentrations of oxygen induce lung inflammation and the release of chemotactic factors which attract pulmonary leucocytes to the lung, leading to the release of more inflammatory mediators and proteolytic enzymes. The preterm infant has lower levels of antiproteases, and of antioxidant enzymes, and therefore is more susceptible to oxygen toxicity and to CLD than is the full-term infant.
- There is a correlation between the development of CLD and the severity of the initial lung disease, partly because infants with the most severe lung disease require the highest ventilator pressures. 'Barotrauma' is the term used for pressure-induced injury. Recent studies, however, suggest that excessive variations in lung volumes during mechanical ventilation are the principal mechanism of iatrogenic lung injury. This mechanism is known as 'volutrauma'.
- Several other factors contribute to the pathogenesis of CLD. The presence of a symptomatic patent ductus arteriosus, excessive fluid administration early in the neonatal course, pulmonary air leak, vitamins A and E deficiency, early intravenous

fat infusions, family history of asthma, intrauterine and postnatal infection, with *Ureaplasma urealyticum*, male gender, and white race have all been postulated.

- The currently favoured mechanism involves the interaction of all the above risk factors. Simply put, intermittent positive pressure ventilation (IPPV) produces shearing and stretching forces which disrupt the pulmonary epithelium, exposing the subepithelial connective tissue and vascular bed to oxidative damage. The accompanying release of chemotactic mediators recruits inflammatory cells, which cause further damage by releasing lysosomal proteases. This leads to extensive damage to the pulmonary epithelium, endothelium, and extracellular lung matrix. The resulting proliferation of fibroblasts and collagen deposition produce alveolar and interstitial destruction with marked architectural remodelling of the lung.

- Histopathology shows alveolar type II cell hyperplasia, intra-alveolar and interstitial fibrosis, alveolar wall rupture, peribronchial and peribronchiolar fibrosis, obliterative fibroproliferative bronchiolitis, and areas of hyperinflated sacs alternating with dispersed foci of atelectasis. The overall picture indicates a process of simultaneous acute and chronic lung destruction, progressing to an abnormal healing phase with fibroproliferative lung damage, diminished alveolisation, and increased pulmonary vascular resistance.

Clinical features

Respiratory system
- tachypnoea with elevated minute ventilation
- increased work of breathing and oxygen consumption
- relative hypoxia with CO_2 retention
- lobar emphysema and atelectasis resulting from air trapping
- large airway collapse from tracheobronchomalacia
- increased pulmonary resistance and reduced compliance
- ventilation-perfusion mismatch
- bronchial hyperreactivity and wheezing attacks.

General and systemic
- growth failure (lower energy intake and high energy expenditure)
- modest elevation of systemic blood pressure
- pulmonary hypertension (and eventually cor pulmonale)
- increased incidence of central and obstructive apnoeas
- increased incidence of late sudden death (up to sevenfold).

During infancy, gross motor delay is common, and this may improve in line with improvements in the respiratory status and somatic growth.

In later childhood, there is a greater risk of more adverse neuropsychological and educational outcomes, including lower verbal and performance IQ, increased hyperactivity, and worse fine motor function, receptive vocabulary, visual-perceptual integration, and memory.

Prevention

- The most effective way of preventing CLD is avoiding preterm delivery and RDS.
- Antenatal steroids decrease the incidence of RDS and requirement for assisted ventilation by 40–60%, increase the concentration of antioxidant enzymes in the preterm lung, and thus decrease the incidence of CLD.
- Surfactant therapy decreases mortality with little effect on the frequency of CLD.
- Early postnatal steroids commencing at 12h of age for 1–12 days, or between seven and 14 days of age, have reduced the incidence of, and deaths from, CLD. However, the effect of steroids on long-term neurodevelopmental outcome remains uncertain, some recent studies suggesting an excess of neuromotor abnormalities in the treated infants.
- Modes of ventilation may also influence the development of CLD. The use of early nasal continuous positive airway pressure (CPAP) and tolerance of high $PaCO_2$ significantly reduces the incidence of CLD. 'Gentler' ventilation with virtually no upper limit to allowable levels of arterial CO_2 tension (permissive hypercapnia) has a tendency to decrease the incidence of CLD.

Management

General

- Once a diagnosis of CLD is established, use the lowest peak inflation pressures and rates to reduce ongoing lung injury in infants receiving assisted ventilation. As hypoxia increases pulmonary vascular resistance and right ventricular strain, maintain adequate oxygenation ($PaO_2 > 7$ kPa or saturations over 95%). Allow $PaCO_2$ to rise as long as the pH is satisfactory (>7.25).
- Transfuse packed red cells if haematocrit falls below 40% (haemoglobin <12 g/dl).
- Nursing in prone position improves oxygenation and decreases pulmonary resistance. Following extubation, those requiring ≤30% may receive their supplemental oxygen via a nasal cannula connected to a low-flow meter, starting at 0.2–0.5 l/min and reducing progressively to less than 0.05 l/min before discontinuing oxygen therapy.
- If necessary, infants may be discharged home on oxygen therapy which reduces hospital stay and treatment costs.
- Gastrooesophageal reflux (GOR) is common and should be managed expectantly.
- Severe bronchiolitis and pneumonia caused by respiratory syncytial virus (RSV) can be life-threatening. Prophylaxis with RSV immunoglobulin (RSVIG) (Synagis, Abbott Laboratories), though expensive, reduces the incidence of RSV infection in infants with CLD. However, prophylactic RSVIG has to be administered by i.m. injection (15 mg/kg into the anterolateral thigh) once each month, during the season for RSV at a cost of £2000—3500 per infant per season.
- Infants with CLD are at increased risk of excess morbidity and mortality from influenza virus infections and invasive pneumococcal disease. It is therefore recommended that they receive annual influenza immunisation and full doses of the heptavalent pneumococcal polysaccharide-conjugated vaccine (Prevenar, Wyeth Pharmaceuticals), beginning at two months of age and continuing up to the age of two years.

Steroids

- Inflammation has an important early role in the pathogenesis of CLD.
- Steroids exert their effect by reducing the tracheobronchial alveolar inflammatory response and pulmonary oedema, thereby facilitating gas exchange, improving airway patency and lung compliance, and facilitating weaning from assisted ventilation. Additional potential benefits include increased surfactant synthesis, enhanced β-adrenergic activity, increased antioxidant production, stabilisation of cell lysosomal membranes, and inhibition of prostaglandin and leukotriene synthesis. Recent trials in which preterm infants at <48 h have been treated with ≥4-day courses of dexamethasone have shown a significant decrease in the risk of death or CLD at 36 weeks' PCA.
- The recommended starting dose of dexamethasone is in the region of 0.5–0.6 mg/kg per day, gradually tapered over 1–6 weeks. More than one course may be given.
- Steroids are associated with several complications including glucose intolerance, elevated blood pressure, impaired growth (decrease in weight, length, and head circumference), myocardial hypertrophy, gastroduodenal perforation (especially when dexamethasone is used at <48 h of life), leucocytosis (especially neutrophilia), suppression of the hypothalamo-pituitary-adrenal axis, and risk of developing renal calcification and nephrocalcinosis (especially in conjunction with frusemide), and they possibly cause new periventricular echodensities.
- After steroids are withdrawn, catch-up growth is usual, the cardiac hypertrophy resolves, and adrenal responsiveness is regained.
- More recent follow-up studies, involving large numbers of subjects, have raised concerns that dexamethasone treatment of preterm infants may be associated with an increased risk of cerebral palsy (CP) or abnormal neuromotor development. Current evidence suggests that treatment early in the course of disease (<7 days of life) is associated with the greatest risk of adverse effects. In addition, the beneficial effect of dexamethasone in decreasing CLD is more apparent in infants with severe lung disease. On the basis of current evidence, dexamethasone treatment cannot be recommended for widespread use among preterm infants, but it should be focused only on severe life-threatening lung disease, starting perhaps at 7–14 days of life, and for the shortest possible duration (minimum ≥4 days) to achieve the desired effect. The minimum effective dose of dexamethasone is yet to be determined. It is also possible that other corticosteroids, such as hydrocortisone, may be associated with decreased adverse effects, and studies comparing hydrocortisone to dexamethasone are needed.

Diuretics

- There is significant interstitial pulmonary oedema in CLD.
- The reported benefits of diuretic therapy include improvements in minute and alveolar ventilation, oxygenation, lung compliance, pulmonary resistance, duration of oxygen and ventilator therapy, and hospital mortality.
- Furosemide causes potent diuresis with associated electrolyte imbalance, hypercalciuria, nephrocalcinosis, nephrolithiasis, and secondary hyperparathyroidism. The renal calcification resolves after cessation of frusemide therapy. Alternate-day therapy may be as effective but without the adverse metabolic consequences.
- Thiazides are less potent diuretics which also improve lung mechanics and are

preferred for maintenance therapy. Chlorothiazide or hydrochlorothiazide with spironolactone, given twice daily, is generally used. Amiloride should be avoided, as it inhibits the pulmonary transepithelial Na^+ transport mechanism.
- Diuretics are probably best used to wean the oxygen-dependent near-term infants off oxygen.

Bronchodilators
- The rationale for using bronchodilators is that infants with CLD have reactive airways disease and bronchiolar smooth muscle hypertrophy.
- Both β-agonists (such as salbutamol) and muscarinic antagonists (such as ipratropium bromide) improve lung mechanics (compliance and resistance) and oxygenation in the short term.

Nutrition
- As growth failure is common in infants with CLD, nutritional intervention is of major importance.
- The input of dieticians is often necessary to provide energy intakes of ≥150 kcal/kg per day.
- Lung repair is impaired by undernutrition.

Long-term outlook

- Most postneonatal hospital deaths in VLBW infants occur in infants with CLD.
- Up to 50% of those still ventilator-dependent at six months will die.
- The mortality following discharge from hospital is 11–20%, and the risk of sudden infant death is sevenfold that of controls without CLD.
- There is a tendency for lung mechanics (compliance and resistance) to improve with age as the airways grow and new alveoli are formed. The risk for developing chronic obstruction or reactive airways disease remains in later life.
- There is clear evidence of adverse cardiovascular sequelae in infants with severe CLD. There may be transient systemic hypertension responsive to antihypertensive therapy, or severe systemic hypertension associated with increased mortality. Some infants develop pulmonary hypertension, right ventricular hypertrophy, and eventually cor pulmonale, which can be readily monitored by echocardiography and angiography. Pulmonary hypertension is a serious complication but may be ameliorated by oral hydralazine or nifedipine.
- Growth failure proportional to the duration and severity of CLD is also common (found in 30–40%) due mainly to the increased work of breathing, chronic hypoxia, diuretic and steroid therapy, and reduced calorie intakes.
- Neurodevelopmental problems may be identified in up to 40% of infants, but this is not related to the duration of oxygen or ventilator therapy. The effects of corticosteroids in ELBW infants (at highest risk of mortality from severe lung disease) and on long-term pulmonary and neurodevelopmental outcome deserves additional study.
- The potential effect of dexamethasone on the preterm infant's risk of diseases of adulthood, such as hypertension, diabetes, or coronary heart disease, is currently unknown and requires further study.

- CLD remains a major cause of neonatal morbidity and mortality; it is associated with chronic respiratory insufficiency, repeated hospitalisations, growth failure, and neurodevelopmental problems. The physiological basis of the adverse effect of CLD on neurodevelopmental outcome is unknown, but recurrent hypoxaemia, lack of specific nutrients and malnutrition, toxic effects of drug therapies (including steroids), and reduced environmental stimulation may all contribute to the altered brain growth, development, and function. Clearly, other approaches to the prevention and treatment of CLD should be explored.

Further reading

Abman SH, Groothius JR. Pathophysiology and treatment of bronchopulmonary dysplasia. *Pediatric Clinics of North America* (1994) **41:**277.

American Academy of Pediatrics, Committee on the Fetus and Newborn. Postnatal corticosteroids to treat or prevent chronic lung disease in preterm infants. *Pediatrics* (2002) **109:**330–8.

Bancalari E (ed.). Bronchopulmonary dysplasia. *Seminars in Neonatology* (2003) **8:**(1).

Banks BA. Postnatal dexamethasone for bronchopulmonary dysplasia. *NeoReviews* (2002) **3:**e24.

Barrington KJ, Finer NN. Treatment of bronchopulmonary dysplasia. *Clinics in Perinatology* (1998) **25:**177–202.

Baud O. Postnatal steroid treatment and brain development. *Archives of Disease in Childhood Fetal and Neonatal Edition* (2004) **89:**F96–100.

Bhutta T, Ohlsson A. Systematic review and meta-analysis of early postnatal dexamethasone for prevention of chronic lung disease. *Archives of Disease in Childhood Fetal and Neonatal Edition* (1998) **79:**F26–33.

Farrell PA, Fiascone JM. Bronchopulmonary dysplasia and chronic lung disease of infancy. In: TJ David (ed.). *Recent Advances in Paediatrics*, 17. Edinburgh: Churchill Livingstone, 1999: 17–34.

Greenough A, Milner AD (eds). *Neonatal Respiratory Disorders*, 2nd edn. London: Arnold, 2003.

Related topics of interest

- complications of mechanical ventilation
- extreme prematurity
- gastrooesophageal reflux
- home oxygen therapy
- mechanical ventilation
- outcome of neonatal intensive care
- pulmonary air leaks
- respiratory distress syndrome.

Complications of mechanical ventilation

While artificial mechanical ventilation has been life-saving for infants with respiratory failure and a variety of other conditions, it is associated with a significant morbidity and several potential complications. The incidence of complications varies between centres due partly to differences in patient demographics and the indications for assisted ventilation. Overall complication rates of 8–24% are reported. Complications may occur both in the short term and after prolonged periods of ventilation.

Short-term complications

- pneumothorax
- tube blockage
- pneumoperitoneum
- pneumomediastinum
- oropharyngeal trauma
- right upper lobe collapse
- subcutaneous emphysema
- pulmonary interstitial emphysema (PIE)
- iatrogenic hypotension (excessive ventilatory pressures).

Clinical presentation
- gradual worsening of gas exchange (PIE)
- oropharyngeal bleeding or pulmonary haemorrhage
- abdominal distension of rapid onset (pneumoperitoneum)
- acute collapse/shock (pneumothorax and/or pneumopericardium)
- sudden deterioration after a period of stability (tube blockage/pneumothorax).

Investigations
- chest radiograph
- arterial blood gases
- chest transillumination.

Management
Chest transillumination allows rapid detection of significant pulmonary air leaks, especially if unilateral. If the situation is not clear, a chest radiograph should be performed. In emergencies, the chest should be needled and a chest drain inserted if a symptomatic air leak is detected. While very small pneumothoraces and pneumomediastinal air collections may be observed, all other symptomatic air leaks should be drained. PIE may be managed by adopting a low-pressure, fast-rate strategy including high-frequency oscillatory ventilation. A collapsed right upper lobe may be re-expanded by withdrawing the endotracheal (ET) tube from the right main bronchus. In rapid acute deteriorations associated with bradycardia and hypoxaemia, it is worth changing the ET tube electively in case it has become blocked or dislodged.

Long-term complications

- CLD
- pneumothorax
- accidental extubation
- vocal cord palsy
- postextubation stridor
- dysphonia
- poor somatic growth
- laryngotracheomalacia
- bronchocutaneous fistula
- periventricular leucomalacia
- tracheal traumatic granulomas
- repeated pulmonary infections
- palatal deformities (oral intubation)
- nasal deformities (nasal intubation)
- endobronchial intubation and atelectasis
- side effects of prolonged sedation and medication.

Clinical presentation

Acquired airway narrowing (as in subglottic stenosis) frequently presents as postextubation stridor and/or failed extubation (with respiratory distress and apnoeas). Vocal cord palsies may present with postextubation respiratory distress or dysphonia. CLD often presents as an insidious prolonged ventilator and oxygen dependency. Early persistent hypocapnia in preterm infants is now recognised to be a risk factor for developing CLD, severe intraventricular haemorrhage, cystic periventricular leucomalacia, and cerebral palsy.

Management

Significant orofacial deformities may require plastic surgery and should be referred for expert opinion. Steroids (dexamethasone) may be tried for postextubation stridor as 1–2 mg/kg per day p.o. or IV given 6-hourly, beginning 24 h prior to extubation and continuing 24–48 h afterwards. If this is unsuccessful, an ear, nose, and throat (ENT) opinion should be obtained with a view to laryngoscopy and possible surgery. Apart from the orofacial deformities from prolonged intubation, which may require plastic surgery, many of the acquired airway problems (such as vocal cord palsy and dysphonia) tend to resolve with time.

Further reading

Contencin P, Narcy P. Size of endotracheal tube and neonatal acquired subglottic stenosis. Study Group for Neonatology and Pediatric Emergencies in the Parisian Area. *Archives of Otolaryngology, Head and Neck Surgery* (1993) **119**:815–19.

Gannon CM, Wiswell TE, Spitzer AR. Volutrauma, $PaCO_2$ levels, and neurodevelopmental sequelae following assisted ventilation. *Clinics in Perinatology* (1998) **25**:159–75.

Goldsmith JP, Karotkin E. *Assisted Ventilation of the Neonate*, 4th edn. Philadelphia: WB Saunders, 2003.

Jobe AH. Hypocarbia and bronchopulmonary dysplasia. *Archives of Pediatrics and Adolescent Medicine* (1995) **149:**615.

Richardson ME. *Otolaryngology*, 3rd edn. *Pediatric Volume*, 3rd edn. St Louis, MO: Mosby, 1998.

Rivera R, Tibballs J. Complications of endotracheal intubation and mechanical ventilation in infants and children. *Critical Care Medicine* (1992) **20:**193–9.

Scottile FD. Complications of mechanical ventilation. In: PD Lumb, CW Bryan-Brown (eds). *Complications in Critical Care Medicine*. Chicago: Year Book Medical Publishers, 1988: 27–33.

Related topics of interest

- chronic lung disease
- intubation
- mechanical ventilation
- respiratory distress
- respiratory distress syndrome
- resuscitation
- stridor.

Congenital diaphragmatic hernia

Congenital diaphragmatic hernia (CDH) has been described, studied, and treated for over four centuries. Despite the great advances made in the care of infants with CDH, the mortality remains high at 30–60%, and survival averages 60%. Approximately 4–10% of all infant deaths from congenital anomalies are caused by CDH. The reported incidence ranges from one in 1000 to one in 12000 (prevalence 3.3 per 10000 births). Chromosomal anomalies are present in 5–30% of cases. Left-sided defects are six times more common than right-sided ones.

Associated malformations are found in 40–50% of cases, structural cardiac anomalies being the commonest (seen in 30%). Renal and genital anomalies are predominant in males, while CNS, heart, gastrointestinal, and liver defects are more common in females. However, the cause of CDH is still largely unknown.

Pathophysiology

CDH results in a diaphragmatic defect and lung hypoplasia. Both lungs are structurally affected, the ipsilateral more severely than the contralateral lung. There are fewer bronchi, respiratory bronchi, and alveoli, resulting in a global reduction in the gas-exchange area. As vascular branching parallels development of the airways, the arterial branches in CDH are also reduced. Thus, in CDH, there is a reduction in the cross-sectional area of the pulmonary vascular bed and an increase in muscularisation of these vessels, leading to the development of a persistent pulmonary hypertension that adversely affects the outcome. Functionally, the surfactant system and ability of CDH lungs to deal with oxygen free radicals are also impaired.

Prenatal diagnosis

A low maternal serum alpha-fetoprotein (AFP) level may be associated with CDH (and also trisomy 18 and 21). The reference standard for antenatal diagnosis of CDH is now a level 3 ultrasound examination. Once CDH is diagnosed, look for associated anomalies, as these alter the prognosis. Amniocentesis should also be performed, as up to 20% of cases may have chromosomal defects (from microdeletions to trisomy 18, 13 and 12p tetrasomy).

Predictors of mortality

- polyhydramnios
- a gestational age of <25 weeks at diagnosis
- a small lung-to-thoracic transverse area ratio
- a preoperative functional residual capacity (FRC) of <9 ml/kg
- a chromosomal anomaly (prognosis depends on the chromosomal defect)
- the presence of a structural cardiac anomaly, especially when detected prenatally
- a contralateral lung-to-head circumference ratio less than 0.62 (corrected for gestational age)

- the presence of an intrathoracic stomach is associated with increased mortality of up to tenfold
- prenatally diagnosed CDH may have a higher incidence of associated anomalies and therefore a poorer prognosis
- left ventricular hypoplasia, a reduced left-to-right ventricular size (left ventricular mass index); a calculated left ventricular mass of <2 g/kg is predictive of death.

Presentation

This depends on the severity of the defect and the side affected. Large left-sided defects present in the immediate postnatal period with respiratory distress (grunting, tachypnoea, recession, and cyanosis) and a scaphoid abdomen. Right-sided defects tend to be less severe, as the liver 'plugs' the defect, preventing abdominal contents from entering the chest. Bowel sounds are present in the chest, and the apex beat is displaced in left-sided defects. Small right hernias may be chance findings on a chest radiograph, and right-sided CDH may also be associated with late-onset GBS infection.

Postnatal diagnosis

The chest radiograph is diagnostic with dilated loops of bowel in the left hemithorax or an opaque hemithorax (before the bowel is filled with air). The main differential diagnosis is cystic adenomatoid malformation of the lung, especially if radiographic findings are right-sided or position of stomach is below diaphragm.

Management

At birth

Avoid mask ventilation during resuscitation, as this will result in visceral distension compromising ventilation and cardiac function. Intubate and ventilate if respiratory distress is present. Use the lowest possible airway pressure to maintain a preductal saturation of $\geq 90\%$. Pass a large bore tube to decompress the stomach.

Administration of prophylactic surfactant therapy is beneficial in patients who have had CDH diagnosed prenatally, as is prenatal steroid (betamethasone) therapy. Secure umbilical arterial and central venous access for pressure monitoring and drug infusions.

Preoperative stabilisation

Confirm the diagnosis by a chest radiograph. Ensure circulatory adequacy and normo-glycaemia. Correct hypovolaemic and/or metabolic acidosis with 4.5% albumin, THAM (tris-hydroxymethyl-aminomethane), or bicarbonate therapy. If ventilation is needed, intubate, paralyse, sedate, and provide analgesia (IV infusion of morphine or fentanyl). Use the lowest airway pressure compatible with adequate oxygenation. Maintain preductal saturations of 85–90%, keeping peak airway pressure at <30 cm H_2O. The strategy of hyperventilation-induced alkalosis (raising pH above 7.5 and reducing $PaCO_2$ to <30 mmHg (4 kPa) should be abandoned, as it produces iatrogenic lung injury. It has also been associated with adverse neurological outcome. Less aggressive mechanical ventilation should be used to avoid overdistending the contralateral lung and the secondary effects of barotrauma. As long as pH can be buffered with bicarbonate or THAM, ignore $PaCO_2$. This strategy of 'permissive hypercapnia' is currently favoured, as it is associated with improved survival and decreased extracorporeal membrane oxygenation (ECMO) utilisation.

High-frequency oscillatory ventilation (HFOV) and high-frequency jet ventilation (HFJV) may at times offer additional benefit, though this is inconsistent. It may be preferable to use HFOV for infants with hypoxaemia and hypercapnia unresponsive to conventional ventilation or responsive only to high-pressure ventilation (peak airway pressure of >30 cm H_2O).

All infants should have a cardiac echocardiogram to exclude congenital heart defects, measure the left-ventricular mass index, and determine the direction of ductal shunting. Right-to-left or bidirectional shunting suggests pulmonary hypertension which may respond to systemic pressor therapy and inhaled nitric oxide (NO) therapy. To date, however, there is no convincing evidence that inhaled NO improves the outcome in CDH.

Infants with persistent pulmonary hypertension of the newborn (PPHN) and severe respiratory failure non-responsive to maximal medical treatment may be referred to ECMO support, provided they do not have severe pulmonary hypoplasia. ECMO may be used, before, during, and after surgical repair of the defect. However, surgical repair on ECMO is associated with a greater mortality from haemorrhagic complications. Although there is a broad opinion that ECMO improves the outcome in CDH, this has not been proven. The UK ECMO trial showed no significant difference in survival between the ECMO-treated infants and those receiving conventional therapy.

As surgical repair of the diaphragmatic defect commonly produces a deterioration in lung compliance and gas exchange, most centres now adopt a strategy of nonurgent or deferred repair. Infants are no longer repaired on an emergency basis, and much greater emphasis is placed on preoperative ventilation and stabilisation up to and including ECMO support. Deferred surgery does not improve survival but helps to select survivors from nonsurvivors prior to undergoing the expense and stress of surgical repair. The timing of surgery depends on the degree of stability or liability of the pulmonary vascular bed. Repair may be deferred for several days, and documenting resolution of pulmonary hypertension (by Doppler echocardiography) may suggest an optimal time for repair. Finally, prior to transfer for surgery, other associated anomalies (including chromosomal) should be excluded.

Operative repair

This is often done through a subcostal oblique incision, and a primary repair is often possible. If the defect is too large, a synthetic patch may be used. Closures that create undue tension compromise the surgical repair, complicate the postoperative ventilatory management, result in reherniation of the diaphragm, and cause dehiscence or wound hernias. Foetal surgery including in utero tracheal ligation, endoscopic intrauterine surgery, and open surgery, is still very experimental. Lung transplantation for severe pulmonary hypoplasia is a distant option.

Long-term outcome

Many survivors of CDH experience considerable morbidity as a consequence of their abnormal pulmonary development, severe respiratory failure, and surgical repair of their defects. Foregut dismotility is common (20–89%), manifest as delayed gastric emptying and gastrooesophageal reflux (GOR) (10–60%). There is a high incidence of chronic lung disease (up to 60%) secondary to the primary lung hypoplasia, barotrauma and oxygen toxicity, chronic aspiration from GOR, and development of reactive airways disease, all resulting in frequent hospitalisation. Somatic growth failure is common (chronic lung disease, GOR, and poor oral intake), 30–40% remaining below the 5th percentile for weight. Short-term neurodevelopmental delay has also been noted. Postsurgical complications include adhesive bowel obstruction and recurrence of the hernia defect.

Further reading

D'Agostino JD, Berbaum JC, Gerdes M et al. Outcome for infants with congenital diaphragmatic hernia requiring extracorporeal membrane oxygenation: the first year. *Journal of Pediatric Surgery* (1995) **30:**10.

Davis CF, Sabharwal AJ. Management of congenital diaphragmatic hernia. *Archives of Disease in Childhood Foetal and Neonatal Edition* (1998) **79:**1–3.

Davis PJ, Firmin RK, Manktelow B et al. Long-term outcome following extracorporeal membrane oxygenation for congenital diaphragmatic hernia: The UK experience. *Journal of Pediatrics* (2004) **144:**309–15.

Downard CD, Wilson JM. Current therapy of infants with congenital diaphragmatic hernia. *Seminars in Neonatology* (2003) **8:**215–21.

Jaffray B, MacKinlay GA. Real and apparent mortality from congenital diaphragmatic hernia. *British Journal of Surgery* (1996) **83:**79–82.

Katz AL, Wiswell TE, Baumgart S. Contemporary controversies in the management of congenital diaphragmatic hernia. *Clinics in Perinatology* (1998) **25:**219–48.

Puri P (ed.). *Newborn Surgery*, 2nd edn. London: Arnold, 2003.

Sweed Y, Puri P. Congenital diaphragmatic hernia: influence of associated malformations on survival. *Archives of Disease in Childhood* (1993) **69:**68–70.

Useful website

www.emedicine.com/ped/topic_2603.htm
Part of the largest and most current online clinical knowledge base available to health professionals.

Related topics of interest

- congenital malformations and birth defects
- extracorporeal membrane oxygenation
- persistent pulmonary hypertension of the newborn
- prenatal diagnosis
- pulmonary hypoplasia
- respiratory distress.

Congenital heart disease—congestive heart failure

Milind Chaudhari

Congestive heart failure (CHF) is a clinical syndrome characterised by the inability of the heart to pump enough blood to meet the metabolic requirements of the tissues. Severe CHF results in inadequate perfusion of vital organs, culminating in cardiovascular collapse or shock.

Clinical features of CHF in neonates

History
Feeding difficulty
- slowness to feed (>30 min)
- pallor and sweating with feeding
- breathlessness and irritability during feeding
- failure to gain weight.

Physical examination
Signs of impaired myocardial function and compromised tissue perfusion
- tachycardia (heart rate of >150/min), gallop rhythm, and weak and thready pulse
- cardiomegaly (clinical and radiographic)
- reduced urine output (<1 ml/kg per h)
- metabolic acidosis
- vascular collapse/shock: pale, mottled skin, cold extremities, prolonged capillary refill time (>3 s), increased toe-core temperature difference (>2 °C), and impalpable pulses.

Signs of pulmonary congestion
- tachypnoea (respiratory rate of >60/min)
- subcostal or intercostal recession
- wet lung fields on chest radiograph
- frank pulmonary oedema
- wheezing or basal rales
- cyanosis.

Signs of systemic venous congestion
- hepatomegaly (>3 cm or progressive)
- excess weight gain (>30 gm/24 h) despite feeding difficulties.

Differential diagnosis of CHF in neonates

Noncardiac causes
- anaemia
- asphyxia

- septicaemia
- fluid overload
- polycythaemia
- hypoglycaemia
- arteriovenous fistulae.

Cardiac causes
Left ventricular outflow tract obstruction
- coarctation of the aorta
- interrupted aortic arch
- critical aortic stenosis
- hypoplastic left heart syndrome (HLHS).

Neonates with these conditions are usually normal at birth, as systemic perfusion and pulses are maintained by the patent ductus arteriosus (PDA). Cardiac failure and cardiogenic shock sets in with postnatal constriction of the ductus, as systemic and coronary perfusion is impaired. Severe heart failure is usually seen in the first week of life.

Left-to-right shunts
- large PDA
- large VSD
- truncus arteriosus
- atrioventricular septal defects (AVSD)
- total anomalous pulmonary venous connection (nonobstructed).

Presentation is beyond the first week of life as pulmonary vascular resistance falls. Features of increased pulmonary blood flow and sympathetic overstimulation are predominant.

Structurally normal heart with left ventricular dysfunction
- cardiac arrhythmias
- transient myocardial ischaemia (TMI) of the newborn
- cardiomyopathies (infective, storage disorders, endocardial fibroelastosis, and infant of diabetic mother).

Evaluation of a neonate with CHF

1. Perform A-B-C of neonatal cardiopulmonary resuscitation.
2. Correct electrolyte and acid–base abnormalities.
3. Exclude noncardiac causes.
4. Determine possible underlying cardiac aetiology and mechanism of CHF.

A schematic representation of the evaluation of an infant with CHF is given in Fig. 1.

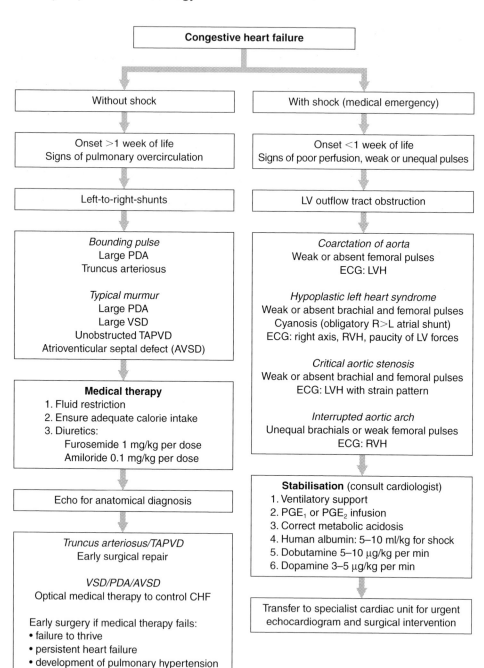

Figure 1 Evaluation of an infant with CHF—a schematic representation.
AVSD: atrioventricular septal defect, LV: left ventricle. LVH: left ventricular hypertrophy, PDA: patent ductus arteriosus, RVH: right ventricular hypertrophy, TAPVD: total anomalous pulmonary venous drainage, VSD: ventricular septal defect.

Further reading

Allen HD, Gutgesell HP, Clark EB et al (eds). *Moss and Adams' Heart Disease in Infants, Children, and Adolescents*, 6th edn. Philadelphia: Lippincott, Williams & Wilkins, 2000.

Anderson R, Baker E, Rigby M et al (eds). *Pediatric Cardiology*, 2nd edn. Edinburgh: Churchill Livingstone, 1998.

Burton DA, Cabalka AK. Cardiac evaluation of infants. *Pediatric Clinics of North America* (1994) **41:**991–1011.

Evans N, Archer N (eds). Perinatal cardiology. *Seminars in Neonatology* (2001) **6**(1).

Park MK. *Pediatric Cardiology for Practitioners*, 4th edn. St Louis, MO: Mosby, 2002.

Silove ED. Assessment and management of congenital heart disease in the newborn by the district paediatrician. *Archives of Disease in Childhood* (1994) **70:**F71–4.

Skinner J, Alverson D, Hunter S (eds). *Echocardiography for the Neonatologist.* Edinburgh: Churchill Livingstone, 2000.

Wernovsky G, Rubenstein SD (eds). Cardiovascular disorders in the neonate. *Clinics in Perinatology* (2001) **28**(1).

Related topics of interest

- acute collapse
- cardiac arrhythmias
- congenital heart disease—cyanotic defects
- heart murmurs in neonates
- shock.

Congenital heart disease—cyanotic defects

Milind Chaudhari

The incidence of congenital heart disease (CHD) is about eight per 1000 live births, and one-third of these cases present in the neonatal period. The common modes of presentation are as follows:

- cyanosis
- heart murmur
- cardiac arrhythmias
- congestive cardiac failure/vascular collapse.

Symptomatic heart disease in the neonate presents as cyanosis, cardiac failure, or cardiovascular collapse. Asymptomatic heart disease is usually diagnosed when incidental finding of a heart murmur, abnormal pulses, or abnormal heart rhythm leads to detailed cardiac evaluation. Routine cardiac screening in cases of various dysmorphic syndromes, chromosomal abnormalities, or congenital abnormalities of the gastrointestinal tract also enables early diagnosis of asymptomatic heart disease. The initial evaluation should be aimed at the recognition of the cardiac problem and its severity, and should be followed by stabilisation of the neonate for safe and timely transfer to a specialist cardiac unit.

Cyanotic heart defects

Cyanosis refers to blue discoloration of the skin and the mucous membranes due to presence of more than 4–5 g/dl of reduced haemoglobin in circulation. Clinically, it is usually apparent at oxygen saturations of 85% or below. It is one of the most significant signs of serious cardiac abnormality; hence, prompt recognition and diagnostic evaluation are mandatory. Central cyanosis results from arterial desaturation or an abnormal haemoglobin and affects the tongue, mucous membranes, and peripheral skin. Peripheral cyanosis results from prolongation of the circulation time and an increase in tissue oxygen extraction, and is confined to the extremities. It is typically seen in neonates with poor cardiac output, sepsis, polycythaemia, or metabolic acidosis. The arterial oxygen saturation and PaO_2 are normal in peripheral cyanosis.

Differential cyanosis (lower limbs more cyanosed than upper limbs) is seen in neonates with right-to-left ductal shunting associated with PPHN or an aortic arch obstruction. Reversed differential cyanosis (upper limbs more cyanosed than lower limbs) is seen in the setting of ventriculoarterial discordance and right-to-left ductal shunting.

Features of cyanosis due to CHD

- differential cyanosis
- worsening of cyanosis with crying/agitation
- central cyanosis with minimal respiratory distress
- arterial blood gas analysis: low PaO_2 with normal $PaCO_2$

- no response to challenge with 100% inspired oxygen (hyperoxia test)
- abnormalities on cardiovascular examination: precordial hyperactivity, heart murmur, and unequal peripheral pulses
- chest radiograph: abnormal cardiac size/shape and abnormal pulmonary vascularity
- abnormal ECG (normal ECG does not exclude serious cardiac abnormality in neonates).

The most important differential of cardiac cyanosis is cyanosis due to respiratory disorders, which is accompanied by signs of respiratory distress. It is also characterised by CO_2 retention on blood gas analysis. Typically, in response to 100% inspired oxygen, the saturation improves and PaO_2 is raised above 150 mmHg (20 kPa). In addition, there is evidence of parenchymal lung disease on chest radiograph. Rarely, both the pulmonary and cardiac components may contribute to cyanosis, as seen in obstructed anomalous pulmonary venous connection, with pulmonary oedema making the distinction more difficult.

Initial evaluation

Investigations
- FBC—check haemoglobin, white cell count, platelets, and markers of sepsis.
- Biochemistry—urea, creatinine, electrolytes, calcium, and blood glucose.
- Chest radiograph—heart size/shape, and pulmonary vascularity (N/↓/↑).
- ECG—note cardiac rhythm, QRS axis, and ventricular hypertrophy (right/left/both).
- Blood gases—arterial sample from the right radial or temporal arteries to avoid the effect of right to left ductal shunt. Additional postductal arterial sample from lower limb in case of differential cyanosis. Capillary samples from a warmed heel can be reliably used for estimation of acidosis and $PaCO_2$.
- Hyperoxia test—measurement of arterial blood gas tensions and pH in room air and after administration of 100% oxygen for 5–10 min aids in the differential diagnosis of central cyanosis. Little or no change in oxygen tension is suggestive of cyanotic heart disease. PaO_2 over 20 kPa makes it less likely and PaO_2 over 30 kPa excludes cyanotic CHD.

Monitoring
Careful monitoring of the following parameters is mandatory during stabilisation and transfer:

- blood pressure
- heart rate and rhythm
- respiratory rate and pattern
- oxygen saturation by pulse oximetry
- body temperature (toe-core differential)
- blood gases with electrolytes and blood glucose
- urine output.

Stabilisation

The *ABCD* of neonatal cardiopulmonary resuscitation is as follows:

- *Airway.* Secure airway; monitor for apnoea if airway is not secured.

- *Breathing.* Ventilatory support in presence of pulmonary oedema or persistent acidosis.

- *Circulation:* Volume expansion (5–10 ml/kg of 4.5% human albumin) if hypovolaemic.

- *Drugs.*

  1. To ensure ductal patency, prostaglandin E_1 or E_2 infusion. Recommended dilution: 500 μg in 500 ml of 5% dextrose, that is 1 μg/ml. Starting dose—0.3 ml/kg per h = 0.005 μg/kg per min. Double the dose in 20 min if SaO_2 is unchanged. Apnoea is a recognised side effect.
  2. Correction of metabolic acidosis. Sodium bicarbonate: half-correction, dose guided by the base deficit.
  3. Inotropic support. Dobutamine infusion (5–10 μg/kg per min) via peripheral IV canula.
  4. To improve renal perfusion, dopamine infusion (3–5 μg/kg per min) via central venous canula.
  5. Diuretics. Furosemide 1 mg/kg IV if in cardiac failure (but not circulatory failure!) to reduce the increased extravascular fluid volume.

Differential diagnosis of cyanotic CHD in neonates

CHD with decreased pulmonary blood flow

Lesions characterised by obstruction to pulmonary blood flow (PBF) with right to left shunt at atrial or ventricular level (see Fig. 1).

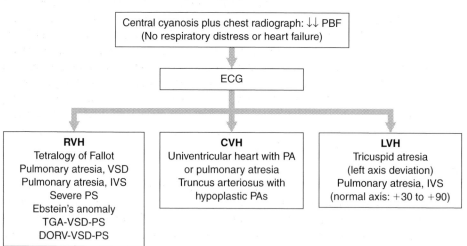

Figure 1
CVH: combined ventricular hypertrophy, DORV: double outlet right ventricle, IVS: intact ventricular septum, LVH: left ventricular hypertrophy, PA: pulmonary artery, PBF: pulmonary blood flow, PS: pulmonary stenosis, RVH: right ventricular hypertrophy, TGA: transposition of the great arteries, VSD: ventricular septal defect.

CHD with normal or increased pulmonary blood flow

Transposition of the great arteries (TGA) is the commonest lesion of this type (see Figure 2).

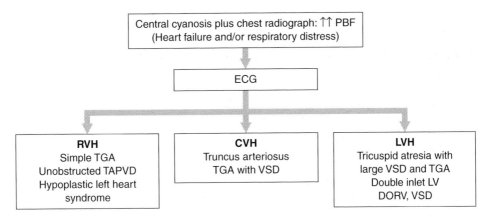

Figure 2
CVH: combined ventricular hypertrophy, DORV: double outlet right ventricle, LV: left ventricle, LVH: left ventricular hypertrophy, PBF: pulmonary blood flow, RVH: right ventricular hypertrophy, TAPVD: total anomalous pulmonary venous drainage, TGA: transposition of the great arteries, VSD: ventricular septal defect.

Structurally normal hearts with right to left shunts

Persistent pulmonary hypertension of the newborn (PPHN)

In this condition, the normal fall in pulmonary vascular resistance at birth is delayed. This results in persistence of pulmonary hypertension, which leads to a right-to-left shunt through the patent ductus arteriosus and foramen ovale, causing arterial desaturation. A right-to-left ductal shunt results in typical differential cyanosis (lower limbs vs upper limbs), whereas a predominantly atrial shunt results in generalised central cyanosis, making distinction from structural heart disease more difficult. Association with precipitating conditions such as meconium aspiration, perinatal asphyxia, or sepsis, and increase in the postductal PaO_2 in response to hyperventilation, causing hypocapnia and respiratory alkalosis, help to distinguish PPHN from structural heart defects. Echocardiographic evaluation is essential to confirm structurally normal heart with right-to-left ductal and/or atrial shunt.

Transient myocardial ischaemia (TMI)

This condition is characterised by ischaemic myocardial dysfunction and presents either with cyanosis or with congestive cardiac failure and a low output state. A preceding history of perinatal hypoxia and/or hypoglycaemia is common. A right-to-left atrial shunt results in central cyanosis and global myocardial dysfunction, causing heart failure. The condition may coexist with PPHN. The ECG shows ischaemic S-T and T-wave changes (S-T depression and T-wave inversion) and at times anterior or inferior infarct patterns. Echocardiography reveals dilated, poorly contractile left and right ventricles with a right-to-left atrial shunt on colour Doppler. Treatment is supportive and aimed at controlling heart failure.

Further reading

Allen HD, Gutgesell HP, Clark EB et al (eds). *Moss and Adams' Heart Disease in Infants, Children, and Adolescents*, 6th edn. Philadelphia: Lippincott, Williams & Wilkins, 2000.

Anderson R, Baker E, Rigby M et al (eds). *Pediatric Cardiology*, 2nd edn. Edinburgh: Churchill Livingstone, 1998.

Burton DA, Cabalka AK. Cardiac evaluation of infants. *Pediatric Clinics of North America* (1994) **41:**991–1011.

Evans N, Archer N (eds). Perinatal cardiology. *Seminars in Neonatology* (2001) **6**(1).

Park MK. *Pediatric Cardiology for Practitioners*, 4th edn. St Louis, MO: Mosby, 2002.

Silove ED. Assessment and management of congenital heart disease in the newborn by the district paediatrician. *Archives of Disease in Childhood* (1994) **70:**F71–4.

Snider AR, Serwer GA. *Echocardiography in Pediatric Heart Disease*. St Louis, MO: Mosby Year Book, 1990.

Stark J, de Leval M (eds). *Surgery for Congenital Heart Defects*, 2nd edn. Philadelphia: WB Saunders, 1994.

Wernovsky G, Rubenstein SD (eds). Cardiovascular disorders in the neonate. *Clinics in Perinatology* (2001) **28**(1).

Related topics of interest

- acute collapse
- cardiac arrhythmias
- congenital heart disease—congestive heart failure
- heart murmurs in neonates.

Congenital malformations and birth defects

The assessment of a dysmorphic newborn infant requires a systematic approach in order to make a correct diagnosis, implement appropriate management, and provide the parents with an accurate prognosis and appropriate genetic counselling. Congenital malformations are present in approximately 2.5% of the general population. Most of these occur as single minor abnormalities, but they occur with increased frequency in infants with other major malformations.

Certain definitions are important at the onset. A *birth defect* is a fault or disorder present or arising at birth. A *malformation* arises during embryonic life as an abnormal developmental process. A *deformation* is a mechanical alteration in the form or shape of a part of the body with previous normal development (as in talipes). A *disruption* is an interruption of normal development resulting in destruction of the body part (as in limb loss from amniotic band).

A single insult that results in a cascade of secondary consequences is a *malformation sequence*. If an insult causes multiple defects not causally related, the term 'malformations syndrome' may be used. A *syndrome* is a pattern of malformations thought to be pathogenically related. An *association* is a nonrandom occurrence of several anomalies not known to be a syndrome or sequence. Malformation syndromes may be chromosomal, inherited, or environmentally induced, whereas disruptions and deformations rarely have a genetic basis.

Clinical approach

Obtain a detailed history, with reference to the following risk factors:

- elderly mother
- affected family members
- oligo- or polyhydramnios
- intrauterine growth restriction
- multiple miscarriages/stillbirths
- prolonged premature rupture of membranes
- breech presentation (? neuromuscular disorder)
- family history of malformations with a genetic basis
- reduced foetal movements (? neuromuscular disorder)
- parental consanguinity (autosomal recessive disorders)
- exposure to alcohol, drugs, radiation, and infection during pregnancy.

Examination

This should be detailed and include careful examination of any physical abnormalities.

- Describe abnormal signs accurately.
- Obtain photographic records if possible.
- Are the malformations present part of a recognised syndrome (such as Down's syndrome) or sequence (such as Pierre Robin sequence)?

If immediate recognition is not possible, identify some well-defined, unusual physical signs as 'handles' (such as ptosis, microcephaly, polydactyly, short limbs, or hypogenitalia) and use the handle or a combination of them to scroll through the possible diagnoses. This process may be facilitated by the use of computerised databases.

Investigations

- chromosome analysis
- haematological (TAR syndrome)
- ultrasound imaging (of head or abdomen)
- skeletal radiographs (osteogenesis imperfecta congenita)
- biochemical analysis (amino aciduria and renal tubular acidosis in Lowe's syndrome)
- specialised genetic techniques (such as DNA probes for DiGeorge or Williams syndromes)
- cytogenetic analysis of specific tissue samples (as in skin fibroblast culture for the diagnosis of 12 p tetrasomy—Killian–Pallister syndrome).

Management

- Depending on the malformations/deformations present, specialist teams may be required: for example, ophthalmologists for ocular defects, ENT surgeons for ear and nose defects, maxillofacial and plastic surgeons for facial anomalies (such as cleft lip and palate), and orthopaedic surgeons and physiotherapists for limb malformations and deformations.
- If diagnosis remains uncertain, always seek review by a clinical geneticist. Genetic counselling is vital in most cases (recurrence risks and possible future antenatal diagnosis).
- Infants with feeding difficulties may require input from dietitians, and speech and language therapists, and the assistance of community nurses.
- Neurodevelopmental follow-up will be required.
- Where appropriate, put the parents in touch with the appropriate parents' self-help organisations (such as the Association for Spina Bifida and Hydrocephalus, the Cleft Lip and Palate Association, and STEPS).

Family support groups and information

Association for Spina Bifida and Hydrocephalus
42 Park Road
Peterborough PE1 2UQ, UK
Tel: 01733 555988
Fax: 01733 555985
www.asbah.org

CLAPA – Cleft Lip and Palate Association
235–237 Finchley Road
London NW3 6LS, UK
Tel: 020 7431 0033
www.clapa.com

STEPS
Association for People with Lower Limb Abnormalities
Lymm Court
11 Eagle Brow
Lymm
Cheshire WA13 0LP, UK
Tel: 0871 717 0044
www.steps-charity.org.uk

Contact a Family
209–211 City Road
London EC1V 1JN, UK
Tel: 020 7608 8700
Helpline: 0808 808 3555
www.cafamily.org.uk

Useful website

www.ncbi.nlm.nih.gov/Omim/
Online Mendelian Inheritance in Man. A mine of information, fully referenced and
with a gene map.

Further reading

Baraister M, Winter RM. *Colour Atlas of Congenital Malformation Syndromes*. London:
    Mosby-Wolfe, 1996.
D'Alton M, Malone F (eds). Congenital anomalies. *Clinics in Perinatology* (2000) **27**(4).
Fletcher MA. *Physical Diagnosis in Neonatology*. Philadelphia: Lippincott, Williams & Wilkins,
    1997.
Gilbert P. *The A–Z Reference Book of Syndromes and Inherited Disorders*, 2nd edn. London:
    Chapman & Hall, 1996.
Goodman RM, Gorlin RJ. *The Malformed Infant and Child. An Illustrated Guide*. New York:
    Oxford University Press, 1983.
Graham JM (ed.). *Smith's Recognizable Patterns of Human Deformation*, 2nd edn. Philadelphia:
    WB Saunders, 1988.
Jones KL (ed.). *Smith's Recognizable Patterns of Human Malformation*, 5th edn. Philadelphia:
    WB Saunders, 1997.
Tabyi H, Lachman RS (eds). *Radiology of Syndromes, Metabolic Disorders, and Skeletal
    Dysplasias*, 3rd edn. Chicago: Year Book Medical Publishers, 1990.
Wiedemann H-R, Kunze J. *Clinical Syndromes*, 3rd edn. London: Mosby-Wolfe, 1997.

Related topics of interest

- chromosomal abnormalities
- death of a baby
- hydrocephalus
- neural tube defects.

The death of a baby

The care of a dead or dying baby and his family has been called the neglected side of neonatal care. It is a daunting task that must be carried out sensitively and empathetically. Most parents need a lot of time to deal with the issues, and on a busy neonatal unit, staff must be careful not to rush them.

In major neonatal units, 5–10% of all admissions die, including approximately 20% of those in intensive care. Common causes of death include extreme prematurity, lethal anatomical and biochemical abnormalities, and birth asphyxia. In some, death will be completely unexpected: the parents may have never even contemplated it. For others, the congenital abnormality may have been diagnosed before birth, or the parents may have witnessed a heroic fight to save their very preterm baby against all odds. If time permits, it is best to ask the parents whether they want any religious blessing or naming of their baby when the critical nature of the illness is recognised, rather than waiting until death is imminent. It is also the time to take a first set of photographs.

Whatever the circumstances, most parents instinctively feel that their baby should not die 'alone' in a mass of tubes and wires. They want to cuddle their dying baby, even though they may be very afraid of this at first. In some circumstances, continuation of intensive care is to prolong death, not to sustain life. Staff must therefore help them recognise that nothing more can be done to save their baby. Parents then usually accept discontinuation of intensive care so long as full nursing care continues while they hold their baby and say goodbye. It is unethical to let the baby suffer in any way during this period—and parents are both acutely and persistently upset if their baby is distressed. It is a period of intensive nursing care—and doctors must be involved! The baby should be dressed in clothes of the parents' choice and taken to them in a quiet and entirely private room. At this point, the baby is usually still alive.

While the parents are holding their baby, they should be asked whether they wish to have photographs taken of the three of them together. Skilled carers can often point out some beautiful features of the baby—the hair, ears, face, and hands—to help parents really look at and remember their baby, whose face may have previously been hidden behind ventilator apparatus. Even very dysmorphic babies have fine features for parents to remember—wriggly toes and long fingers perhaps! The moment of death—when the heart stops—cannot be recognised by parents as the baby quietly passes away after a period of apnoea. The heart may beat for 20–30 min after the final breath. Parents are comforted to be told that death will not be a cataclysm, but a quiet fading of life while their baby is unconscious and unaware of the change.

After the death, the parents may wish to be alone with their baby. If so, they must be given as much time as they desire—sometimes several hours. They should have free access to a telephone to contact relatives, and the extended family should be allowed to gather with the baby and parents if that is what they wish. Staff should pop in and out from time to time to ensure that they are coping and to offer support if needed. When they are ready to leave, they must go to an environment where on-going support is available. This may be a special bereavement suite on the postnatal ward where neonatal staff and midwife counsellors can help, or it may be at home with the support of grandparents, other relatives, and other health professionals. The parents should know where their baby is going next, and should be advised that they can see him again at any time.

For the staff, there are practical things to do and achieve. A most useful checklist published by the Royal College of Obstetricians and Gynaecologists is used in many units. A modified list of tasks (some of which have been covered above) based on that checklist includes:

- mother and father informed of death
- parents given opportunity to handle the baby
- religious adviser notified if parents wish
- religious service requested/arranged
- footprints and handprints of baby taken
- other keepsakes collected: parents advised of book of remembrance
- photographs taken of baby—with parents if wished
- consultant paediatrician and consultant obstetrician informed
- general practitioner informed
- community midwives and/or health visitor informed
- consent for postmortem (PM) requested—given/refused
- parents offered *Guide to the Post-Mortem Examination*
- PM form completed: date and time of PM confirmed
- death/stillbirth certificate completed and given to parents
- information about funeral arrangements given to parents
- parents offered booklet *Saying Goodbye to Your Baby*
- parents told about support groups and given contact telephone numbers
- parents seen by counsellor/social worker
- parents seen by consultant obstetrician/paediatrician
- preliminary results of PM explained to parents
- follow-up visits arranged.

Some of the items on this list must be dealt with promptly—the family doctor and community midwife must know of the death before grieving relatives call them. If religious beliefs allow, discussion about the PM and funeral may be left to the following day, when the parents will be more able to absorb what is said to them.

Follow-up meetings must be arranged. The paediatrician should have clear goals for such visits. At a first meeting, the tasks of the paediatrician include:

- Reviewing the baby's medical problems and answering all questions about them.
- Discussing the findings of the PM if one was performed.
- Ensuring that appropriate postnatal follow-up is in place, including an appointment with a consultant obstetrician if necessary.
- Assessing how the couple are grieving.
  — Can they talk to each other about the baby, using his/her first name?
  — Have they had a funeral and said goodbye?
  — Are they grieving differently—is the father buried in work while the mother weeps at home?
  — Are they eating and sleeping reasonably under the circumstances?
- Reminding the parents of support groups and encouraging contact if appropriate.
- Helping them to begin to look to the future.
- Considering whether genetic counselling is needed.

- Asking whether the parents are thinking about the next pregnancy. Could there be an unplanned early conception—would this be a problem if it happened?
- Explaining the risks of the same thing happening again.
- Counselling the parents that it is normal to feel sad for many months after such a loss, but that they should seek help if symptoms worsen or persist too long.

It is virtually impossible to achieve all this at one visit soon after the death. The paediatrician or a counsellor may need sessions with the parents over a period of several months, and these may be best held away from the hospital.

Last but not least is the question of caring for the carers. Junior nurses and doctors find perinatal deaths extremely distressing and must be given time to reflect on the issues surrounding an individual death, particularly if they feel guilt as part of their grief. Senior colleagues must support and counsel them. These same senior staff who may have been involved in very distressing conversations and procedures must learn to turn to each other for help, or be confident of strong support outside the neonatal unit. The stress of dealing with a neonatal death is one of the experiences known to contribute to psychological 'burn-out' of neonatologists. Its impact should not be dismissed lightly.

Parent support groups and information

Stillbirth and Neonatal Death Society
28 Portland Place
London W1N 4DE, UK
Tel: 020 7436 5881 (Helpline)
         020 7436 7940 (Administration)
www.uk-sands.org

Further reading

American Academy of Pediatrics. The initiation or withdrawal of treatment for high-risk newborns (RE9532). *Pediatrics* (1995) **96:**362–3.
Guide to the Post-Mortem Examination. London: Department of Health, 1994.
Hindmarch C. *On the Death of a Child*, 2nd edn. Oxford: Radcliffe Medical Press, 2000.
Laing IA. Clinical aspects of neonatal death and autopsy. *Seminars in Neonatology* (2004) **9:**247–54.
McHaffie HE. *Crucial Decisions at the Beginning of Life: Parents' Experience of Treatment Withdrawal from Infants*. Oxford: Radcliffe Medical Press, 2001.
McIntosh N, Eldridge C. Neonatal death—the neglected side of neonatal care? *Archives of Disease in Childhood* (1984) **59:**585–7.
Royal College of Paediatrics and Child Health. *Withholding or Withdrawing Life Saving Treatment in Children*. London: Royal College of Paediatrics and Child Health, 1997.
Saying Goodbye to Your Baby. London: Stillbirth and Neonatal Death Society, 1997.

Related topics of interest

- congenital malformations and birth defects
- extreme prematurity
- hypoxic ischaemic encephalopathy
- inherited metabolic disease—investigation and management.

Discharge planning and follow-up

There are three main groups of infants to consider.

1. the otherwise well term or near-term newborn infant following a hospital delivery
2. term or near-term infants with proven or suspected disorders, such as congenital anomaly, which require medical intervention(s) in the perinatal period
3. preterm infants who have required varying periods of care on the neonatal unit.

The well term or near-term newborn infant

There is no consensus on the optimum postpartum length of stay for healthy term infants. There is a worldwide variation in policies and guidelines on the perinatal stay. Generally, the usual stay for a vaginal delivery in most countries is 1–3 days and up to seven days after a caesarean section. Discharges may, however, be done as early as 6–8 h, depending on, among other things, social and financial factors. The timing of each discharge is probably best individualised for each infant, depending on the individual medical, social, and economic aspects. Prior to discharge, however, the following important points should be noted:

- The infant is feeding well.
- The infant has voided urine and passed stools.
- The physical examination is normal.
- There is no evidence of clinical jaundice in the first 24 h.
- The mother is well and capable of looking after her newborn infant(s).
- There are no adverse social, environmental, or familial factors which would jeopardise the safety or well-being of the infant following discharge (such as history of domestic violence, drug or child abuse, or homelessness).
- Any necessary vaccinations (such as for hepatitis B or BCG have been administered).

The problematic term or near-term infant

These infants may be discharged once their problems (such as transient tachypnoea) have resolved or once appropriate investigations or therapies (such as renal scan for antenatally diagnosed hydronephrosis) have been instituted and follow-up appointment(s) have been made.

The ex-preterm infant

The discharge of infants who have required neonatal care for prematurity and related disorders requires more planning. Once it looks likely that the infant's discharge is imminent, the parent(s) should be notified so they can prepare themselves for their baby's home coming. This enables the parents to receive a comprehensive training which reduces parental anxiety and increases their satisfaction. The following should be addressed.

Social and environmental factors
- Assess adequacy of home environment and domestic arrangements and obtain a home visit by the health visitor if necessary.
- If home oxygen therapy will be required, make arrangements for the appropriate equipment to be installed.
- Check that there are no concerns regarding child protection matters (such as parental drug or alcohol abuse, maternal postnatal depression, or other adverse factors) that would prejudice the infant's care.

Parental factors
- Instruct parents on the special requirements of their infant (such as general routine infant care after discharge, positioning, avoidance of overheating, risk of cot death, and avoidance of smoking indoors especially with home oxygen therapy).
- Inform parents of the common signs of illness and when to obtain assistance for their infant.
- Assess adequacy of parenting skills and teach parents where appropriate (for example, cardiopulmonary resuscitation training for infants on supplemental oxygen therapy).
- The mother should be invited to 'room-in' on the neonatal unit to familiarise herself with her infant's care requirements (especially first-time mothers), and this also gives the NICU staff an opportunity to assess parental skills and competency.

Infant factors
- Temperature should be maintained in an open cot.
- The infant should be feeding well with a steady weight gain (10–30 g/day).
- There should be no recent apnoea or bradycardia for at least 5–8 days before discharge.
- Infants at risk of retinopathy of prematurity (ROP) should have been screened for this and any outstanding follow-up appointments formalised.
- High-risk infants (such as those at risk of severe jaundice, neonatal meningitis, congenital rubella or cytomegalovirus [CMV], or family history of deafness) should have a formal audiological examination.
- No absolute discharge weight requirements exist, though most infants weigh ≥1800 g and are of ≥35 weeks' gestation at discharge. Infants of birth weight under 1000 g are generally older at discharge (≥37 weeks' gestation) due to associated problems of prematurity.
- Earlier home discharges are possible in the presence of comprehensive support in the community by dedicated and skilled neonatal nurses, competent parents who have been adequately prepared prior to discharge.

On discharge home
- Ascertain that the parents are clear on how to administer any necessary medications and how to obtain further supplies.
- Document any immunisations given in the parent-held record.
- Give written records of any follow-up appointments or hospital visits.
- Send summary of hospital course, medications, and follow-up plans to the general

practitioner and any other relevant primary care workers (such as health visitor and community midwife) with copies to the relevant hospital records.

Who needs follow-up?

Conditions needing follow-up are numerous and partly depend on the available resources and expertise. While a complete list would be inappropriate for every setting, some of the common reasons include:

- prolonged jaundice
- infants at risk of child abuse
- infants of drug-abusing mothers
- infants who had severe sepsis (such as meningitis)
- infants with known congenital infections (such as CMV)
- infants with haematological disorders (such as thalassaemia)
- complications of neonatal intensive care (such as CLD, IVH, and ROP)
- infants with metabolic or endocrine disorders (such as suspected hypothyroidism)
- congenital malformations and birth defects (such as renal and urinary tract disorders)
- infants who experienced significant perinatal complications (such as birth injuries and asphyxia).

Further reading

American Academy of Pediatrics, Committee on Fetus and Newborn. Hospital discharge of the high-risk neonate: proposed guidelines. *Pediatrics* (1998) **102:**411–17.

Britton JR (ed.). Early perinatal hospital discharge: issues and concerns. *Clinics in Perinatology* (1998) **25**(2).

Casiro OG, McKenzie ME, McFadyen L et al. Early discharge with community-based intervention for low birth weight infants: a randomised trial. *Pediatrics* (1993) **92:**128–34.

Friedman MA, Spitzer AR. Discharge criteria for the term newborn. *Pediatric Clinics of North America* (2004) **51:**599–618.

Primhak R, Smith M (eds). Community neonatology: the continuing care of NICU graduates after hospital discharge. *Seminars in Neonatology* (2003) **8**(2).

Rawlings J, Scott J. Post-conceptional age of surviving low birth weight preterm infants at hospital discharge. *Archives of Pediatrics and Adolescent Medicine* (1996) **150:**260–2.

Samuels MP, Southall DP. Home oxygen therapy. In: TJ David (ed.). *Recent Advances in Paediatrics*. No. 14. Edinburgh: Churchill Livingstone, 1995: 37–51.

Related topics of interest

- chronic lung disease
- home oxygen therapy
- postnatal examination
- retinopathy of prematurity.

Extracorporeal membrane oxygenation

Extracorporeal membrane oxygenation (ECMO) is a technique for treating severe respiratory failure from which the patient can be expected to recover within 1–2 weeks. It may be used in the treatment of term babies with MAS, CDH, PPHN, or pneumonia. Contraindications to ECMO include major congenital abnormalities, IVH, irreversible cardiopulmonary disease, NEC, and a period of asystole. Before starting ECMO, each baby should have echocardiography to exclude cyanotic CHD (particularly total anomalous pulmonary venous drainage) and an ultrasound scan of the brain. Prolonged high-pressure ventilation causes lung damage, so babies need to be transferred onto ECMO ideally after less than 7–10 days' conventional ventilation. It is used only in babies of ≥35 weeks' gestation and at least 2 kg body weight, as the heparinisation could cause severe intracranial haemorrhage in the more immature infants.

The right internal jugular vein is cannulated and blood flows into a primed heparinised circuit with a pump, membrane oxygenator, and bubble trap before being returned to the baby, either via the carotid artery (venoarterial ECMO) or right atrium (venovenous ECMO). More recently, venovenous ECMO, in which the right internal jugular vein is cannulated with a double lumen cannula (VVDL ECMO), has become the technique of choice in the UK as it avoids the need to tie off the cannulated carotid artery and then relying on anastomoses to maintain the circulation from the contralateral carotid artery. VVDL ECMO cannulae are now increasingly being inserted percutaneously. During treatment, the baby is gently ventilated to maintain lung inflation, but the main source of gas exchange is the membrane oxygenator. Following promising reports of trials on small numbers of babies, over 75 ECMO centres opened in the USA, and submitted data to the Extracorporeal Life Support Organisation Registry. Currently, over 18000 infants have been treated, with an overall 80% survival, but 95% survival for meconium aspiration syndrome. These infants would have had expected mortality rates of approximately 80% (see Table 1).

In the UK, a more circumspect approach was taken, as fewer term babies were seen with respiratory failure. In a multicentre, randomised trial of 185 term babies, 30 of 93 babies allocated to ECMO died, compared with 55 of the 92 allocated to conventional management (CM). The relative risk was 0.55 (95% CI 0.39–0.77), equivalent to one extra survivor for every 3–4 babies allocated ECMO. However, outcome in those with diaphragmatic hernia was poor: all 17 in the CM group died, as did 14 of the 18

Table 1 Extracorporeal Life Support Organisation Registry survival data through January 2000.

Diagnosis	Survival (%)	n
Meconium aspiration syndrome (MAS)	94	5329
RDS	84	1289
PPHN	79	2154
Sepsis	76	2107
Other diagnoses	67	811
Congenital diaphragmatic hernia (CDH)	54	3290

allocated ECMO. More data are needed to help understand the role of ECMO in infants with diaphragmatic hernias. When that group was excluded, the survival was 79% in the ECMO group, and 51% in those allocated CM. Of the 124 initially followed to 1 year, 51% of those allocated to ECMO were alive with no signs of impairment (74% of survivors), compared with only 28% of those allocated CM (71% of survivors).

ECMO therefore has a clearly established role in the treatment of term babies with severe respiratory failure. Technical problems of cannulation make it difficult to use this technique in smaller babies. The development of tubing with heparin bonded onto the walls may enable a reduction in systemic heparinisation. Treatment with inhaled nitric oxide (NO) in babies who would normally qualify for ECMO reduces the need for ECMO by about 60%. Pleasing as this is, it does mean that neonatal transport incubators will need NO circuits in the future to transfer babies who have become NO dependent but still need to be transported to an ECMO centre.

There remains the question as to the threshold for starting ECMO in babies with meconium aspiration, pneumonia, persistent pulmonary hypertension of the newborn (PPHN), and indeed diaphragmatic hernia. The criterion that is usually considered is the oxygenation index (OI) which is calculated as:

$$\text{Mean airway pressure (cmH}_2\text{O)} \times \text{FiO}_2\,(\%) \div \text{postductal } PaO_2 \text{ (mmHg)}$$

or

$$\text{Mean airway pressure (cmH}_2\text{O)} \times \text{FiO}_2\,(\%) \times 0.13 \div \text{postductal } PaO_2 \text{ (kPa)}$$

An alternative parameter is the alveolar-arterial oxygen ($AaDO_2$) gradient calculated as:

$$AaDO_2 = FiO_2\,(P-47) - PaO_2 - PaCO_2\,[FiO_2 + (1 - FiO_2)/R]$$

where P is the barometric pressure, 47 is the partial pressure of water vapour, R is the respiratory quotient (0.8), FiO_2 is the fractional inspired oxygen concentration, PaO_2 is the arterial PO_2, and $PaCO_2$ is the arterial $PaCO_2$. When FiO_2 is 100%, and assuming P_ACO_2 (alveolar PCO_2) is equivalent to $PaCO_2$, the equation reduces to:

$$AaDO_2 = 713 - (PaO_2 + PaCO_2), \text{ where P} = 760\,\text{mmHg (sea level)}$$

An $AaDO_2$ gradient of greater than 620, or an OI of greater than 40, for 8h correlates with an 80% predicted mortality. The $AaDO_2$ and OI are equally effective predictors of outcome.

In the UK trial, the entry criterion was an OI of ≥ 40, or a $PaCO_2 > 12\,$kPa for 3h. In view of the success of ECMO, it may be best to lower the threshold to an OI of 30 or even 25, a view supported by survival and morbidity data, and increasing use of the relatively noninvasive techniques such as percutaneous VVDL ECMO. Recent experience has also shown that ECMO referral after more than 72h of ventilation is associated with longer ECMO runs. Another recent study reported that all neonates with an OI of ≥ 25 after 72h of inhaled NO or HFOV therapy eventually required ECMO (sensitivity 91%, specificity 100%). The UK trial also clearly showed that referral of very ill infants to ECMO centres resulted in some infants dying before ECMO could be instituted.

The collaborative UK ECMO Trial 1-year follow-up data show that ECMO support reduces the risk of mortality without a major concomitant rise in severe disability by about 45%, regardless of the severity of the infant's condition. The results of the economic evaluation, carried out alongside the trial, based on the principal endpoint of death or severe disability at age one year, found the additional cost of ECMO per additional survivor to be within the range of other life-extending technologies such as renal transplantation.

Summary of eligibility criteria for ECMO

- gestational age of ≥34 weeks and weight over 2000 g
- absence of intracranial haemorrhage
- absence of congenital heart disease
- reversible lung disease
- fewer than 10–14 days of mechanical ventilation
- failure of maximal medical treatment (that is, supporting cardiac output with volume expansion or pressor support and respiratory support, which includes surfactant therapy, inhaled NO, and, where relevant, HFOV).

Useful website

www.elso.med.umich.edu
The Extracorporeal Life Support Organisation site with details of the ELSO Registry and educational programmes.

Further reading

Bennett C, Johnson A, Field D et al. UK collaborative randomised trial of neonatal extracorporeal membrane oxygenation: follow-up to age four years. *Lancet* (2001) **357**:1094.

Elbourne D, Field D, Mugford M. Extracorporeal membrane oxygenation for severe respiratory failure in infants (*Cochrane Methodology Review*). In: The Cochrane Library, Issue 4. Chichester: Wiley, 2003.

Graziani LJ, Gringlas M, Baumgart S. Cerebrovascular complications and neurodevelopmental sequelae of neonatal ECMO. *Clinics in Perinatology* (1997) **24**:655–75.

Kossel H, Bauer K, Kewitz G et al. Do we need new indications for ECMO in neonates pretreated with high-frequency ventilation and/or inhaled nitric oxide? *Intensive Care Medicine* (2000) **26**:1489–95.

UK Collaborative ECMO Trial Group. UK collaborative randomised trial of neonatal extracorporeal membrane oxygenation. *Lancet* (1996) **348**:75–82.

UK Collaborative ECMO Group. The Collaborative UK ECMO Trial: follow-up to 1 year of age. *Pediatrics* (1998) **101**(4).

Walker GM, Coutts JAP, Skeoch C et al. Paediatricians' perception of the use of extracorporeal membrane oxygenation to treat meconium aspiration syndrome. *Archives of Disease in Childhood Fetal and Neonatal Edition* (2003) **88**:F70–1.

Related topics of interest

- congenital diaphragmatic hernia
- meconium aspiration syndrome
- nitric oxide therapy
- persistent pulmonary hypertension of the newborn.

Extreme prematurity

The last 30 years has witnessed remarkable improvements in the survival of small preterm infants. For instance, US data show a 70-fold increase in the number of survivors per 1000 live births between 1960 and 1983. Further improvements in survival were noted in the 1990s with the introduction of surfactants, increased use of antenatal corticosteroids, and other technological advances, particularly in assisted ventilation. However, there has been no concomitant reduction in the neurodevelopmental morbidity, particularly in the lowest birth weight, where survival had previously been exceptionally low. The threshold of viability has been retreating to the currently perceived limit of extrauterine survival (22–23 weeks). The term 'extreme prematurity' (or 'threshold of viability') is now used to refer to infants of <26 completed weeks' gestation. Such infants constitute less than 1% of all live births, comprise approximately 5% of all NICU admissions, but account for almost one-third of all NICU deaths. Most of the complex medical, social, and ethical decisions encountered on the NICU surrounds the decisions to forego, initiate, or withdraw intensive care in these tiny babies. It is worth summarising the following important facts about this group of infants:

- Pregnancies which terminate at <26 weeks' gestation have a high intrapartum and immediate postnatal mortality rate.
- Gestational age is a better predictor of neonatal mortality than birth weight, since organ maturity at birth is the ultimate determinant of outcome.
- Gender, gestational age, and intrauterine growth rate have a marked influence on mortality and the likelihood of survival.
- Female infants have a survival advantage equivalent to almost one additional gestational week.
- The survival rate increases with each additional half-week of gestation.
- Nonsurvivors die early; approximately 80% of ELBW deaths occur in the first three days of life—consequently, once an infant survives this initial period, the likelihood of survival (actuarial survival) improves dramatically (approximately doubles, regardless of birth weight or gestational age), although a significant risk of late death remains in the smallest infants.
- Individual mortality is difficult to predict (although morbidity may not be).
- If the infant survives, there is an almost equal risk of impairment or normal outcome at <26 weeks' gestation.
- In extremely preterm infants, morbidity is inversely related to birth weight and gestational age.
- The incidence of moderate or severe disability at age 18–30 months is high (30–50%) and does not appear to change significantly between 23 and 25 weeks' gestation, with many infants having more than one disability.

Many valuable data on the outcome of extremely preterm infants have been compiled by the EPICure study, National Institute of Child Health and Human Development (NICHD) Research Network Centres 1995–6, and the French Epipage study, each with an initial cohort of over 4000. The EPICure Study evaluated the outcome for all infants born before 26 weeks of gestation in the UK and Ireland during nine months in 1995. This is displayed in Table 1 alongside data from the current world literature.

Table 1 Summary of survival and morbidity data on regional populations of ELBW infants.

| | Summary of world literature on regional populations of ELBW infants | | | | EPICure study | | |
| Gestational age | Survival | Neonatal morbidity | | | Survival % (95% CI) | Neonatal morbidity | |
		CLD	CNS	ROP		CLD (%, 95% CI)	ROP (%, 95%CI)
<23	0–9%				9%(0–21)	86% (67–96)	26% (11–46)
23	12–35%	57–86%	10–83%	25–50%	20% (13–27)	86% (67–96)	26% (11–46)
24	17–62%	33–89%	9–64%	13–33%	34% (28–39)	77% (68–85)	20% (13–29)
25	35–72%	16–71%	7–22%	10–17%	52% (47–57)	70% (63–76)	10% (6–15)

CLD: chronic lung disease, oxygen requirement at 36 weeks' postmenstrual age; CNS: central nervous system injury (severe cerebral ultrasound abnormality); ROP: severe retinopathy of prematurity requiring laser or cryotherapy.

Table 2 The Epipage study, a population based cohort study of all births between 22 and 32 weeks during 1997 in nine regions covering a third of all births in France.

Gestation (weeks)	Stillbirths % (Percentage of all births)	Live births (Percentage of all births)	Labour ward deaths (Percentage of live births)	Admitted to NICU (Percentage of live births)	Survival to discharge (Percentage of live births)
<23	84	16	100	0	0
23	78	22	80	20	0
24	63	37	36	64	31
25	42	58	21	79	50

Table 3 Neonatal survival and morbidity by gestational age and birth weight among infants born in the NICHD neonatal centres, 1995–6.

Gestation (weeks)	Survival (%)	Birth weight (g)	Survival rate (%)	Moderate or severe disability (%)
<23	–	401–500	11	–
23	30	501–600	27	29
24	52	601–700	63	30
25	76	701–800	74	28

Table 4 Neonatal morbidities in infants of birth weight <750 g in the NICHD neonatal centres, 1995–6.

Condition	Frequency (%) of morbidities (range)
Respiratory distress syndrome	78 (54–97)
Oxygen needed at 28 days after birth	81 (64–92)
Chronic lung disease*	52 (8–86)
Necrotising enterocolitis	14 (9–38)
Septicaemia	48 (30–64)
Grade 3 intraventricular haemorrhage	13 (6–29)
Grade 4 intraventricular haemorrhage	13 (3–26)
Periventricular leucomalacia	7 (2–30)
Growth failure†	100 (92–100)

*Oxygen requirement at 36 weeks' postmenstrual age.
†Weight <10th centile at 36 weeks' postmenstrual age.

The Epipage study reported on the outcome of all births and late terminations of pregnancy occurring from 22 to 32 completed weeks gestation in nine regions covering a third of all births in France during 1997 (Table 2). The NICHD neonatal centres, 1995–6 study evaluated the outcome for infants weighing 401–1500 g at birth (Table 3) with morbidity data in Table 4. Using survival data which include stillbirths in the denominator, the EPICure study quotes an intrapartum and labour ward mortality rate of 79% (Table 5), whereas survival data based only on the number of live births in the denominator show a 32% mortality on the labour ward (Table 5).

Infants weighing less than 500 g

The chances of survival free of handicap at birth weight of <500 g are extremely slim. One study of a large regional experience from Alberta, Canada, reported 70% of 382 live birth infants having died in the delivery room and only 5% of all live births surviving to be discharged home. At the time of discharge from hospital, 90% of the survivors had CLD and half were still on oxygen therapy. At three years of age, survival was down to 3% of all live births, and 69% of the survivors had one or more disabilities including CP, mental retardation, blindness, and deafness. Handicap-free survival at

Table 5 EPICure Study.

Outcome of pregnancies ending between 20 and 25 weeks	
Prenatal or intrapartum death	70%
Death on labour ward	9%
Death on neonatal unit	12%
Survival to discharge	8%
Death between discharge and $2\frac{1}{2}$ years	<1%
Neurodevelopmental normality at $2\frac{1}{2}$ years	4%
Outcome of live births between 20 and 25 weeks	
Death on labour ward	32%
Death on the neonatal unit	42%
Survival to discharge	26%
Neurodevelopmental normality at $2\frac{1}{2}$ years (as % of live births)	13%
Severe disability at $2\frac{1}{2}$ years (as % of live births)	6%

Table 6 Actuarial survival.

Gestation (weeks)	Probability of survival to discharge (%)		
	Chronological age (days)		
	Day 0	Day 7	Day 28
<23	20 (13–27)	48 (35–60)	68 (54–83)
24	34 (28–39)	60 (53–67)	78 (70–85)
25	52 (47–57)	75 (69–80)	89 (85–93)

three years was therefore approximately 1%. Apart from Japanese reports that appear more promising, most of the world literature gives similar poor survival and neurodevelopmental outcomes for infants with birth weight of <500 g. The few survivors have tended to be female and small for gestational age.

Counselling parents

Parents should be counselled that the probability of survival and neonatal management plans made before delivery may have to be altered according to the baby's condition at birth, its response to resuscitation measures, and its subsequent progress. Parents should receive clear and consistent accounts of care that will be required to support their infant soon after birth. A panoramic view of the commonest complications encountered during neonatal intensive care, survival rates, and the potential long-term outcomes, including the range of disabilities, should also be provided. The counselling physician should be knowledgeable about contemporaneous local and comparative population-based data on survival and long-term outcomes of extremely preterm infants. Survival figures given to parents should vary according to the timing of the counselling, that is, whether before birth or after birth, or according to postnatal age. Once an infant has been delivered and admitted to the NICU, survival data based on live births only should be offered (Table 6). Survival statistics should also be based on gestational age rather than birth weight.

Counselling should be sensitive to ethnic and cultural differences, and, where necessary, an interpreter should be made available. There should be ongoing assessment of the condition and prognosis of the infant, and the parents should be given accurate updates. Whenever possible, parents should be participants in the decision-making process of their infant's care and management. Should the decision be made to discontinue or withhold resuscitation, or withdraw life support, humane care must be provided to the infant, and the family treated with compassion in a setting that maintains dignity. Life-prolonging treatment should not be continued when treatment is judged to be futile—but parents may need time to accept the futility of such treatment. The family should receive support beyond the time of the infant's death; ideally, a follow-up bereavement appointment should be made with the parents to review the medical events surrounding the infant's death, any postmortem reports, or other outstanding issues.

Management at birth

As ethical considerations of infants at the margins of viability will vary in time and place, individual units should draw up their own guidelines. In the light of published survival and morbidity rates, infants born at ≤22 weeks with a birth weight of <500 g should probably receive only comfort care, whereas resuscitation should be offered to infants of ≥25 weeks' gestation. For infants born at 23–24 weeks, a policy of flexibility with regard to resuscitation is suggested, taking into account the parents' views and the condition of the infant at birth. The presence of oligohydramnios, intrauterine growth restriction, or reversed end diastolic flow (EDF) may further reduce the chances of survival. When circumstances do not permit a full discussion and assessment before birth, resuscitation is the rule. The baby could be several weeks older than the mother thinks.

The decision to offer resuscitation and commence intensive care is not an unconditional commitment to prolonged intensive care. If the likelihood of severe neurological handicap becomes very high, there is always the option of discontinuing intensive care and offering palliative nursing care. At least two experienced paediatricians should attend the birth of an extremely preterm infant to determine whether the neonate is viable and how aggressive resuscitation should be. If the infant is stillborn, no resuscitation should be offered. For infants with poor respiratory effort or bradycardia, resuscitate with T-piece and mask (or bag and mask) ventilation. If a satisfactory response is observed, proceed to intubation and ventilation with prophylactic surfactant administration. Prolonged resuscitation of infants who do not respond does not change mortality but merely delays death. Where the infant is vigorous, proceed with intubation, surfactant administration and ventilation, and then transfer to the NICU. Take great care to avoid hypothermia; for example, place infants immediately into a transparent polyethylene bag, which greatly reduces evaporative heat loss.

Parent information and support group

BLISS
68 South Lambeth Road
London SW8 1RL, UK
Parent support helpline: Freephone 0500 618140
www.bliss.org.uk
The premature baby charity.

Useful websites

www.aap.org
American Academy of Pediatrics.

www.bapm.org
British Association of Perinatal Medicine.

www.marchofdimes.com/prematurily
March of Dimes Birth Defects Foundation – a US based charity concerned with birth defects, low birthweight and prematurity.

Further reading

Costelo K, Hennessy E, Gibson AT et al. The EPICure Study: outcomes to discharge from hospital for infants born at the threshold of viability. *Pediatrics* (2000) **106:**659–71.
Doron MW, Veness-Meehan KA, Margolis LH et al. Delivery room resuscitation decisions for extremely premature infants. *Pediatrics* (1998) **102:**574–82.
Hack M, Fanaroff AA. Outcomes of children of extremely low birthweight and gestational age in the 1990s. *Seminars in Neonatology* (2000) **5:**89–106.
Larroque B, Breart G, Kaminski M et al on behalf of the Epipage Study group. Survival of very preterm infants: Epipage, a population based cohort study. *Archives of Disease in Childhood Fetal and Neonatal Edition* (2004) **89:**F139–44.
Lemons JA, Bauer CR, Oh W et al. Very low birth weight outcomes of the National Institute of Child Health and Human Development Neonatal Research Network, January 1995 through December 1996. *Pediatrics* (2001) **107:**e1.
Lorenz JM. Management decisions in extremely premature infants. *Seminars in Neonatology* (2003) **8:**475–82.
MacDonald H and American Academy of Pediatrics. Committee on Foetus and Newborn. Perinatal care at the threshold of viability. *Pediatrics* (2002) **110:**1024–7.
Meadow W, Reimshisel T, Lantos I. Birth weight-specific mortality for extremely low birth weight infants vanishes by four days of life: epidemiology and ethics in the neonatal intensive care unit. *Pediatrics* (1996) **97:**636–43.

Related topics of interest

- chronic lung disease
- death of a baby
- outcomes of neonatal intensive care
- resuscitation.

Feeding difficulties

Feeding difficulties are extremely common in the newborn period. These may be categorised as transient or persistent. Transient feeding difficulties invariably are related to perinatal factors and commonly resolve within the first few days or weeks of life. Persistent feeding difficulties suggest an underlying organic cause and require careful evaluation to determine the correct aetiology and therefore appropriate management. For transient feeding difficulties, both maternal and infant factors can be identified.

Transient feeding difficulties

Maternal factors
- inexperienced, first-time mother(s)
- pregnancy-related maternal illness (such as severe pre-eclampsia, eclampsia, delivery complications, and postnatal depression)
- pre-existing chronic maternal illness (such as rheumatoid arthritis and multiple sclerosis)
- breast abnormalities in breast-feeding mothers (such as inverted nipples and previous breast surgery or injury)
- maternal medication—drugs taken during pregnancy and/or delivery may adversely affect the infant; for example, benzodiazepines (drowsy infant) and methadone (neonatal drug withdrawal syndrome)
- maternal anxiety.

Infant factors
- prematurity (immature suck-and-swallow reflex)
- traumatic delivery (instrumental delivery with facial injury)
- hypoglycaemia
- birth asphyxia
- cold stress
- intrauterine growth restriction (IUGR)
- sepsis.

With appropriate support from the midwifery and neonatal staff, most mothers and their infants can be successfully supported through the initial transitional period to feed their infants by their preferred method. If feeding is particularly poor, capillary blood glucose should be monitored regularly (until they are persistently above 3 mmol/l). Nasogastric tube feeds may be required in the preterm, small for gestational age, or large infants of diabetic mothers.

Persistent feeding difficulties

A careful search often reveals a cause in most of these infants. As listed below, the possible causes are numerous.

Neurological abnormalities
- local (as in facial nerve palsy, bulbar and suprabulbar palsy, and vocal cord palsy)
- central (as in CNS malformations, severe intracranial haemorrhage, severe hydrocephalus, and seizures).

Neuromuscular disorders
- spinal muscular atrophy
- myotonic dystrophy and other muscular dystrophies
- Prader-Willi syndrome
- myasthenia gravis.

Syndromic disorders
- Down's syndrome
- Möbius's syndrome
- Pierre Robin sequence
- Roberts syndrome
- Beckwith–Wiedemann syndrome.

Anatomic defects
- cleft lip and palate
- submucous cleft
- choanal atresia/stenosis
- hiatus hernia
- oesophageal atresia (associated polyhydramnios)
- tracheoesophageal fistula
- laryngeal webs and clefts
- oesophageal compression (as in vascular rings)
- gut malrotation
- oropharyngeal vascular malformations (as in carvenous haemangioma)
- tumours.

Metabolic disorders
- galactosemia
- hypothyroidism
- organic and amino acidopathies (such as propionic acidaemia and nonketotic hyperglycinaemia)
- urea cycle defects
- other inherited metabolic disorders.

Miscellaneous disorders
- isolated swallowing disorders with pharyngeal and cricopharyngeal incoordination
- chalasia or achalasia of oesophagus
- choanal atresia
- stomatitis
- oesophagitis.

Investigations

- pH monitoring (reflux oesophagitis)
- endoscopy (reflux oesophagitis)
- barium swallow and follow through (hiatus hernia and malrotation)
- chromosomes (dysmorphic infants)
- laryngoscopy
- video fluoroscopy
- cranial ultrasound
- cranial CT/MRI.

Management

- oropharyngeal stimulation (nonnutritive sucking)
- use of special teats and bottles (cleft lip/palate)
- orthodontic devices (cleft lip/palate)
- nasogastric tube feeding
- gastrostomy (persistent difficulties especially in the neurologically impaired)
- Nissen fundoplication (especially in neurologically impaired infants).

Multidisciplinary teams are often required in managing these infants. Infants with anatomic defects (such as cleft lip and palate and oesophageal atresia) may require the input of plastic surgeons, orthodontists, faciomaxillary surgeons, speech therapists, and dietitians. Even in the absence of anatomic defects requiring surgery, speech and language therapists and dietitians are often required to optimise the calorie intake of such infants. Similarly, a paediatric neurologist and clinical geneticist may offer valuable advice in infants with suspected neurologic disorders and dysmorphic features, respectively. Remember to exclude feed intolerance, especially with a family history of atopy, cow's milk protein intolerance, or other, rarer metabolic disorders.

Further reading

Arvedson JC, Brodsky L. *Paediatric Swallowing and Feeding Assessment and Management.* London: Whurr Publishers, 1993.

Cooper PJ, Stein A (eds). *Feeding Problems and Eating Disorders in Children and Adolescence.* Reading: Academic Publishers, 1992.

Hyman P. Gastroesophageal reflux: one reason why baby won't eat. *Journal of Pediatrics* (1994) **125:**S103–9.

Related topics of interest

- congenital malformations and birth defects
- hypoxic-ischaemic encephalopathy
- nutrition.

Fluid and electrolyte therapy

The management of fluids and electrolyte administration is vital in the management of sick newborn infants. The handling of water and solute by the immature kidneys is impaired, and this is often compounded by large water losses through the highly permeable immature skin. To maintain normal fluid and electrolyte balance, it is necessary therefore to control their administration accurately.

Water balance

Approximately 75% of the total body weight is water, half of which is extracellular fluid. A reduction of the extracellular space occurs during the first week of life, accounting for most of the 10–15% reduction in body weight; inadequate calorie intake accounts for the remainder of the weight loss. Respiratory distress syndrome (RDS) is associated with delayed contraction of the extracellular fluid volume, and this contraction occurs with resolution of RDS.

Factors associated with increased water loss

- use of radiant warmers
- phototherapy
- preterm thin skin
- poor humidification of respiratory gases
- watery stools
- high ileostomy losses
- osmotic diuresis as in glycosuria
- low ambient humidity.

Factors associated with water overload

- excess fluid administration
- inappropriate sodium administration
- conditions (such as pneumonia and RDS) associated with the syndrome of inappropriate antidiuretic hormone (SIADH) secretion.

Remedial steps to maintain optimal water balance

- Avoid nursing very preterm infants under radiant warmers.
- Cover infants with plastic sheeting to reduce fluid losses.
- Nurse newborn infants in a humid environment.
- Humidify respiratory gases adequately for infants receiving respiratory support.

Adverse effects of fluid overload

- persistence of ductus arteriosus

- chronic lung disease
- increased mortality.

Electrolyte balance

The main extracellular and intracellular cations are sodium and potassium, respectively. Sodium absorption is under the influence of renin-angiotensin-aldosterone, while potassium (K^+) absorption is influenced by mineralocorticoids, K^+ being exchanged for H^+ in the kidneys. Potassium excretion is greatly reduced in renal failure. Sodium supplementation is not required until after the reduction of extracellular fluid space (24–48 h), but thereafter sodium may be supplemented at 4 mmol/kg per day (or more depending on serum sodium) in preterm infants and 2 mmol/kg per day in term infants. Aim to keep sodium at 135–140 mmol/l. Potassium is supplemented at 2 mmol/kg per day if urine output is satisfactory.

While calcium is predominantly stored in bone, 40% of that in the extracellular fluid is bound to albumin, the rest (approximately 1.25 mmol/l) being free ionised Ca^{2+} (ionised calcium falls with rising pH). For every 10 g fall in albumin below 40 g/l, the total calcium is reduced by 0.05 mmol/l.

Calcium homeostasis is under the influence of calcitonin, parathormone, and vitamin D (1,25-dihydroxyvitamin D). Parathormone increases calcium absorption from the gut and kidneys. Intravenous supplementation should provide 2 mmol/kg per day and oral supplementation 1.75–3.5 mmol/kg per day (with a calcium:phosphate ratio of 1.4–2:1). Avoid rapid IV administration of calcium (as calcium gluconate), as this causes bradycardia, and beware of extravasation (produces unsightly scars).

Phosphate, like calcium, is a major constituent of bone, and its absorption from the gut and kidneys is influenced by vitamin D and parathormone. Intravenous supplements of 1 mmol/kg per day are appropriate with oral supplements of 1.6 mmol per 100 kcal. Human milk contains low phosphorus levels (0.4 mmol/l), making it mandatory to supplement preterm infants fed on breast milk.

Magnesium is mainly an intracellular ion excreted by kidneys and absorbed from the gut. Always check serum magnesium when hypocalcaemia is present. For urgent replacement, give a slow infusion of 25% magnesium sulphate at 0.5 mmol/kg or intramuscularly as 0.2 ml/kg of 50% magnesium sulphate. For oral supplementation, give as 10% magnesium chloride once daily. Diuretics may cause hypomagnesaemia.

Chloride is an extracellular ion whose requirements are usually met from the normal dietary chloride.

Monitoring fluid and electrolyte therapy

Changes in weight relate well to total body water in newborns. Daily weights are a valuable aid in fluid management. Similarly, urine output should be monitored (minimum 1 ml/kg per h and maximum 7 ml/kg per h).

- Measure serum sodium, potassium, urea, creatinine, and calcium daily in sick infants.
- With abnormal electrolytes and/or large fluid requirements, six-hourly electrolyte determinations may be required.

- Paired measurements of plasma and urine osmolality are helpful in diagnosing SIADH secretion. Plasma osmolality = (2 × sodium) + (2 × potassium) + glucose + urea; (all values in mmol/l). Suspect SIADH if urine is not maximally dilute <100 mOsmol/kg H_2O with serum osmolality <270 mOsmol/kg H_2O. To diagnose SIADH, urine osmolality need only be inappropriately elevated and not necessarily greater than the corresponding serum osmolality.

Analyte	Reference range
Sodium	132–145 mmol/l
Potassium	3.6–5.9 mmol/l
Urea	1–5 mmol/l
Creatinine	<20–150 μmol/l
Chloride	90–110 mmol/l
Calcium	
Total	1.9–2.85 mmol/l
Ionised	1.12–1.52 mmol/l
Magnesium	0.71–1.1 mmol/l
Phosphate	1.4–3.0 mmol/l
Glucose	2.6–7 mmol/l
Plasma osmolality	280–300 mOsmol/kg H_2O
Urine osmolality	50–700 mOsmol/kg H_2O

Further reading

Modi N. Sodium intake and preterm babies. *Archives of Disease in Childhood* (1995) **69**:87–91.
Modi N. Management of fluid balance in the very immature neonate. *Archives of Disease in Childhood Fetal and Neonatal Edition* (2004) **89**:F108–11.
Modi N. Fluid balance and renal function. *Seminars in Neonatology* (2003) **8**(4).
Morgan JB, Dickerson JWT (eds). *Nutrition in Early Life*. Indianapolis, IN: Wiley, 2003.
Polin RA, Fox WW, Abman SH (eds). *Foetal and Neonatal Physiology*, 3rd edn. Philadelphia. WB Saunders, 2003.
Sedin G. Fluid management in the extremely preterm infant. In: TN Hansen, N McIntosh (eds). *Current Topics in Neonatology*, No. 1. London: WB Saunders, 1996: 50–66.
Shaffer SG, Weisman DN. Fluid requirements in the preterm infant. *Clinics in Perinatology* (1992) **19**:233–46.
Taeusch HW, Ballard R, Gleason CA (eds). *Avery's Disease of the Newborn*, 8th edn. Philadelphia: WB Saunders, 2004.

Related topics of interest

- nutrition
- patent ductus arteriosus
- trace minerals and vitamins.

Gastrooesophageal reflux

Gastrooesophageal reflux (GOR) is one of the commonest symptomatic clinical disorders affecting the gastrointestinal tract of infants and children. In recent years, GOR has been recognised more frequently because of the increased awareness of the condition and the more sophisticated diagnostic techniques that have been developed for both identifying and quantifying the disorder. It must be appreciated, however, that virtually all infants have some degree of GOR, though the severity of symptoms varies from the occasional posset to persistent vomiting. In the vast majority of infants with GOR, the symptoms improve spontaneously between the ages of nine to 24 months. Most infants with GOR are healthy and thriving, and require no diagnostic or therapeutic interventions, other than a careful history and examination with appropriate reassurance being given to the parents.

Aetiology

GOR is commonly due to a weakness of the gastrooesophageal junction sphincter. In addition, there may be an associated hiatus hernia. Chronic respiratory disorders, particularly CLD, are associated with an increased incidence of GOR, as are some neuromuscular disorders. It is also more common following some forms of thoraco-abdominal surgery (such as repair of oesophageal atresia and congenital diaphragmatic hernia). Conditions which delay gastric emptying encourage GOR. Methylxanthines may also promote GOR, as they reduce lower oesophageal sphincter tone. Overfeeding may also encourage reflux.

Clinical features

- reflex apnoeas refractory to other therapies
- 'unexplained' deteriorations in respiratory status
- repeated aspirations and aspiration pneumonias
- frequent small vomits to severe vomiting after feeds
- persistent small or large vomits which continue long after feeds
- difficulty with feeds and crying during feeds from associated oesophagitis.

Some infants with GOR exhibit abnormal behaviour and posturing, with tilting of the head to one side and bizarre contortions of the trunk, which has been labelled Sandifer's syndrome.

Investigations

1. *Chest radiograph.* Look for the radiographic changes of aspiration.
2. *Barium swallow.* Look for oesophageal anomalies, reflux, malrotation, and hiatus hernia.
3. *pH monitoring.* Oesophageal pH monitoring for 12–24h is the most sensitive investigation for detecting, quantifying, and monitoring GOR. The pH should be less than 4.0 for <5% of the study time. Values of $\geq15\%$ denote severe GOR.

4. *Endoscopy*. The availability of small fibre-optic endoscopes in recent years has made it possible for small infants and children with GOR to undergo endoscopy in order to visualise directly the oesophageal mucosa and take biopsies to determine the severity of reflux oesophagitis.

Management

Postural

Keep infant prone with head elevated (anti-Trendelenburg position). Do *not* nurse infant sitting at an angle of 60°, as this is associated with worse reflux. The right lateral position is associated with more reflux than positioning the infant in the prone or left lateral positions.

Feeding

Give small frequent feeds. Nasogastric feeds may also be helpful, as may food thickening agents such as Carobel (Cow & Gate) or Nestargel (Nestlé). Food thickeners, however, are not suitable for small preterm infants; although they may produce symptomatic relief, they do not improve reflux. Thickeners may also increase episodic coughing.

Drugs

- Antacids such as Gaviscon may be beneficial.
- H_2-antagonists (such as cimetidine or ranitidine) may relieve associated oesophagitis.
- Gastrokinetic agents (such as domperidone) are agents which improve gastrooesophageal motility and gastric emptying. Gastric emptying is accelerated by an increase in gastric and duodenal contractility. Gastric reflux into the oesophagus is decreased through a mechanism of increasing oesophageal peristaltic activity and enhancing oesophageal sphincter tone. Studies report decreased gastric residuals, decreased incidence of vomiting, a decrease in all reflux parameters measured, and improved weight gain in infants with vomiting. The average dose used in most studies is 200 µg/kg (range 200–400 µg/kg), 6–8-hourly.
- Proton pump inhibitors (such as omeprazole) are relatively new agents which inhibit the final step (H^+/K^+ ATPase) in gastric acid release from the parietal cell. They not only increase the pH of the refluxate, but also decrease total gastric secretion volume, thereby facilitating gastric emptying. Omeprazole is an effective therapy for histamine receptor type 2 antagonist-resistant peptic oesophagitis and relieves most symptoms and signs of GOR, even those that surgery has not helped. It is safe for short-term use (3–6 months) at doses of 20–40 mg/m^2 per day (0.5 mg/kg once daily = 20 mg/m^2 per day).

Surgery

When medical therapy has failed in infants with severe symptoms, especially in the presence of severe chronic lung disease, Nissen fundoplication may be required. It is worth remembering, however, that antireflux surgery has a significant failure and complication rate and occasional mortality, particularly in the neurologically impaired. In one study, over 30% of neurologically impaired children had major complications or died within 30 days of surgery; within a mean follow-up of 3.5 years,

25% had documented operative failure, and, overall, 71% had return of one or more preoperative symptoms of GOR. Increasing use of proton pump inhibitors may decrease the need for surgery.

Further reading

Alliet P, Raes M, Bruneel E et al. Omeprazole in infants with cimetidine-resistant peptic oesophagitis. *Journal of Pediatrics* (1998) **132:**352–4.

Ashcraft KW. Gastroesophageal reflux. In: KW Ashcraft, TM Holder (eds). *Pediatric Surgery*, 2nd edn. Philadelphia: WB Saunders, 1993: 270–88.

Berseth CL (ed.). Neonatal gastroenterology and nutrition. *Clinics in Perinatology* (2002) **29**(1).

del Rosario JF, Orenstein SR. Gastroesophageal reflux. In: TJ David (ed.). *Recent Advances in Paediatrics*, No. 17. Edinburgh: Churchill Livingstone, 1999: 161–72.

Gunasekaran TS, Hassall E. Efficacy and safety of omeprazole for severe gastroesophageal reflux in children. *Journal of Paediatrics* (1993) **124:**148–54.

Hassall E. Wrap session: is the Nissen slipping? Can medical treatment replace surgery for severe gastroesophageal reflux in children? *American Journal of Gastroenterology* (1995) **90:**1212–20.

Hillemeier AC. Gastroesophageal reflux: diagnosis and therapeutic approaches. *Pediatric Clinics of North America* (1996) **43:**197–212.

Hyman P. Gastroesophageal reflux: one reason why baby won't eat. *Journal of Pediatrics* (1994) **125:**S103–9.

Newell SJ, Booth IW, Morgan MEI et al. Gastro-oesophageal reflux in preterm infants. *Archives of Disease in Childhood* (1989) **6:**780–6.

Related topics of interest

- apnoeas and bradycardias
- chronic lung disease
- feeding difficulties
- vomiting.

Germinal matrix-intraventricular haemorrhage

The last two decades have witnessed a striking improvement in the survival of very premature infants, due mainly to the major improvements in perinatal medicine. There has also been a reassuring fall in the incidence of germinal matrix-intraventricular haemorrhage (IVH) from 40–50% to 20% in infants of birth weight less than 1500 g. However, IVH remains very common in the extremely preterm infant. The two major sequelae of IVH are posthaemorrhagic hydrocephalus (PHH) and periventricular haemorrhagic infarction. In contrast to the declining incidence of IVH, recent studies suggest that the prevalence of PHH has remained constant or may be increasing.

Incidence

IVH occurs primarily in the preterm infant requiring mechanical ventilation for RDS. The incidence of IVH is inversely related to gestation, being approximately 40% in infants of 30 weeks' gestation but rising to ~70–80% in the extremely preterm infants (<26 weeks' gestation). Ultrasound studies suggest that it may occur asymptomatically in approximately 5% of term infants.

Aetiology

The germinal matrix is a transient zone of the brain found in various periventricular sites, but which is most abundant in the caudate nucleus, where only a single layer of ependymal cells separates it from the lateral ventricles. In the germinal matrix, mitosis is active, and neurones then migrate to their final position within the brain. At the end of the second trimester, it is one of the most metabolically active areas of the brain, and has a rich vascular network. The vessels have thin epithelial cell walls and no muscular layer; it is hard to distinguish arterioles, capillaries, and veins, and they are particularly prone to bleed. The germinal matrix slowly involutes until 33–34 weeks' gestation.

Bleeding from the germinal matrix is thought of as an initial bleed which is then followed by its extension. IVH is essentially a postnatal event, although prenatal haemorrhage is well documented but uncommon. Approximately 30% of IVH has occurred by 6 h of age and more than 50% occurs during the first 24 h of life. Onset after 72 h of age is unusual. This high incidence of bleeds in the early hours of life in unstable preterm babies with respiratory distress has led to the view that haemodynamic instability and vessel wall immaturity are the major risk factors for IVH. Thus, the aetiology of the bleeding is considered under the following heads:

1. changes in cerebral haemodynamics
2. the wall of the blood vessels
3. coagulation abnormalities.

The cerebral blood flow (CBF) of preterm babies is pressure dependent; that is, if the blood pressure rises or falls, so does the CBF, including that through the germinal matrix. Increases in CBF may lead to vessel rupture and hence IVH. Situations known to acutely raise blood pressure include pneumothoraces, breathing against (fighting) the ventilator, painful procedures, endotracheal suction, and rapid infusions of blood or plasma. Hypercapnia—such as seen during a pneumothorax—is a potent cerebral vasodilator and an independent risk factor for IVH.

The thin capillary endothelial cell wall may be at risk of free radical damage. If so, administering a free radical scavenger, such as vitamin E, should reduce the risk of haemorrhage. Conflicting evidence exists as to whether this is so. If IVH is a very early postnatal phenomenon, it may be hard to give therapeutic doses of free radical scavengers prior to the onset of bleeding.

Once vessel rupture has occurred, bleeding is more likely to continue or recur if coagulation abnormalities exist. Conflicting evidence exists as to whether the administration of clotting factors in fresh-frozen plasma (FFP) is beneficial in preventing or reducing the extent of haemorrhages. Studies looking at clotting factor status at birth as a predictor of IVH have also produced conflicting evidence.

Classification

The extent of the bleeding has been classified by a number of authors. One classification frequently used in the UK is that of Papile:

grade I: isolated germinal matrix haemorrhage
grade II: rupture of the haemorrhage into the ventricle but without ventricular dilation
grade III: rupture of the haemorrhage into the ventricle with ventricular dilation
grade IV: IVH with parenchymal extension.

Prevention

If a preterm delivery cannot be avoided, the single most effective intervention is antenatal corticosteroids, which benefits the infant both by reducing RDS, and by an independent effect in reducing IVH, probably by improving capillary wall stability. Postnatal prevention of IVH is based on the recognition of the associated risk factors. Meticulous attention should be paid to rapid but gentle stabilisation of the sick preterm baby with RDS. Ventilation to achieve desired $PaCO_2$ should be achieved early with low peak pressures, with the baby not fighting the ventilator. Surfactant should be administered early, preferably during resuscitation on the labour ward, for the extremely premature baby at greatest risk. Humidification of the airway reduces the risk of tube blockage and associated hypercapnia. If the baby is hypotensive, blood pressure should be raised slowly and smoothly. Although the role of prophylactic FFP in reducing haemorrhage is unproven, many neonatologists use fresh-frozen plasma 'prophylactically' if colloid is needed for volume expansion. Severe thrombocytopaenia or coagulopathy should be treated without causing rapid volume overload.

A number of drug treatments have been attempted (such as that with phenobarbital). As yet, none have consistently shown benefit in both reducing the extent of haemorrhage and preventing later handicap.

Consequences

Periventricular haemorrhagic infarction
This is thought to occur when a clot distending the lateral ventricle obstructs the medullary veins draining into the subependymal veins. This stasis leads to haemorrhage and infarction. Extension of sonographic echodensities from an IVH into the parenchyma is difficult to interpret. They may represent direct extension, venous infarction, or bleeding into an ischaemic infarction of periventricular leucomalacia.

Posthaemorrhagic hydrocephalus
Defined as a ventricular index above the 97th percentile, this occurs in 20–40% of babies after IVH. The ventricular index is the distance from the midline to the most lateral point of the ventricle in the coronal plane at the level of the hippocampal gyrus. Such dilation is usually transient, and only 15–20% of patients need shunting for progressive hydrocephalus.

Death
Over 50% of babies with parenchymal extension of their IVH die. These babies usually have the worst respiratory problems, and the IVH is not always the principal cause of death.

Neurodevelopmental handicap
This is most common in those with parenchymal involvement. The most potent predictor of handicap is ultrasonographic abnormalities of the white matter, best imaged by MRI. Two-thirds of babies left with periventricular cysts after grade IV IVH or periventricular leucomalacia develop cerebral palsy. PHH also increases the risk of severe neurologic sequelae to 50–60%. This may be related more to cerebral atrophy after parenchymal infarction and/or haemorrhage than to the hydrocephalus *per se*. Preterm babies with only grade I and II IVHs have handicap rates of 4–5%, little different from the risk of about 2% for babies of the same gestation with normal scans.

Further reading

Govaert P. Cranial haemorrhage in the term newborn infant. In: *Clinics in Developmental Medicine*, No. 129. London: MacKeith Press, 1994.

Govaert P, de Vries LS. *An Atlas of Neonatal Brain Sonography*. London: MacKeith Press, 1997.

Levene MI, Chervenak FA, Whittle M (eds). *Fetal and Neonatal Neurology and Neurosurgery*, 3rd edn. Edinburgh: Churchill Livingstone, 2001.

Paneth N, Rudelli R, Kazam E et al. Brain damage in the preterm infant. In: *Clinics in Developmental Medicine*, No. 131. London: MacKeith Press, 1994.

Perlman J (ed.). Perinatal brain injury. *Clinics in Perinatology* (2002) **29**(4).

Rennie JM. *Neonatal Cerebral Ultrasound*. Cambridge: Cambridge University Press, 1997.

Saliba E (ed.). Perinatal brain injury. *Seminars in Neonatology* (2001) **6**(2).

Stevenson DK, Benitz WE, Sunshine P (eds). *Fetal and Neonatal Brain Injury: Mechanisms, Management and the Risks of Practice*, 3rd edn. Cambridge: Cambridge University Press, 2003.

Related topics of interest

- bleeding disorders
- death of a baby
- hypoxic-ischaemic encephalopathy
- hydrocephalus
- periventricular leucomalacia.

Haemolytic disease

Haemolytic disease may have adverse but transient effects on the developing foetus and the newborn infant but also the potential to cause permanent adverse sequelae. Timely antenatal diagnosis and appropriate treatment may prevent many of these unfavourable effects.

In the foetus

In haemolytic disease, antibodies acquired transplacentally from a sensitised mother destroy foetal red cells. Several blood group antigens can cause problems in pregnancy, but rhesus incompatibility still accounts for the majority of severe disease. It is diagnosed antenatally by rising maternal antibody titres, and then monitored at the following three levels of increasing complexity and risk:

1. antibody titres in maternal serum in pregnancy
2. optical density of the amniotic fluid
3. cordocentesis to measure foetal haemoglobin.

Most affected pregnancies are managed expectantly and monitored by serum antibody levels alone. Unfortunately, these have a poor predictive value for foetal disease, and when severe foetal disease is suspected, invasive monitoring and treatment are indicated. Liley's curves of optical density at 450 nm, the absorption wavelength of bilirubin, are used to predict the severity of the disease from 27 weeks onwards. They have been extended and modified by others. If very severe disease is present, either delivery—if the baby is definitely viable—or cordocentesis and intrauterine transfusion are indicated. The transfused cells must be compatible with maternal serum. This does not stop the haemolysis of foetal cells, but maintains an adequate haemoglobin until delivery is possible.

Rhesus haemolytic disease can develop only after maternal exposure to foetal cells at birth, as in an abortion, APH, or amniocentesis, or after an incompatible transfusion. About 90% of rhesus-incompatible pregnancies cause no reaction, either because the innoculum is small, or because ABO incompatibility protects the foetus. Usually, first pregnancies are unaffected, and the disease worsens in second and later pregnancies after recurrent exposure of the mother's immune system to foreign red cell proteins. The risk of rhesus sensitisation and hence disease is greatly reduced by the administration of anti-D immunoglobulin to affected mothers at 28 weeks and again within 24 h of delivery. Overall, the incidence of severe disease has now fallen to about one per 1000 births.

Other red cell antigen incompatibilities, notably ABO, can cause haemolysis. ABO incompatibilities can occur in a first pregnancy, as the AB red cell markers are strongly antigenic. Early severe jaundice can result, but haemolysis and anaemia are generally mild. Haemolysis in babies can also result from the following:

- infection
- hereditary spherocytosis
- vitamin E deficiency in preterm babies some weeks after birth

- deficiencies of enzymes such as glucose-6-phosphate dehydrogenase (G6PD) and pyruvate kinase.

The second and last factors may result in anaemia and prolonged jaundice, starting soon after birth.

Foetal assessment
In the present pregnancy, check the antibody titres and amniotic fluid optical density, and, if necessary, perform cordocentesis. Monitor biophysical profile for foetal well-being, and if preterm delivery is likely, give the mother corticosteroids.

In the neonate

Many babies will have only mild disease, needing either no treatment or only photo-therapy and tests to exclude anaemia. When a neonate is at risk of severe disease, early assessment and treatment are essential.

Assessment at birth
History
Check previous pregnancies and their outcome.

Physical examination
The main features are as follows:

- pallor
- jaundice
- tachycardia
- hepatosplenomegaly
- respiratory distress
- oedema, ascites, and effusions.

Laboratory tests on the cord blood
- FBC
- U and E
- clotting screen
- serum bilirubin
- serum albumin
- liver function tests
- blood group and Coombs' test
- blood glucose and blood gases.

Treatment at birth

Prompt cardiorespiratory resuscitation and stabilisation may be necessary if severe rhesus disease and hydrops fetalis are expected. Intubation, ventilation, insertion of an umbilical venous catheter (UVC), and drainage of effusions and ascites may be necessary on the labour ward. If there is heart failure, the UVC can facilitate central venous pressure measurement. If necessary, a negative balance partial exchange with mother-compatible cytomegalovirus (CMV)-negative O-negative blood performed within minutes of birth can reduce the circulating volume and begin to correct the anaemia. Other complications such as hypoglycaemia, thrombocytopenia (with or without DIC), hypoalbuminaemia, and surfactant deficiency may also require prompt attention.

Early treatment

After initial stabilisation, the major concerns are to control hyperbilirubinaemia and prevent kernicterus, and to correct the anaemia further if necessary. Cord haemoglobin and bilirubin have been suggested as a guide to when early exchange transfusion (that is, one initiated within an hour or so of birth solely on the basis of cord blood values) should be performed. There is poor correlation between these single cord blood values and the need for early exchange. The advent of more effective phototherapy has further undermined these old criteria. However, a rise in bilirubin of over 8 µmol/l per h is indicative of a need for an early exchange transfusion, particularly if the cord bilirubin was over 95 µmol/l. These crude guidelines need to be interpreted against a knowledge of the output and effectiveness of the phototherapy unit used on an individual baby.

The criteria for later exchange transfusions in haemolytic disease have been debated, but most authorities still consider a total bilirubin level of >340 µmol/l to be the threshold. Exchange transfusions and phototherapy are considered further in the chapter 'Jaundice'.

Later treatment

Late anaemia, at 3–8 weeks of age, is a frequent complication of haemolytic disease. Top-up transfusion should be considered if the infant is lethargic or feeding poorly rather than on a specific haemoglobin concentration, though if the latter falls below 6 g/dl, most practitioners would then transfuse. Erythropoietin is currently being researched as an adjunct to therapy, but it cannot yet be recommended on a routine basis.

Outcome for rhesus haemolytic disease is good. More research is needed to establish whether paediatricians should remain 'vigintiphobic', that is, afraid of letting the bilirubin level rise above 20 mg/dl (340 µmol/l), or whether higher levels in well term babies with haemolysis can be tolerated without fear of long-term neurologic sequelae.

Further reading

Ahlfors CE. Criteria for exchange transfusion in jaundiced newborns. *Pediatrics* (1994) **93**:488–94.

Fanaroff AA, Martin RJ. *Neonatal-Perinatal Medicine: Diseases of the Fetus and Infant*, 7th edn. St Louis, MO: Mosby, 2001.

Gollin YG, Copel JA. Management of the Rh-sensitized mother. *Clinics in Perinatology* (1995) **22**:545–59.

Maisels MJ, Watchko JF. *Neonatal Jaundice*. London: Martin Dunitz, 2000.

Nathan DG, Orkin SH, Look T et al (eds). *Nathan and Oski's Hematology of Infancy and Childhood*, 6th edn. Philadelphia: WB Saunders, 2003.

Peterec SM. Management of neonatal Rh disease. *Clinics in Perinatology* (1995) **22**:561–92.

Related topics of interest

- anaemia
- hydrops fetalis
- jaundice
- prenatal diagnosis.

Head size

The size of the head in the newborn infant is an important physical sign, as a small or large head may be indicative of an underlying malformation, antenatal infection, or metabolic or chromosomal disorder, often with resultant cerebral damage. An occipito-frontal head circumference above the 90th percentile or below the 10th percentile (especially if unduly disproportionate compared to the birth weight) should make one consider possible pathologic causes for the discrepant head size. The infant may otherwise look normal or have a number of malformations which might be recognisable as a specific disorder or syndrome. It is therefore important to evaluate carefully any dysmorphic features in an infant with an abnormally sized head, as this will help achieve the correct diagnosis and management plans.

Large head

Aetiology
Hydrocephalus
- posthaemorrhagic (as in alloimmune thrombocytopenia)
- postinfection (as in TORCH infections)
- malformations (as in spina bifida and Dandy–Walker cyst)
- X-linked
- syndromic (as in neurofibromatosis).

Hydranencephaly

Megalencephaly (as in Sotos syndrome or familial megalencephaly)

Clinical features
- obviously large head with large anterior fontanelle, widely separated sutures, and open posterior fontanelle at term
- head circumference greater than 97th percentile by $\geq 2\,cm$
- sunsetting
- head freely transilluminates (hydranencephaly or severe hydrocephalus)
- accompanying dysmorphic features or malformations when part of a syndrome or malformation sequence (as in myelomeningocele)
- depressible 'springy' membranous bones of the cranial vault (craniolacunae).

Investigations
- cranial ultrasound
- CT scan
- MRI scan (best resolution)
- coagulation studies (unusual haemorrhages)
- search for congenital infections (signs of prenatal infection evident).

Management
- Hydrocephalus is treated by insertion of ventriculoperitoneal shunt.
- Repeated lumbar or ventricular punctures are not appropriate for congenital hydrocephalus.

- Rectify coagulation defect(s) where appropriate.
- If syndromic, address accompanying problems appropriately.
- Treat congenital infections if appropriate (as in toxoplasmosis).
- Provide genetic counselling where indicated.

Small head

Aetiology
- chromosomal abnormalities
- syndromic
- hereditary—autosomal recessive and x-linked
- antenatal developmental malformations
- metabolic disorder (phenylketonuria—late)
- intrauterine infections such as TORCH.

Clinical features
- head circumference below 2nd percentile
- forehead slopes backwards
- accompanying dysmorphic features or malformations if syndromic
- other signs of congenital infection (such as cataracts and chorioretinitis).

Investigations
- ultrasound scan
- CT scan (intracranial calcification)
- MRI scan (for congenital malformations)
- chromosomal analysis
- family history
- review by clinical geneticist/syndromologist
- audiology assessment (exclude deafness)
- ophthalmology assessment (congenital malformation).

Management
- Isolate infants with congenital infection (such as CMV).
- Counsel parents on prognosis and recurrence.
- Arrange appropriate developmental follow-up.
- Treat congenital infections if appropriate.

Family support group and information

Association for Spina Bifida and Hydrocephalus
42 Park Road
Peterborough PE1 2UQ, UK
Tel: 01733 555 988
www.asbah.org

Further reading

Aicardi J. *Diseases of the Nervous System in Childhood.* Cambridge: Cambridge University Press, 1998.

Garton HJL, Piatt JH. Hydrocephalus. *Pediatric Clinics of North America* (2004) **51:**305–25.

Levene M, Chervenak FA, Whittle M (eds). *Fetal and Neonatal Neurology and Neurosurgery,* 3rd edn. Edinburgh: Churchill Livingstone, 2001.

Volpe JJ. *Neurology of the Newborn*, 4th edn. Philadelphia: WB Saunders, 2001.

Related topics of interest

- congenital malformations and birth defects
- infection—prenatal
- neural tube defects.

Hearing screening

Infants have had their hearing screened in the UK since the early 1960s with the Health Visitor Distraction Test (HVDT). The HVDT is performed when the child is 7–8 months old. The test consists of identifying responses to low-level sounds presented to the child by a tester while the child's attention is manipulated by a second tester. By the early 1970s, however, professionals were questioning the effectiveness of this test in terms of its ability to reach and screen all infants, and its ability to identify the majority of infants with congenital hearing impairment.

By the 1980s, more robust screening techniques had been developed, that is, automated auditory brainstem response (AABR) and automated otoacoustic emission (AOAE), which are capable of screening the hearing of newborn babies. As a result, the Department of Health commissioned a comprehensive survey of current pre-school hearing screening provision in the UK coupled with a health economics study of hearing screening costs. The Health Technology Assessment review (1997) highlighted major problems with the current information system. It revealed that the screening performance of the HVDT had poor sensitivity and specificity with a relatively low yield. For those screened only by the health visitor, identification was, on average, at about 26 months of age (median age 12–20 months), with intervention at about 32 months, on average. By contrast, neonatal hearing screening methods (AOAE and AABR) showed a high test sensitivity (>90%) and specificity (~95%). Pilot universal neonatal screening programmes would have a greater coverage (>90%), yields of 11.3 per 1000, and a median identification age for those screened at about two months. Universal neonatal screening appeared to have lower associated initial costs than HVDT per child screened. The cost per case found is several magnitudes lower with universal neonatal screening.

Epidemiology

Approximately 840 children a year (or one in 842 newborns) are born in the UK with moderate to profound hearing impairment (hearing impairment on the better ear of over 40 dB HL over the frequencies 0.5, 1.2, and 4 kHz). Present services (mainly HVDT) are not sensitive enough to identify about 400 of these by the time they are one-and-a-half years old, and 200 of these until the age of three-and-a-half years. This significantly delays the child's acquisition of language and communication skills, with consequent longer-term risk to education achievement, general behaviour, and quality of life. There is also increased benefit for the family, as appropriate support and guidance is given to the family at the earliest opportunity.

The UK National Screening Committee, the body that advises the government on all aspects of screening policy, has accepted the recommendations of the Health Technology Review. The Newborn Hearing Screening Programme (NHSP) will be gradually rolled-out across the country, with all areas of England being covered by 2006. The programme will implement the hearing screen for all newborn babies in England.

Newborn Hearing Screening Programme (NHSP)

This offers universal hearing screening by the otoacoustic emissions tests and/or auditory brainstem response carried out in the first days of life by holding a device in the child's ear to measure sound emissions. The screening programme will be hospital based, allowing babies missed at birth to be tested at 4–6 weeks. Infants without clear responses on AOAE testing go on to AABR testing. If clear responses in one or both ears are still not obtained, a formal hearing assessment (ABR) is performed. Where this shows a raised hearing threshold, audiological follow-up is required, and should the hearing threshold not be raised, appropriate child health surveillance follows.

Deafness

Deafness may be classified as *conductive* deafness or *sensorineural* deafness (nerve deafness). Conductive deafness is less severe and is often amenable to medical or surgical treatment. In developed countries, bilateral significant sensorineural deafness occurs in one in 1000 live births. 'Significant loss' is a loss of between 25–35 dB in the better ear. High frequency loss is more important. If the loss in the better ear is at a level of 30 dB when averaged over the four frequencies 500 Hz, 1 kHz, 2 kHz, and 4 kHz, some kind of amplification will be required for the child to attain normal speech and language. Causes for significant bilateral sensorineural loss are identifiable in only 50% of cases.

Causes of sensorineural deafness

Hereditary prenatal causes
Isolated genetic
The genetic causes may be autosomal recessive, autosomal dominant, or sex-linked.

Associated syndromes
- *Waardenburg syndrome*: autosomal dominant disorder with variable expression, comprising some or all of the following traits: unilateral or bilateral perceptive deafness; hypertrichosis of the eyebrows, which meet in the midline; heterochromia of the irises; or a white forelock.
- *Klippel-Feil syndrome*: a short neck which limits head movements with low hairline at back, paralysis of the external rectus muscle in one or both eyes, and perceptive hearing loss, which may be severe.
- *Alport's syndrome*: X-linked dominant affecting boys more severely than girls. There is severe, progressive glomerulonephritis and a progressive sensorineural loss, which normally manifests after the age of ten years.
- *Pendred's syndrome*: autosomal recessive. Causes simple goitre at about 4–5 years and severe deafness.
- *Jervell and Lange-Nielsen syndrome*: autosomal recessive with cardiac arrhythmia (prolonged QT interval) and severe deafness.
- *Usher's syndrome*: autosomal recessive. Retinitis pigmentosa with contraction of the visual fields and severe sensorineural deafness, which may be progressive.

- *Refsum's syndrome*: icthyosis, ataxia, retinitis pigmentosa, mental retardation, and deafness.

Nonhereditary prenatal (sensorineural) deafness
- maternal illness (especially first trimester) due to TORCH infections (toxoplasmosis exerts most effect in the last trimester), glandular fever, and syphilis
- maternal administration of ototoxic drugs (such as aminoglycosides, quinine, and alcohol).

Perinatal and postnatal (sensorineural) deafness
- Perinatal hypoxia, including hypoxica ischaemic encephalopathy (HIE) (the cochlea is especially sensitive to hypoxia). PPHN is highly associated with sensorineural hearing loss, up to 4–21% of survivors being reported as having hearing loss.
- Bilirubin encephalopathy (kernicterus) causes a high-frequency sensorineural deafness.
- Bacterial meningitis is the single most important cause of acquired sensorineural hearing loss in childhood, neonates being especially vulnerable.
- Toxicity (as of antibiotics such as aminoglycosides and streptomycin).

Management of sensorineural deafness
- Evidence of prenatal infection should be sought.
- In view of the associated syndromes, genetic counselling should be provided.
- The mainstay of treatment remains amplification by some form of hearing aid. Children with severe (65–80 dB) to profound (85 dB) hearing loss derive most benefit from a radio transmission aid where the amplified output of the remote microphone is transmitted to the child by frequency modulated radio transmission (the phonic ear).
- Cochlear implants are the latest and most powerful forms of hearing aids. These devices are inserted into the inner ear of a totally deaf person to introduce or restore perception of sound.

Parent information and support groups
National Deaf Children's Society
15 Dufferin Street
London EC1Y 8UR, UK
Tel: 020 7490 8656
www.ndcs.org.uk

Royal National Institute for Deaf People (RNID)
19–23 Featherstone Street
London EC1Y 8SL, UK
Tel: 020 7296 8001
www.rnid.org.uk

Useful websites

www.nsc.nhs.uk
The UK National Screening Committee website.

www.nhsp.info
The NHS Newborn Hearing Screening Programme website.

Further reading

Cunningham M, Cox EO. Hearing assessment in infants and children: recommendations beyond neonatal screening. *Pediatrics* (2003) **111:**436–40.
Hone SW, Smith RJH. Genetics of hearing impairment. *Seminars in Neonatology* (2001) **6:**531–41.
Johnson KC. Audiologic assessment of children with suspected hearing loss. *Otolaryngology Clinics of North America* (2002) **35:**711–32.
Kerschner JE. Neonatal hearing screening: to do or not to do. *Pediatric Clinics of North America* (2004) **51:**725–36.
Ramsden R, Graham J. Cochlear implantation. *British Medical Journal* (1995) **311:**1588.
Sirimanna KS. Management of hearing impaired infant. *Seminars in Neonatology* (2001) **6:**511–19.
Watkin PM. Neonatal screening for hearing impairment. *Seminars in Neonatology* (2001) **6:**501–9.

Related topics of interest

- discharge planning and follow-up
- extreme prematurity
- postnatal examination.

Heart murmurs in neonates

Milind Chaudhari

Neonatal heart murmurs are extremely variable due to the postnatal cardiopulmonary adaptations. The intensity and the character of the murmur may not bear any relation to the severity of the underlying cardiac malformation, and distinction between innocent and pathological murmurs is often difficult on clinical grounds only.

Innocent cardiac murmurs in neonates

Transient murmurs are common in neonatal period. Two-thirds of normal neonates will have an innocent murmur in the first few days of life. These neonates are entirely asymptomatic from the cardiac viewpoint, and there are no abnormal physical findings on examination. The ECG and chest radiograph are normal. The commonest innocent murmurs in neonates are discussed below.

Pulmonary flow murmur of the newborn

This murmur is common in preterm and small for gestational age infants. The murmur is soft, grade 2/6 or less in intensity. This is best heard in the pulmonary area and may radiate over both lung fields, the axillae, and the back. This murmur is thought to be largely due to a physiological pulmonary branch stenosis, which resolves in two-thirds of infants by six weeks and in almost all infants by six months.

Transient systolic murmur of the patent ductus arteriosus (PDA)

This murmur presents due to delayed closure of the PDA and is best heard beneath the left infraclavicular area. The murmur is soft, systolic, and grade 2/6 or less in intensity, and it usually disappears a few days after birth as the PDA closes. PDA murmurs may be detected in up to 60% of healthy infants at term within the first 48 h of life. By six weeks of age, however, most, if not all, PDAs should have closed.

Transient systolic murmur of tricuspid regurgitation

This soft systolic murmur localised to the left sternal edge is due to mild tricuspid regurgitation in the presence of high pulmonary vascular resistance (PVR). It disappears in the first few days of life as PVR falls to normal values.

Murmurs persisting beyond the neonatal period require further cardiac evaluation.

Pathological heart murmurs in neonates

In contrast to innocent murmurs, pathological heart murmurs are louder in intensity (grade 3/6 or more), longer in duration, and less variable. The presence of a diastolic component points to the pathological nature of a murmur. In general, murmurs audible soon after birth are due to obstructive lesions, such as pulmonary stenosis, aortic stenosis, coarctation of aorta, and other lesions, whereas murmurs due to left-to-right shunts are audible a few days later when PVR is sufficiently lowered. Evaluation in an asymptomatic and otherwise well neonate should include detailed cardiac examination with recording of four limb blood pressure, pulse oximetry, ECG and chest radiograph. The echocardiogram is essential for anatomical diagnosis and also to plan subsequent therapy and follow-up. A neonate with cardiac symptoms and associated dysmorphic features or congenital anomalies of other organ systems requires a complete evaluation by the paediatric cardiologist.

Further reading

Allen HD, Gutgesell HP, Clark EB et al. *Moss and Adams' Heart Disease in Infants, Children, and Adolescents*, 6th edn. Philadelphia: Lippincott, Williams & Wilkins, 2000.

Arlettaz R, Archer N, Wilkinson AR. Natural history of innocent heart murmurs in newborn babies: controlled echocardiographic study. *Archives of Disease in Childhood Fetal and Neonatal Edition* (1998) **78:**F166–70.

Burton DA. Cabalka AK. Cardiac evaluation of infants. *Pediatric Clinics of North America* (1994) **41:**991–1011.

Park MK. *Pediatric Cardiology for Practitioners*, 3rd edn. Chicago: Year Book Medical Publishers, 1996.

Silove ED. Assessment and management of congenital heart disease in the newborn by the district paediatrician. *Archives of Disease in Childhood* (1994) **70:**F71–4.

Related topics of interest

- acute collapse
- cardiac arrhythmias
- congenital heart disease—congestive heart failure
- congenital heart disease—cyanotic defects.

Hepatitis B and C

Hepatitis B infection is a significant global public health problem, with the total number of asymptomatic carriers worldwide being greater than the combined population of Europe. The majority of carriers reside in the developing countries. The prevalence of hepatitis B surface antigen, HBsAg, varies from 0.1% in parts of Europe to 20% in the Far East. Hepatitis B is transmitted parenterally (blood-to-blood contact or injury with contaminated sharp instruments), by perinatal transmission from mother to child, or sexually. Transplacental infection is uncommon, and most infants acquire the infection at birth from their carrier mothers or later during childhood. Susceptibility to infection and perinatal transmission vary with ethnicity, being highest in the Chinese. Expression of 'e' antigen (HBeAg) markedly increases risk of infection in the baby. The risk is low when the mother is e-antibody positive (anti-HBe positive) and e-antigen negative, and intermediate when neither the e-antigen nor antibody is detectable. Transfusion-associated infection is now rare in the UK.

Following infection, the HBsAg appears in the infant's blood after 6–16 weeks, with most infants (90%) becoming chronic asymptomatic carriers in contrast to 2–10% of those infected as adults. A few may develop severe and fatal hepatitis. Currently, the carrier status, once developed, is permanent and is significantly associated with fatal chronic liver disease and carcinoma in adulthood. Prevention of hepatitis B by immunisation is therefore particularly important. All medical and nursing staff should be immunised against hepatitis B.

Risk factors

- maternal hepatitis B carriage (HBsAg positive), especially HBeAg positivity
- parent(s) having been resident in certain high-risk institutions (such as prison and mental institutions)
- parent(s) frequent traveller(s) to areas of high hepatitis B prevalence
- parent(s) originating from region with high prevalence of hepatitis B
- parent(s) with recent hepatitis infection or chronic liver disease
- parent(s) changing sexual partners frequently
- parent(s) being intravenous drug abuser
- parent(s) being haemophiliac.

Treat all patients as potential hepatitis B carriers!

Investigations

Screen all mothers or those in at-risk groups for presence of serologic markers of hepatitis B virus (HBV) infection (HBsAg and HBeAg). Offer human immunodeficiency virus (HIV) screening for HBsAg-positive drug abusers.

Prevention

Take appropriate precautions at the delivery and resuscitation of all infants, but especially where mothers are known hepatitis B carriers or one of the parents has the risk factors above. Breast-feeding by hepatitis B carrier mothers is discouraged because of a small risk of infecting the infant, but in developing countries the dangers of not breast-feeding may be greater than the risks of continuing breast-feeding.

Immunisation

There are two types of immunisation product—a vaccine that produces an immune response, and a specific hepatitis B immunoglobulin (HBIG) that provides passive immunity, conferring immediate but temporary protection after accidental innoculation or contamination with antigen-positive blood.

Infants of hepatitis B carriers or those at a high risk of infection should be immunised against hepatitis B as follows: hepatitis B vaccine 0.5 ml (10 µg) Engerix B (SmithKline Beecham) or 0.5 ml (5 µg) H-B-Vax II (Pasteur Merieux MSD) i.m. at birth, one month, and two months after the first, with a booster dose at 12 months. If the mother is e-antigen positive but e-antibody negative, or had acute hepatitis B during pregnancy, HBIG 200 mg (200 IU) is also given i.m. (deep thigh injection) within 48 h of birth. Use anterolateral thigh, and not the buttock, as vaccine efficacy may be reduced.

Check for evidence of adequate immunity at one year. Individuals producing antibodies to HBsAg (anti-HBs) at levels of ≥100 mIU/ml are considered immune; poor responders (anti-HBs 10–100 mIU/ml) should receive a booster dose, and nonresponders (anti-HBs <10 mIU/ml should receive a repeat course of vaccine. The duration of antibody persistence is variable, but, generally, a booster dose is required after five years.

The above schedule of active/passive immunisation is highly effective at confirming immunity (nine out of ten immune at one year).

Postexposure prophylaxis

Active/passive immunisation is recommended for all staff who accidentally innoculate themselves or contaminate their eye(s), mouth, fresh cuts, or skin abrasions with blood from a known HBsAg-positive person. The affected area should be washed well with soap and warm water, and HBIG (500 IU adults, 200 IU infants) administered with simultaneous administration of hepatitis B vaccine at a different site. In the previously adequately immunised, only a single booster dose of HB vaccine is required, whereas an accelerated complete course of HB vaccine should be used in the nonimmunised. If, however, infection has already occurred at the time of immunisation, severe illness and the development of the carrier state may still be prevented.

Hepatitis C

With the identification of the hepatitis C virus in 1989, hepatitis C rapidly became a worldwide public health problem. The World Health Organisation estimates that 3%

of the world population has been infected. An estimated 500 000 people are chronically infected in the UK, with at least 100 dying each year. Prevalence of the virus varies around the world (1% in France, 1.8% in the USA, and higher still in Africa, Asia, and the Middle East). The UK has a low prevalence of only 0.5%. In developed countries, transmission is largely related to previous or current injecting drug use (92.3% in the UK), with sexual exposure (1.5%), vertical transmission from mother to baby (0.9%), and skin piercing and tattooing with nonsterile equipment being minor contributors. As blood donors are now screened for hepatitis C, with viral inactivation of blood products, the chances of being infected with hepatitis C through blood transfusion are extremely low. Mother to baby transmission occurs at a rate of 5–6%, mainly in women with high levels of virus and most probably around the time of delivery. In mothers who are coinfected with HIV, hepatitis C transmission to infants is threefold higher at 14–17%. Unlike HIV, breast-feeding does not appear to increase the risk of transmission of infection, and currently there are no drugs that may be offered to reduce the risk of mother to infant transmission of hepatitis C, nor is there an effective vaccine.

The hepatitis C virus (an RNA virus), has six genotypes, an incubation period of 6–9 weeks, and it produces a specific antibody response three months after infection. Initial infection generally produces no symptoms, and 20% of those infected clear the virus in 2–6 months, while 80% become chronically infected. Some 20% of chronically infected people may develop serious liver disease (such as cirrhosis) after 20 years; of these, 1–4% per year develop liver cancer. Hepatitis B is a cofactor for progression of hepatitis C disease. However, antiviral therapy can clear the virus in 50% of individuals showing signs of moderate to severe disease. Most chronically infected children are asymptomatic and hence have normal growth and development. They should, however, be referred to a specialist paediatric hepatology centre for treatment. NICE recommends combination antiviral drug therapy consisting of ribavirin and interferon in patients over the age of 18 years who have moderate to severe hepatitis C. Where ribavirin is contraindicated, interferon monotherapy may be used. Treatment aims to clear the hepatitis C virus and achieve normal liver function tests. In the absence of a safe and effective intervention to prevent mother to infant infection and the limited evidence on the efficacy of treatment of children infected with hepatitis C, antenatal screening for hepatitis C is presently not recommended.

Useful websites

www.cdc.gov/ncidod/diseases/hepatitis
US National Center for Infectious Diseases – Viral Hepatitis.

www.doh.gov.uk/cmo/hcvstrategy
Hepatitis C strategy by the UK Department of Health.

Further reading

Beasley RP, Hwang L-Y, Lee GC-Y et al. Prevention of perinatally transmitted hepatitis B virus infections with hepatitis B immune globulin and hepatitis B vaccine. *Lancet* (1983) **ii:**1099–102.

Booth J, O'Grady J, Neuberger J (on behalf of British Society of Gastroenterology). Clinical guidelines on the management of hepatitis C. *Gut* (2001) **49**(Suppl 1):i1–21.

Broderick AL, Jonas MM. Hepatitis B in children. *Seminars in Liver Disease* (2003) **23**:59–68.

Department of Health. *Hepatitis C: Essential Information for Professionals*. London: Department of Health, 2002.

Dusheiko GM, Khakoo S, Poni S, Grellier L. A rational approach to the management of hepatitis C infection. *British Medical Journal* (1996) **312**:357–64.

Polakoff S, Vandervelde EM. Immunisation of neonates at high risk of hepatitis B in England and Wales. A national surveillance. *British Medical Journal* (1988) **297**:249–53.

Saari TN and the Committee on Infectious Diseases of the American Academy of Pediatrics. Immunization of preterm and low birth weight infants. *Pediatrics* (2003) **112**:193–8.

Salisbury DM, Begg NT (eds). *Immunisation Against Infectious Disease*. London: HMSO, 1996.

Williams IT, Goldstein ST, Tufa J, et al. Long term antibody response to hepatitis B vaccination beginning at birth and to subsequent booster vaccination. *Pediatric Infectious Disease Journal* (2003) **22**:157–63.

Related topics of interest

- HIV/AIDS
- immunisations
- infection—perinatal.

Herniae

Inguinal

A patent processus vaginalis left in the wake of the descending testes predisposes the infant to develop an inguinal hernia. Inguinal hernias are therefore six times more common in boys than girls. The right side is more commonly affected (60%) than the left (30%), with 1:10 being bilateral. The more premature the infant, the greater is the incidence and the more likely are the complications. As the risks of strangulation are highest during the first few months of life, aim to repair hernias before discharge from hospital.

Presentation
- persistent or intermittent mass in the groin
- constant crying or irritability
- abdominal distension
- bilious vomiting
- apnoeic spells.

Diagnosis
- This is made on clinical grounds when a mass is felt overlying the inguinal ring, in the scrotum, or in the labia majora on the affected side.
- The mass enlarges when infant strains or cries.
- A tender discoloured swelling which does not reduce is a surgical emergency.

The differential diagnosis includes an encysted hydrocele of the cord (cyst is non-tender, moves with cord, and is translucent), torsion of the testis (testis is swollen and tender), superficial inguinal lymphadenitis, and localised inguinal abscess (located below and lateral to the external inguinal ring).

Management
- Herniae should be repaired when the respiratory status is optimal—usually before discharge from hospital.
- Spinal anaesthesia reduces respiratory morbidity.
- Exploring the contralateral side may be beneficial, as the processus may be patent in up to 50%.
- In female patients, the surgeon should ascertain that the hernia does not contain male gonads.

Oxygen requirements frequently come down following inguinal hernia repair in infants with CLD who are oxygen dependent.

Umbilical hernia

Umbilical hernias are fairly common and result from failure of the umbilical ring to obliterate. In infants, the hernia may be quite large, giving the skin a blue hue. They are always reducible and cause no symptoms, although they may be blamed for 'colic'.

Even large herniae tend to resolve spontaneously as the umbilical cicatrix contracts over the first few years of life, so repair should be delayed for at least one year and probably up to the age of three years. The main indication for surgery is cosmetic appearance, as strangulation is almost unknown in children.

Epigastric hernia

An epigastric hernia occurs when extraperitoneal fat bulges through a small defect in the linea alba, commonly midway between the xiphisternum and umbilicus. The fat arises from within the falciform ligament, and the hernia presents as a midline small lump between the xiphisternum and umbilicus. The lump is usually irreducible but rarely causes symptoms (discomfort after meals). Bowel or peritoneum never protrudes through the defect (commonly only 1–2 mm diameter). Surgery is required only if they cause discomfort or for cosmetic reasons.

Further reading

Beasley SW, Hutson JM, Auldist AW. *Essential Paediatric Surgery*. London: Arnold, 1996.
Black JA, Whitfield MF. *Neonatal Emergencies: Early Detection and Management*, 2nd edn. Oxford: Butterworth-Heinemann, 1991.
Donnellan WL, Kimura K, Schafer JC et al. *Abdominal Surgery of Infancy and Childhood*. London: Martin Dunitz, 1996.
Liebert PS. *Color Atlas of Pediatric Surgery*, 2nd edn. Philadelphia: WB Saunders, 1997.
Puri P (ed.). *Newborn Surgery*, 2nd edn. London: Arnold, 2003.

Related topics of interest

- abdominal distension
- congenital diaphragmatic hernia
- neonatal surgery
- surgical emergencies
- vomiting.

Hirschsprung's disease

Hirschsprung's disease or congenital aganglionic megacolon, was first accurately described by Harald Hirschsprung of Copenhagen in 1886, though this disorder had been recognised almost some 200 years earlier. It is the commonest cause of intestinal obstruction in the neonate (80–90% of patients present in the neonatal period), with an incidence of one in 5000 births. Seventy-five per cent of patients have short-segment disease confined to the rectosigmoid, 14% have involvement of the transverse and descending colon (long-segment disease), and in 5–10% of patients the entire colon is affected (Zeulzer–Wilson syndrome).

There is a male to female preponderance both in the more common short-segment disease (4:1) and the long-segment disease (2:1). There is an increased familial incidence, with a family risk of 9–12.5% in the long-segment disease and 2% in the short-segment disease, and a genetic influence giving a risk of 7.6% for siblings of a female patient and 2.5–6% for siblings of a male patient. Approximately 4% of patients with Hirschsprung's disease have associated genitourinary abnormalities, and 5–9% have trisomy 21; an association with Waardenburg, Laurence–Moon–Bardet–Biedl and congenital central hypoventilation syndrome (Ondine's curse) has also been noted. Five to ten per cent of infants with Hirschsprung's disease are preterm.

Pathophysiology

Hirschsprung's disease is due to an arrest of neuroblast migration from the proximal bowel (oesophagus) to the distal hindgut, resulting in abnormal innervation of the affected distal segment. There is a total absence of ganglion cells in the affected, segment of the intestine and an overgrowth of large nerve trunks in the intermuscular and submucosal zones. The distal rectum is always affected and this extends to variable lengths of the more proximal gut.

The classical gross pathological picture is one of a narrow, contracted, aganglionic segment which extends proximally into a markedly dilated, thickened, hypertrophied, and normally innervated but functionally obstructed colon. A cone-shaped 'transitional' zone is noted between the dilated and contracted intestine. Histologically, hypertrophied nerve bundles with a high concentration of acetylcholinesterase between the muscle layers and submucosa are noted, with an absence of ganglion cells in the submucosal plexus of Meissner, and hypoganglionosis or aganglionosis in the intermyenteric plexus of Auerbach. More recently, there have been some new insights into the aetiology of Hirschsprung's disease. It appears that a loss of neural cell adhesion molecule could be the cause of neuroblasts failing to migrate to aganglionic segments, and a lack of neuronal NO synthase (and therefore NO) in nerve fibres of aganglionic intestine may contribute to the inability of the smooth muscle to relax and the absence of peristalsis in the aganglionic segment. Some forms of Hirschsprung's disease have also been found to be associated with gene deletions.

Clinical presentation

- Delayed passage of meconium (that is, >24 h after birth) in >90% of cases—99% of term infants pass meconium within 48 h of birth.
- Bilious vomiting, marked abdominal distension, and complete intestinal obstruction.
- Chronic constipation following normal passage of meconium.
- Rectal examination shows normal anal tone and is followed by explosive, foul-smelling stools and gas.
- Meconium plug syndrome: 10–20% of infants with this disorder may have Hirschsprung's disease.
- Enterocolitis (which is most common in the first 2–4 weeks of life). This is the main cause of mortality in Hirschsprung's disease and is a consequence of delayed diagnosis. Inability to pass stools leads to massive abdominal distension, increased intraluminal pressure, decreased intestinal blood flow, and a breach of the mucosal integrity. The stasis also encourages bacterial proliferation (*Clostridium difficile*, anaerobes, and coliforms) and sepsis. The infant presents with profuse mucusy and bloody diarrhoea, abdominal distension, bilious vomiting, hypotension (large fluid losses), and occasionally, shock. Left untreated, 33% of infants with Hirschsprung's disease develop enterocolitis within the first three months of life, and a third of these develop it within 30 days of birth. Once an infant has developed enterocolitis, he or she remains at increased risk of further bouts of enterocolitis even after a successful pull-through procedure.

Diagnosis

Radiology
Plain abdominal films show gas-filled bowel loops throughout the abdomen except for the pelvis, which is devoid of gas. A barium contrast enema in a previously unprepared colon shows a small-calibre aganglionic segment followed by a funnel-shaped 'cone', or 'transitional zone', leading into a normal but dilated proximal colon. However, a barium enema is less accurate in the neonatal period than at any other time, as a transitional zone may not be seen before the age of two weeks, and a megacolon may not be present. Delayed films (after 24 h) show retention of contrast material. A barium enema may, however, reveal other disorders which cause neonatal lower bowel obstruction.

Manometry
Failure of the internal anal sphincter to exhibit a relaxation wave in response to inflation of a balloon inserted into the rectum is diagnostic of Hirschsprung's disease (>90% accuracy), but it cannot be performed in infants under 3 kg in weight (39 weeks' postconceptual age), as the anal relaxation reflex may be physiologically absent. Diagnosis of ultrashort-segment Hirschsprung's disease can be made only with manometry, which shows failure of the internal sphincter to relax, with a seemingly normal suction biopsy.

Biopsy

Suction, punch, or open rectal biopsy is the reference standard for diagnosis. The submucosa must be included in the biopsy specimen to determine the presence or absence of ganglion cells. Absence of ganglion cells or elevated acetylcholinesterase staining is diagnostic of Hirschsprung's disease (91% accuracy). In ultrashort-segment disease, the aganglionic segment is limited to the internal sphincter, so ganglion cells may be present on rectal suction biopsy. Excision of a strip of rectal muscle including the internal sphincter is diagnostic and therapeutic.

Management

Obstruction

This is relieved by gentle rectal washouts using warm saline until various investigations are completed. A defunctioning colostomy sited in the ganglionic bowel is commonly performed initially. Definitive repair is performed at 2–6 months of age by one of five techniques, namely: Swenson's operation (rectosigmoidectomy), Duhamel's procedure (retrorectal pull-through), Soave's procedure (endorectal pull-through), Rehbein's procedure (resection of rectum and aganglionic bowel and dilation of anal sphincter), and rectal myomectomy. Duhamel's procedure is probably the best technique when the entire colon is affected.

Enterocolitis

These infants may be critically ill from massive fluid and electrolyte losses. Resuscitate with fluid expansion (for example, 20 ml/kg of FFP or albumin), correct acid–base imbalance, replace fluid and electrolytes, and commence broad-spectrum antibiotics (including vancomycin and metronidazole). Emergency colostomy is contraindicated.

Long-term outcome

In the majority (85%), the outcome for surgically treated Hirschsprung's disease is satisfactory. Complications include disturbances of micturition (4%), anastomotic leaks (2%), anal stenosis (5–14%), prolapse, perianal abscesses, incontinence and soiling. Once enterocolitis occurs, the patient is at increased risk of recurrence, even years after a successful definitive repair operation. The current mortality rate is 1–3%. Note, however, that Hirschsprung's disease is only one of several disorders with abnormalities of the neuronal intestinal network. In neuronal intestinal dysplasia, ganglion cells are present but in an ectopic site. The submucosal and intermyenteric plexuses are also hypertrophied. Approximately 25% of patients with Hirschsprung's disease may have concomitant neuronal intestinal dysplasia.

Further reading

Doody DP, Donahoe PK. Hirschsprung's disease. In: PJ Morris, RA Malt (eds). *Oxford Textbook of Surgery*. Oxford: Oxford University Press, 1994: 2048–52.

Holschneider AM, Puri P (eds). *Hirschsprung's Disease and Allied Disorders*. London: Martin Dunitz, 2000.

Kusafuka T, Puri P. Altered mRNA expression of the neuronal nitric oxide synthase gene in Hirschsprung's disease. *Journal of Pediatric Surgery* (1997) **32:**1054–8.

Teitelbaum DH. Hirschsprung's disease in children. *Current Opinion in Pediatrics* (1995) **7:**316–22.

Tomita R, Munakata K, Kurosu Y et al. A role of nitric oxide in Hirschsprung's disease. *Journal of Pediatric Surgery* (1995) **30:**437–40.

Related topics of interest

- abdominal distension
- neonatal surgery
- postnatal examination
- shock
- vomiting.

HIV and AIDS

UNAIDS, the United Nations programme on HIV/AIDS, estimates that currently over 40 million individuals (2.5 million children) are infected with HIV. More than 22 million people have died from AIDS since it was identified in 1982. The HIV/AIDS epidemic now represents a formidable public-health burden, particularly for the developing countries. Africa has the largest number of affected individuals, with some 30% of those living with HIV/AIDS residing in sub-Saharan Africa. Current statistics show Eastern Europe as the fastest-growing area for the epidemic worldwide. There is evidence that HIV is moving into poorer communities in high-income countries and that young adults face greater risks of infection than they did five years ago. The prevalence of HIV infection among pregnant women varies from below 1.5 cases per 1000 in the developed nations to almost one in three in some developing nations. The rate of mother-to-child (vertical) transmission of HIV is also lower in the industrialised countries (14–33%) than in developing countries (22–40%).

It is a misconception that HIV is no longer a problem in the UK. The public-health laboratory service (PHLS) communicable disease surveillance centre estimated there were 33500 people living with HIV at the end of the year 2000, just under a third of whom were diagnosed, and the number is set to rise by almost 50% by 2005. Since the year 2000, the number of heterosexual diagnoses has exceeded diagnoses in gay men. Three-quarters of new cases of HIV are thought to originate abroad, both in people who have gone to live or work abroad and those who have come to live in the UK from countries of higher prevalence. At the turn of the millennium, fewer than 600 HIV-positive infants had been reported to the British Paediatric Surveillance Unit, with half going on to develop AIDS. Most of these infants are of African origin and live in the greater London area. Of the infants diagnosed as having AIDS in the UK in 1996, outside London, approximately three-quarters of the mothers or their partners contracted HIV infection through intravenous drug abuse, in contrast to London, where heterosexual transmission is now more common. Recent data put the prevalence of HIV infection among pregnant women in the UK at 0.19% (one in 520) in Greater London, and 0.02% (one in 5700) elsewhere in the UK. However, over 75% of HIV infections in pregnant women remain undiagnosed at the time of birth, and often women discover they are HIV positive only when their child develops AIDS. Vertical transmission accounts for approximately 85% of cases of paediatric AIDS in the UK. These statistics and the fact that transmission of HIV from an infected mother to her child can be greatly reduced by interventions in pregnancy and in the perinatal period were recently highlighted in the 'Recommendations of an Intercollegiate Working Party for Enhancing Voluntary Confidential HIV Testing in Pregnancy' (Royal College of Paediatrics and Child Health, April 1998).

Risk factors for HIV transmission

Maternal disease status
- decreased CD4$^+$ count
- advanced maternal disease (as in development of clinical symptoms)
- increased viral load (as in p24 antigenaemia and positive HIV blood culture).

Obstetric determinants
- chorioamnionitis
- vaginal delivery
- preterm delivery
- post-term delivery
- prolonged rupture of membranes
- invasive intrapartum procedures.

Maternal immune response
- breast-feeding
- cigarette smoking
- neutralising antibody
- multiple sexual partners.

Timing of HIV transmission

- intrauterine (24–50%)
- intrapartum (~66% in developed countries, in the absence of breast-feeding)—ingestion of blood or maternal secretion and also maternal-foetal transmission
- postnatal (14%) mainly via breast-feeding.

HIV is present in the cell-free and cellular portions of human milk, and its highest concentration is in colostrum. Breast-feeding doubles the rate of transmission. Reported rates of vertical transmission range from 14% in Europe, 20–30% in the USA, to ≥40% in parts of Africa. Transmission to infants occurs at a higher rate if the mother has a primary HIV infection during breast-feeding. In industrialised countries, HIV-exposed infants should be formula-fed but breast-feeding may still be safer in some developing countries. Combined breast-feeding and bottle-feeding carries a higher risk of HIV transmission than exclusive breast-feeding.

Prevention of perinatal transmission

- Zidovudine (azidothymidine; AZT or ZDV) therapy from early pregnancy through labour and for the newborn infant in HIV-infected women can reduce perinatal transmission by up to 67% to around 5%. Other potentially useful anti-retrovirals, as single agents or as combination therapy, are currently undergoing evaluation. The aim is to reduce the viral load to under 50 viral copies per ml. One recent study (the NVAZ trial conducted in Malawi) reported on the efficacy of a single dose of nevirapine (2 mg/kg) or one dose of nevirapine (2 mg/kg) plus one week of treatment with AZT (4 mg/kg twice daily) in infants whose mothers were not treated during pregnancy or labour. Mother-to-child transmission was reduced from 28% to 12.1% with nevirapine alone, and to 7.7% in the nevirapine/AZT group.
- Intact foetal membranes may decrease the risk of vertical transmission, and so may delivery by caesarean section.
- Invasive procedures (such as scalp sampling and operative vaginal delivery) in HIV-seropositive labouring women should be avoided.

- Passive immunisation of mother and infant with HIV hyperimmune intravenous immunoglobulin (ACTG 185) is advised.
- Maternal vitamin A supplementation is recommended.
- HIV-seropositive mothers should not breast-feed.
- Ongoing trials of reverse-transcriptase inhibitors (such as didanosine) and active immunisation of mother and infant are awaited.

Clinical manifestations of HIV infection

Signs and symptoms, listed as follows, are rarely present in the newborn period or first few weeks of life.

1. *General.* IUGR, hepatosplenomegaly, lymphadenopathy, and failure to thrive.
2. *Respiratory.* Pneumocystis carinii pneumonia (PCP) and lymphoid interstitial pneumonia/pulmonary lymphoid hyperplasia (LIP/PLH).
3. *Dermatological.* Fungal, bacterial, and viral skin infections, severe seborrhoeic dermatitis, vasculitis, and drug eruptions.
4. *Gastrointestinal.* Oral candidiasis, aphthous ulcers, parotid gland swellings, and diarrhoea.
5. *Cardiovascular.* Myocarditis, cardiac dysrythmias, pericardial effusions, and cardiomyopathy.
6. *Neurological.* Developmental delay or regression, spastic weakness of extremities, microcephaly, cerebral atrophy, basal ganglia calcification, HIV encephalopathy, and seizures.
7. *Renal.* Proteinuria, renal failure, and nephrotic syndrome.
8. *Haematological.* Thrombocytopenia, anaemia, and leucopenia.
9. *Infection.* Recurrent bacterial infections, especially *Streptococcus pneumoniae*, *Salmonella* sp., *Staphylococcus aureus*, and *Haemophilus influenzae*, type b.

Diagnosis of HIV infection

Early diagnosis is important for the family's peace of mind and has implications for decisions concerning prophylaxis for opportunistic infections, intercurrent illnesses, and therapeutic medications including antiretroviral agents. However, standard HIV serological tests are not useful during the first 18 months because of the presence of transplacentally passed maternal IgG. Infection in infancy can be diagnosed by either direct (detecting virus or viral products) or indirect assays (detecting host response to virus). Direct tests include HIV culture (reference standard), PCR for detection of HIV proviral DNA, and p24 antigen detection after immune complex dissociation (p24–ICD)—a technique of freeing p24 antigen from immune complexes. Indirect assays detect intrinsically produced anti-HIV antibodies (such as anti-HIV IgA). The sensitivity of anti-HIV IgA and IgM for diagnosing HIV infection during infancy is debatable. Direct assays are more widely used. However, in the first week of life, these assays have a sensitivity of only 50%, but by the age of one month, HIV culture and PCR have a sensitivity and a specificity greater than 90%.

Practical approach to an HIV-exposed neonate

The primary aims are to prevent HIV infection, where possible, and also to ascertain whether the vertical transmission of HIV infection has been successfully prevented. Neonatal antiretroviral prophylaxis with AZT (4 mg/kg orally twice daily, or 2 mg/kg six-hourly, for six weeks) should be commenced within 6 h of birth. Initial screening for HIV infection is also carried out with blood samples obtained from the infant (not cord blood) within the first 48 h of life. The baseline investigations include a full blood count, HIV viral load, p24 antigen, PCR for proviral DNA, liver function tests, T cells, and immunoglobulin levels. Follow-up samples (HIV viral load, p24 antigen, and PCR for proviral DNA) are obtained at six weeks and three months, with a repeat sample if either test is positive. However, combining two tests does not increase sensitivity.

An infant under 18 months old may be considered HIV infected if he or she is HIV seropositive, or was born to an HIV infected mother *and* has positive results on two separate direct tests performed on separate blood samples (not cord blood).

An infant is also considered HIV infected if he or she meets the US Centers for Disease Control and Prevention (CDC) surveillance case definition for AIDS. AIDS-defining conditions include PCP, LIP/PLH, CMV, HIV encephalopathy, recurrent bacterial infections, wasting syndrome, *Candida* oesophagitis, pulmonary candidiasis, cryptosporidiosis, herpes simplex disease, and *Mycobacterium avium–M. intracellulare* complex infection.

Commence PCP prophylaxis at 4–6 weeks of age until at least 12 months of age unless HIV infection has been excluded (two or more negative direct tests performed at ≥1 month of age, either of which is performed at ≥4 months of age). Continue prophylaxis after one year in the presence of severe immunosuppression. Following PCP, maintain life-long prophylaxis. Prophylaxis consists of daily (or alternate day, that is, three days a week) trimethoprim-sulphamethoxazole. Alternatively, oral dapsone and monthly intravenous pentamidine may be given.

Monthly intravenous immunoglobulin (IVIG) may reduce infectious complications in some HIV-infected children though mortality is unaffected.

Treatment

There is no cure for HIV infection, though a number of antiretroviral drugs may slow or stop disease progression and increase life expectancy. Drug therapy for HIV is both toxic and expensive, and requires specialist advice, as HIV management has been changing rapidly (see www.aidsinfo.nih.gov). Antiretrovirals belong to three main groups, nucleoside reverse transcriptase inhibitors (or nucleoside analogues, such as AZT, the first anti-HIV drug), protease inhibitors (such as ritonavir), and non-nucleoside reverse transcriptase inhibitors (such as nevirapine). Symptomatic HIV infection or asymptomatic infection with significant HIV-related immunosuppression is an indication for antiretroviral therapy (currently nucleoside analogues that inhibit viral nucleic acid synthesis by binding to the reverse transcriptase enzyme). The largest experience is with AZT. Didanosine (ddi) is an alternative agent for children with advanced HIV disease and AZT intolerance or deterioration during AZT therapy.

Prognosis

Approximately one in five infants contracting HIV develop AIDS or die in the first year of life. Without antiretroviral therapy and PCP prophylaxis, median survival times for infants with vertically acquired HIV infection is 2–3 years. By age six years, 25% of the children will have died or developed some illness because of HIV infection. PCP especially in the first year of life, candidal oesophagitis, or severe encephalopathy indicate poor prognosis, while low $CD4^+$ lymphocyte counts, poor lymphocyte proliferative responses to mitogens and antigens, and lack of anti-HIV neutralising antibodies indicate rapid disease progression. Survival has improved, however, with antiretrovirals and prophylaxis. While the long-term outcome is not yet known, most infected infants will die from AIDS or AIDS-related illnesses, only a few surviving until adulthood.

Finally, the social and ethical issues surrounding HIV infection are complex. The mother's status may not be known by her partner, immediate family, or her GP. Confidentiality is therefore paramount, and great care should be taken when communicating with the infant's GP and other health-care professionals. These infants may also be at risk from other health problems, including hepatitis B and C, other sexually transmitted diseases, and the neonatal abstinence syndrome.

Useful websites

www.bhiva.org
The British HIV Association website has a mine of information including current treatment guidelines.

www.bhiva.org/chiva
The website for the Children's HIV Association of UK and Ireland, provides information on the diagnosis and treatment of children with HIV and the care of children infected or affected by HIV and their families.

www.aidsinfo.nih.gov
A US Department of Health and Human Services education and resource initiative, with a wealth of data on the latest HIV/AIDS clinical trials, treatment and prevention guidelines, and drug and vaccine developments.

www.aidsmap.com
A useful site with a worldwide perspective on HIV/AIDS developments.

www.unaids.org
Joint United Nations Programme on HIV/AIDS.

www.who.int/hiv/en/
World Health Organisation HIV/AIDS pages.

Further reading

Bardeguez AD. Management of HIV infection for the childbearing age woman. *Clinics in Obstetrics and Gynaecology* (1996) **39:**344.

Chin J. The growing impact of the HIV/AIDS pandemic on children born to HIV infected women. *Clinics in Perinatology* (1994) **21**(1).

Intercollegiate Working Party for Enhancing Voluntary Confidential HIV Testing in Pregnancy. *Reducing Mother to Child Transmission of HIV Infection in the United Kingdom*. London: Royal College of Paediatrics and Child Health, 1998.

Kline MW. Vertical human immunodeficiency virus infection. In: TN Hansen, N McIntosh (eds). *Current Topics in Neonatology*, No. 1. London: WB Saunders, 1996: 195–223.

Lindsay MK, Nesheim SR. Human immunodeficiency virus infection in pregnant women and their newborns. *Clinics in Perinatology* (1997) **24**:161–80.

Pickering LK (ed.). *The Red Book: 2003 Report of the Committee on Infectious Diseases*. 26th edn. Elk Grove Village, IL: American Academy of Pediatrics, 2003.

Pizzo PA, Wilfert CM (eds). *Pediatric AIDS: The Challenge of HIV Infection in Infants, Children, and Adolescents*, 2nd edn. Baltimore, MD: Williams & Wilkins, 1994.

Rogers MF (ed.). HIV/AIDS in infants, children, and adolescents. *Pediatric Clinics of North America* (2000) **47**(1).

Shearer WT. *Medical Management of AIDS in Children*. Philadelphia: WB Saunders, 2003.

Taha TE, Kumwenda NI, Gibbons A et al. Short postexposure prophylaxis in newborn babies to reduce mother-to-child transmission of HIV-1: NVAZ randomised clinical trial. *Lancet* (2003) **362**:1171–7.

Related topics of interest

- infection—perinatal
- hepatitis B and C
- maternal drug abuse.

Home oxygen therapy

Home oxygen therapy enables ex-preterm babies with chronic lung disease to go home from hospital weeks or months before they would do so if all oxygen therapy was hospital based and they had to wait until they were in air all the time. Such babies should have been stable on low-flow nasal oxygen for some weeks, and show no sign of coming out of oxygen in the immediate future.

There are advantages to the baby, the family, and the health service. The baby no longer has multiple caregivers who can offer attention only when their other charges are well or sleeping. Instead, the baby gets to know his/her parents really well for the first time, as they become the regular caregivers. The home environment is more friendly and stimulating, and the baby starts to develop the normal diurnal rhythm missing in the ever-bright lights and noise of a neonatal unit. The parents feel that their baby is truly theirs to care for and bring up in their own fashion, without the 'supervision' of hospital staff. Home oxygen therapy is cost-effective care for the health service, saving considerable sums of money by taking the oxygen-dependent baby out of a hospital cot that then becomes available for another patient.

Concerns about home oxygen therapy focus on the ability of the parents to cope with the 24-hours-a-day therapy, and in particular on their responses to sudden respiratory illnesses or life-threatening events. Babies with CLD are at increased risk of sudden infant death. Before the parents agree to take their baby home, an experienced doctor must have discussed these issues openly and honestly. Usually, the parents will have seen their baby have a series of critical episodes, and be all too aware of what they are taking on. Discharge home should only be with the full support of the family doctor, health visitor, district paediatric nurse, and/or neonatal liaison nurse. A planning meeting to which the parents and these support workers are invited is useful.

The following has to be achieved once it is agreed that the baby should go home in oxygen:

- A home assessment visit is undertaken to ensure the baby can be kept warm, bathed, and cared for while on oxygen therapy.
- The family doctor has to prescribe oxygen via nasal prongs at a specific flow rate.
- An oxygen concentrator with a low-flow meter has to be installed in the home with a number of outlets to enable the baby to be cared for in two or three rooms. This equipment can only be installed once the home oxygen has been prescribed.
- Small portable oxygen cylinders (at least two) with low flow heads are provided. These are to enable brief outings to the shops, relatives, and clinics! Clear arrangements should exist for their replacement when empty, and the supplier must always have some full cylinders.
- Both parents must be shown an ABC of neonatal resuscitation. Simple mucus extractors can be provided to help the parents clear the airway (no risk of HIV transmission here). The parents must practise mouth-to-mouth and nose breathing and know how to check that air is entering the lungs. They should also practise external cardiac massage with intermittent breaths. Baby mannequins provide excellent material for teaching these skills. The only thing they need do with their

own baby is to learn how to find a radial or brachial pulse—rapidly, repeatedly, and reliably.

- A decision must be made as to whether the family should have an apnoea alarm at home (most choose to do so). This would be more for parental reassurance than any proven efficacy at preventing death, and this should be made clear to the parents.
- The family must have a telephone.
- The family must have open access to the children's ward.
- Regular clinic follow-up and assessment is planned.
- Planned follow-up by health visitors and nurses is coordinated so as to avoid conflicting advice over therapy, feeding, and other issues.
- The possibility of qualifying for an attendance allowance should be explored.

Home oxygen therapy should be continued until placing the carefully monitored baby in air for periods of 30–60 min no longer leads to an early desaturation. If the baby's saturations in air remain in the mid-nineties in this situation, oxygen therapy should be continued until an overnight oximetry sleep study in air has been performed. Only if this is satisfactory can the continuous oxygen be stopped. The oxygen concentrator and small cylinders should be retained for a few weeks after that in case of a transient deterioration with a viral infection.

Further reading

Angell C. Equipment requirements for community-based paediatric oxygen treatment. *Archives of Disease in Childhood* (1991) **66:**755.

Primhak R, Smith M. Community neonatology: the continuing care of NICU graduates after hospital discharge. *Seminars in Neonatology* (2003) **8**(4).

Samuels MP, Southall DP. Home oxygen therapy. In: TJ David (ed.). *Recent Advances in Paediatrics*, 14th edn. Edinburgh: Churchill Livingstone, 1995: 37–51.

Sauve RS, McMillan DD, Mitchell I et al. Home oxygen therapy. Outcome of infants discharged from NICU on continuous treatment. *Clinical Pediatrics* (1989) **28:**113–18.

Related topics of interest

- chronic lung disease
- discharge planning and follow-up
- extreme prematurity.

Hydrocephalus

Hydrocephalus may be evident at birth (congenital hydrocephalus) or result from complications in the perinatal or postnatal period. Hydrocephalus is commonly due to obstruction to the CSF pathways (and rarely CSF overproduction) leading to dilation of the ventricles and back pressure proximal to the site of obstruction. The most common sites of obstruction are the aqueduct of Sylvius (between the third and fourth ventricles) and the exit foramina of the fourth ventricle (the central foramen of Magendie and the two lateral foramina of Luschka). In communicating hydrocephalus, CSF can flow out of the ventricular system and reach the subarachnoid space. Communication is easily confirmed clinically by the rise and fall of lumbar CSF pressure on jugular venous compression (Queckenstedt's test).

Aetiology

Congenital hydrocephalus

This may be a single abnormality or be associated with other congenital malformations within or outside the CNS.

- Arnold–Chiari malformation (commonly associated with myelomeningocoele) obstructs fourth ventricle foramina and occasionally the aqueduct of Sylvius
- Dandy–Walker malformation (cystic dilation of fourth ventricle) obstructs fourth ventricle foramina and occasionally the aqueduct of Sylvius
- sex-linked aqueductal stenosis confined to males (associated with flexion and adduction defects of the thumbs)
- post-infection (toxoplasma, rubella, and CMV)—cerebral atrophy may also contribute to hydrocephaly
- cerebral tumours and arteriovenous malformations
- choroid plexus papilloma (hydrocephalus from CSF overproduction, not obstruction—rare).

Secondary hydrocephalus

- posthaemorrhagic (following intraventricular haemorrhage especially in preterm infants), usually communicating but with obstruction of the fourth ventricle foramina may become noncommunicating.
- postinfection (meningitis) due to obstruction of the aqueduct of Sylvius and fourth ventricle foramina as well as cerebral atrophy.

Clinical features

Anterior fontanelle is large or bulging with widely separated sutures and open posterior fontanelle in newborn period. Down-turning eyeballs (sunsetting may be observed), head circumference exceeds 97th percentile by ≥ 2 cm, and head may transilluminate.

Investigations

- Cranial ultrasonography (most useful first-line investigation)—serial scans may be necessary.
- CT scan or MRI may be required for more detailed imaging.
- Congenital infection screen (TORCH titres if intrauterine infection suspected).
- For posthaemorrhagic hydrocephalus in newborn term infants, exclude a bleeding disorder (clotting studies and platelet count) and alloimmune thrombocytopenia (mother produces IgG antibodies to Pl^{A1} antigen on the infant's platelets).

Management

This partly depends on the aetiology. Congenital hydrocephalus is probably best treated surgically by insertion of a ventriculoperitoneal or ventriculoatrial shunt. Repeated lumbar or ventricular taps are not beneficial and are associated with a high risk of infection. However, after posthaemorrhagic hydrocephalus, serial CSF drainage (lumbar or ventricular taps) may be required to control rapid head growth or symptoms (apnoeas and fits) until CSF protein level is below 1 g/l, when a shunt may then be inserted.

Shunt complications include CSF overdrainage, blockage, and infection with low-grade septicaemia (*Staphylococcus albus*). Long-term neurodevelopmental follow-up is required.

Parent support group and information

Association for Spina Bifida and Hydrocephalus
42 Park Road
Peterborough PE1 2UQ, UK
Tel: 01733 555988
www.asbah.org/

Further reading

Bayston R. *Hydrocephalus shunt infections*. London: Chapman and Hall, 1989.
Chumas P, Tyagi A, Livingston J. Hydrocephalus—what's new? *Archives of Disease in Childhood Fetal and Neonatal Edition* (2001) **85:**F149–54.
Fanaroff AA, Martin RJ (eds). *Neonatal-Perinatal Medicine: Disease of the Fetus and Infant*, 7th edn. St Louis, MO: Mosby, 2002.
Levene M, Chervenak FA, Whittle M (eds). *Fetal and Neonatal Neurology and Neurosurgery*, 3rd edn. Edinburgh: Churchill Livingstone, 2001.
Rutherford M. *MRI of the Neonatal Brain*. Philadelphia: WB Saunders, 2001.
Volpe JJ. *Neurology of the Newborn*, 4th edn. Philadelphia: WB Saunders, 2001.

Related topics of interest

- germinal matrix-intraventricular haemorrhage
- head size
- haemorrhagic disorders
- neural tube defects.

Hydrops fetalis

Hydrops is a generalised hypoalbuminaemic oedema of the foetus and neonate. Ascites, pleural and pericardial effusions occur, and heart failure is common. It is diagnosed antenatally by ultrasound scanning with characteristic appearances—a halo of oedema, thickened subcutaneous tissues, ascites, effusions, and hepato-splenomegaly. There are many causes, grouped into 'immune' and 'nonimmune':

Immunological hydrops

This disorder is secondary to haemolytic disease from rhesus or other isoimmunisation. It is now rare, occurring in fewer than one in 10000 deliveries because of improved antenatal care. Treatment is as for severe rhesus haemolytic disease, but with the added issues discussed below under emergency treatment at birth.

Nonimmunological hydrops (known associations)

Chromosomal
- trisomies (13, 15, 18, and 21)
- 45XO (Turner's syndrome)
- XX/XY
- triploidy.

Cardiac
Structural disorders
- septal defects
- hypoplastic left heart
- truncus arteriosus
- pulmonary atresia
- cardiac rhabdomyoma
- premature closure of ductus arteriosus
- pericardial teratoma
- subaortic stenosis with fibroelastosis
- right atrial haemangioma.

Dysrhythmias
- supraventricular tachycardia
- heart block.

Other cardiac disorders
- myocarditis
- cardiomyopathy
- calcification of arteries or myocardium
- asplenia syndrome
- causes of cardiac failure (such as arteriovenous malformation or haemangioma).

Pulmonary
- diaphragmatic hernia
- cystadenomatoid malformation
- tracheooesophageal fistula (TOF)
- sequestered lung.

Infective
- syphilis
- hepatitis
- parvovirus
- toxoplasmosis
- Chagas' disease
- cytomegalovirus.

Maternal/placental
- diabetes
- toxaemia
- true knot in cord/umbilical vein thrombosis
- vascular malformation of the cord or placenta
- multiple births (especially twin–twin transfusion).

Gastrointestinal
- biliary atresia
- jejunal atresia
- volvulus.

Renal
- polycystic kidneys
- renal vein thrombosis
- congenital nephrotic syndrome
- urethral obstruction (posterior urethral valves).

Haematological
- G6PD deficiency
- any foetal anaemia
- alpha thalassaemia
- twin–twin transfusion
- foetomaternal haemorrhage.

Neurological
- encephalocoele
- tuberous sclerosis
- holoprosencephaly
- intracranial haemorrhage
- agenesis of corpus callosum.

Skeletal
- osteogenesis imperfecta
- some dwarfisms.

Congenital tumours
- teratoma
- neuroblastoma
- hepatoblastoma
- choriocarcinoma.

Storage disorders
- Gaucher's disease
- Niemann–Pick disease
- mucopolysaccharidosis.

Miscellaneous
- myotonic dystrophy
- prune belly syndrome
- Neu–Laxova syndrome
- infant of a diabetic mother
- Beckwith–Wiedemann syndrome.

It is important to remember these are some of the associations with nonimmune hydrops, and that they are not necessarily the cause.

Antenatal investigation and management

Isoimmunisation and rhesus disease must be excluded first by investigating ABO, rhesus, and other blood group antigens and haemolysins. If negative, detailed ultrasound scanning is essential, as is karyotyping and TORCH, parvovirus, and venereal disease research laboratory (VDRL) screening. If samples are taken by cordocentesis, the presence of foetal anaemia and abnormal haemoglobin can be detected in addition to the other tests. Treatment as appropriate with maternal antidysrhythmic drugs, supportive transfusions to the foetus, and possibly procedures to drain foetal ascites and pleural effusions should be considered.

Postnatal investigations and management

Emergency treatment at birth
- Intubate and maintain ventilation with high pressures (up to $30\,cmH_2O$).
- Drain pleural effusions and ascites (diagnosed antenatally): keep aspirates for analysis.
- Insert umbilical venous lines to secure vascular access.
- Transfer ventilated patient to the neonatal unit.

On the neonatal unit

- Insert UAC and obtain blood for baseline observations including gases, glucose, albumin, electrolytes, FBC, clotting screen, blood group, and Coombs' test.
- If a pericardial effusion is suspected, perform cardiac echocardiography to confirm and then perform pericardiocentesis under ultrasonic guidance.
- Get chest and abdominal radiographs.
- Assess the baby for congenital abnormalities: plan second-line investigations for diagnoses listed above.
- As first results come back, adjust ventilation to achieve satisfactory gases, maintain blood pressure and circulation, bring central venous pressure down to 6 mmHg, if necessary by withdrawing further aliquots of blood 10 ml at a time, and treat any metabolic acidosis as necessary. Colloid can be given slowly later, when hypoalbuminaemia has been confirmed.

Long-term management

If the baby survives, long-term management begins with the stabilisation of the baby on the ventilator. Once haematological and biochemical abnormalities have been corrected, and heart failure, pleural effusions, and ascites resolved, intensive care is discontinued. If still undiagnosed, further investigations may be necessary, and the parents should be supported and referred to a clinical geneticist. In 50% of cases, no cause is found. Mortality is also 50% or more. If the baby is stillborn or dies later, request a postmortem examination. The parents should be counselled and referred to a clinical geneticist.

Further reading

Avery GB, Fletcher MA, MacDonald M. *Neonatology: Pathophysiology and Management of the Newborn*, 5th edn. Philadelphia: Lippincott Williams & Wilkins, 1999.

Fanaroff AA, Martin RJ. *Neonatal-Perinatal Medicine: Diseases of the Fetus and Infant*, 7th edn. St Louis, MO: Mosby, 2001.

Nathan DG, Orkin SH, Look T et al (eds). *Nathan and Oski's Hematology of Infancy and Childhood*, 6th edn. Philadelphia: WB Saunders, 2003.

Phibbs RH. Hydrops fetalis and other causes of neonatal edema and ascites. In: RA Polin, WW Fox (eds). *Fetal and Neonatal Physiology*, 2nd edn. Philadelphia: WB Saunders, 1998: 1730–6.

Smith OP, Hann IM. *Essential Paediatric Haematology*. London: Martin Dunitz, 2002.

Stephenson T, Zuccollo J, Hohajer M. Diagnosis and management of non-immune hydrops in the newborn. *Archives of Disease in Childhood* (1994) **70:**F151–4.

Related topics of interest

- anaemia
- cardiac arrhythmias
- haemolytic disease
- respiratory distress
- resuscitation.

Hypotonia

Most floppy babies do not have a persistent neuromuscular disorder. They may have benign neonatal hypotonia—characterised by a floppiness with normal strength—or transient hypotonia related to conditions such as prematurity or mild birth asphyxia (stage 1 hypoxic-ischaemic encephalopathy). Hypotonia is classified 'anatomically' in a centrifugal fashion; that is, as central in origin, or from the spinal cord, the peripheral nerves, the neuromuscular junction, or the muscles themselves.

Central hypotonia

Primary
- Down's syndrome.
- Prader–Willi syndrome
- peroxisomal disorders
- cerebral palsy—the hypertonia develops later
- brain malformations.

Secondary
- anaesthesia
- drugs such as maternal benzodiazepines
- sepsis
- respiratory distress
- hypoglycaemia
- metabolic disorders.

Spinal cord disorders

- birth injuries to the cervical spine and cord
- spinal muscular atrophy—type 1 (Werdnig–Hoffmann).

Peripheral nerve abnormalities

A generalised peripheral neuropathy is very rare in neonates. Local palsies secondary to trauma are easily recognised.

Neuromuscular junction disorders

- transient neonatal myasthenia—anti-acetylcholine receptor antibodies cross the placenta
- feeding and respiratory difficulties—usually responsive to neostigmine; ventilation is occasionally needed and improvement after days/weeks
- congenital myasthenic syndromes.

Muscle disease

1. *Congenital muscular dystrophy.* Patient is weak, with contractures/arthrogryposis. Many improve slowly. Several subgroups are now recognised (see 'Neuromuscular disorders—muscular').
2. *Myotonic dystrophy.* The mother is always affected. The symptoms are polyhydramnios secondary to swallowing difficulties in utero, immobile face, triangular mouth, and respiratory difficulties; patient was not myotonic as a baby. Many have learning difficulties and some have gut, and later CNS and endocrine involvement.
3. *Congenital myopathies.* Symptoms include hypotonia, respiratory difficulties, and, later, learning difficulties. Biochemical abnormality has yet to be clarified in many types, and diagnosis is usually by muscle biopsy.

Investigation and management

As is evident from the above lists, the causes of neonatal hypotonia are legion. The approach to investigating hypotonia is determined to a large part by the clinical impression of the suspected underlying cause(s). The investigation and management of the various disorders are outlined under the relevant topics. Detailed accounts on neuromuscular investigations have been set out under 'Neuromuscular disorders'.

Further reading

Crawford TO. Clinical evaluation of the floppy infant. *Pediatric Annals* (1992) **21:**348.
Curran A, Jardine P. The floppy infant. *Current Paediatrics* (1998) **8:**37–42.
Dubowitz V. *The Floppy Infant*, 2nd edn. Clinics in Developmental Medicine No. 76. Cambridge: Cambridge University Press, 1980.
Dubowitz V. *Muscle Disorders in Childhood*, 2nd edn. London: WB Saunders, 1995.
Roper HP. Neuromuscular diseases in children. *British Journal of Hospital Medicine* (1993) **49:**537–45.

Related topics of interest

*   assessment of gestational age
*   birth injuries
*   feeding difficulties
*   hypoxic-ischaemic encephalopathy
*   inherited metabolic disease—investigation and management
*   neurological evaluation
*   neuromuscular disorders—muscular
*   neuromuscular disorders—neurological.

Hypoxic-ischaemic encephalopathy

The term 'birth asphyxia' is poorly defined, but includes decreased oxygen delivery to, and perfusion of, vital organs, particularly the brain. It is associated with metabolic acidosis, low Apgar scores, and end organ damage. Many authorities feel the term should no longer be used, and more objective measures should be recorded (such as umbilical cord-blood gases). Although birth asphyxia is a multisystem disorder, it is the effect on the brain—the postasphyxial encephalopathy—which is of prime importance in the outcome. Postasphyxial or hypoxic-ischaemic encephalopathy (HIE) is a variable constellation of symptoms and signs, including alterations in consciousness and behaviour, feeding difficulties, abnormal tone, convulsions, and failure to maintain regular respiration. About one in 500 term babies has HIE severe enough to cause fits or coma.

Prognostic evaluation

Early prediction of prognosis in each case of perinatal asphyxia and HIE is important. Accurate information should be given to parents, for starting resuscitation or withdrawing therapy, and in the future, the possibility of offering effective neuroprotective therapy. Prognostic statements for infants with HIE are best made from the level of severity of the clinical syndrome. Two main classifications are in use, and their features are summarised in Tables 1 and 2.

Table 1 Sarnat and Sarnat classification of HIE.

	Stage 1	Stage 2	Stage 3
Consciousness	Hyperalert	Lethargic	Stuporous
Seizures	None	Common: focal or multifocal	Uncommon: excluding decerebration
Muscle tone	Normal	Mild hypotonia	Flaccid
Duration	<24h	2–14 days	Hours to weeks
EEG	Normal	Variable changes: seizures of <1–1.5 Hz spike and wave	Periodic pattern with isopotential phases, later totally isopotential

Table 2 Levene et al classification of HIE.

	Mild	Moderate	Severe
Consciousness	Hyperalert	Lethargy	Comatose and fails to maintain ventilation
Seizures	Absent	Present	Present
Muscle tone	Minor disturbances	Abnormal	Profound hypotonia
Duration	Recovering by 48h	Recovering by 7 days	

The authors of these two classifications, Sarnat and Sarnat and Levene et al, respectively (see Tables 1 and 2) reported on the outcome, albeit in slightly different ways.

- All babies with mild or stage 1 HIE did well. Of those with moderate or stage 2 HIE, 75% also did well, but with more severe asphyxia (stage 3 HIE); some 60% died, and a high proportion of the survivors were handicapped.
- In one large American study, neonates with clinically recognised seizures, a 5-min Apgar score of ≤5, and at least one sign compatible with HIE had a 33% risk of death in the first year, and 55% of the survivors had a motor disability.
- At age one year, infants with mild (stage 1) HIE or moderate (stage 2) HIE for less than five days had developed normally. Severe (stage 3) HIE or the persistence of moderate encephalopathy was associated with seizures, and motor and cognitive delay.
- At age eight years, infants who had mild HIE as neonates were free of handicap in motor, cognitive, and school performance. However, infants who had experienced moderate or severe HIE had greater impairment of performance in each of these developmental spheres.
- The likelihood of long-term neurologic sequelae after HIE was increased by the presence of neonatal seizures. Interictal background EEG abnormalities, such as persistently low voltage, isoelectric activity, and burst suppression, correlated with poor outcome.

Management of HIE

Immediate
1. Establish effective ventilation and oxygenation. If intrapartum asphyxia is suspected, an experienced resuscitator should be at the delivery, with the aims of:
   - clearing the airways of meconium if present
   - establishing effective ventilation.
2. Provide circulatory support if necessary:
   - external cardiac massage
   - adrenaline
   - glucose 200 mg/kg as a bolus if there is profound hypoglycaemia (the myocardial glycogen stores are depleted in severe asphyxia).
3. Correct hypoglycaemia, but marked hyperglycaemia may exacerbate brain damage.

Ongoing management
- Restrict fluids by 20–25%. This protects against cerebral oedema and reduces the risk of fluid overload if there is renal failure.
- Monitor urine output and electrolytes.
- Monitor and support blood pressure and perfusion with inotropes. If, after initial resuscitation, hypotension persists, the asphyxiated myocardium may be more contractile on an inotrope such as dopamine (initially 10 μg/kg per min) and if the condition is thought to be hypovolaemic, an infusion of 10–20 ml/kg of human albumin or saline (but beware hazard of fluid overload).

- Ventilate if $PaCO_2$ rises above 7 kPa with spontaneous respiration. A raised $PaCO_2$ causes cerebral vasodilation, may contribute to raised intracranial pressure, and may indicate impending coma.
- If ventilated, maintain $PaCO_2$ at 4.5–5 kPa. This will reduce cerebral oedema. Lower $PaCO_2$ may cause cerebral vasoconstriction to the point of causing further ischaemic damage to compromised parts of the brain. Hyperventilation for HIE is associated with a high risk of pneumothoraces.
- Monitor for cerebral oedema. Following perinatal hypoxic-ischaemic cerebral injury, intracranial pressure may be elevated due to cytotoxic cerebral oedema. However, cerebral perfusion pressure (mean arterial blood pressure minus intracranial pressure) remains within the normal range throughout the postnatal course unless intracranial pressure becomes markedly increased. Trials performed to protect the neonatal brain by reducing this oedema by mannitol, steroids, furosemide, or elective intubation followed by hyperventilation all lack effect on eventual outcome.
- Give anticonvulsants if recurrent or prolonged convulsions occur. Anticonvulsants are generally given to babies with hypoxic-ischaemic fits, though they have not been shown to improve outcome. Fits develop in the first 48 h (75% in the first 24 h) and often settle within another 2–3 days. The concern is that underperfusion or underoxygenation of excited cells will lead to further damage. Reducing cellular metabolism with the following membrane-stabilising anticonvulsant drugs should be beneficial, but this has yet to be confirmed:
  - Phenobarbital, given as a loading dose of 20 mg/kg and then 5–6 mg/kg per day, is the first-line anticonvulsant.
  - Phenytoin, with a loading dose of 20 mg/kg and then 8 mg/kg per day, is also used.
  - Clonazepam is also effective given as a loading dose of 100 μg/kg and then 'titrated' as an infusion starting at 10 μg/kg per h and increasing in 10-μg increments until the fits are controlled.

Hypothermic neural rescue treatment

Over 40 years ago, Westin and colleagues made observational studies suggesting that cooling the brain after a period of hypoxia and ischaemia might ameliorate cerebral injury. Although the initial confirmatory animal studies were unsuccessful, there has been renewed interest in this field, as more recent animal studies have reported that moderate cooling of the brain by 3–4 °C for 12–72 h after experimental hypoxia-ischaemia reduces the severity of brain injury and long-term sequelae. Maximum benefit occurs when treatment is started within 6 h of the insult. While the mechanism of this neuroprotective effect of cooling has not been fully established, it appears, at least in part, to be due to an attenuation of the delayed neuronal cell death (apoptosis) that characterises hypoxic-ischaemic brain injury. Several multicentre clinical trials are currently in progress worldwide to examine the potential therapeutic role of moderate hypothermia in infants who have suffered moderate to severe HIE. One such trial is the Medial Research Council (MRC)-funded UK TOBY trial.

Withdrawal of intensive care

- As up to 93% of infants with severe HIE die or are severely handicapped, withdrawal of life support should be an option.
- Doppler studies and EEG are of value in evaluating the severity of brain injury.
- Severe EEG abnormalities include burst suppression, low-voltage or isoelectric EEGs, and moderate EEG abnormality, including slow-wave activity.
- The overall risk of death or handicap with a severely abnormal early EEG is up to 95%; it is 64% for a moderately abnormal EEG and 3.3% for a mildly abnormal EEG.
- After the first 24 h of life, abnormal Doppler signals from the anterior cerebral artery accurately predict very poor outcome. Doppler cerebral blood-flow velocity studies showing a high diastolic velocity, and therefore a low Pourcelot resistance index (<0.55), predict adverse outcome with a sensitivity of 100% and a specificity of 81%.
- Neuroimaging (MRI or ultrasound) showing bilateral basal ganglia involvement is a poor prognostic sign, as is absence of signal from myelin in the posterior limb of the internal capsule on MRI imaging.
- Discussions with the parents should always be frank, truthful, and to the point to allow them to come to terms with the situation and be prepared for the eventuality of withdrawing life support (see 'Death of a baby').

Birth asphyxia and cerebral palsy

Only about 8% of cases of cerebral palsy (CP) are caused by perinatal factors. The vast majority of these cases are of uncertain antenatal origin.

Further reading

Blennow M, Lagercrantz H. Management of the asphyxiated Infant. In: TN Hansen, N McIntosh (eds). *Current Topics in Neonatology*, No. 2. London: WB Saunders, 1997: 39–64.

Cowan F. Outcome after intrapartum asphyxia in term infants. *Seminars in Neonatology* (2001) **5**:127–40.

Edwards AD, Azzopardi D. Hypothermic neural rescue treatment: from laboratory to cotside? *Archives of Disease in Childhood Fetal and Neonatal Edition* (1998) **78**:F88–91.

Gluckman P, Pinal CS, Gunn AJ. Hypoxic-ischaemic brain injury in the newborn: pathophysiology and potential strategies for intervention. *Seminars in Neonatology* (2001) **6**:109–20.

Perlman J (ed.). Perinatal brain injury. *Clinics in Perinatology* (2002) **29**(4).

Thoresen M. Cooling the newborn after asphyxia—physiological and experimental background and its clinical use. *Seminars in Neonatology* (2000) **5**:61–73.

Volpe JJ. Hypoxic-ischaemic encephalopathy: biochemical and physiological aspects. In: *Neurology of the Newborn*, 4th edn. Philadelphia: WB Saunders, 2001: 217–76.

Related topics of interest

- childbirth complications and foetal outcome
- death of a baby
- germinal matrix-intraventricular haemorrhage
- periventricular leucomalacia
- seizures.

Immunisations

Immunity can be conferred by passive transfer (for short term) or actively (long term). Passive immunity results from the injection of human immunoglobulin and affords immediate but short-lived (a few weeks') protection. There are two types of human immunoglobulin: human normal immunoglobulin (HNIG) and specific immunoglobulins (such as for varicella-zoster or tetanus). Active immunity is induced by using attenuated live organisms (as in oral poliomyelitis vaccine [OPV] and BCG vaccine) or their products (as in tetanus and diphtheria) or inactivated organisms (as in pertussis and inactivated poliomyelitis virus [IPV]). Vaccines produce their protective effect by inducing cell-mediated immunity and serum antibodies, which can be demonstrated by their detection in the serum.

All infants should receive their full complement of immunisations unless valid medical contraindications exist. The date of each immunisation, type of vaccine, batch number, and, for BCG, site of injection should always be recorded on the recipient's record. Where two vaccines are given concurrently, the relevant sites should be recorded to facilitate identification of any untoward reactions. Expired vaccines should not be used, and the expiry date should be noted. The specified routes of administration should be adhered to. With the exception of BCG (given intradermally), OPV, and oral typhoid vaccine, all vaccines should be given by deep i.m. or s.c. injection (anterolateral thigh or upper arm, not buttocks). Allow skin-cleaning agents to dry *before* injecting vaccines, as live vaccines may be inactivated by the disinfecting agents. Live vaccines should not be given within three months of an immunoglobulin injection, as the immune response may be suboptimal. When two or more live vaccines have to be administered at the same time, they should be given at different sites concurrently (unless using a combined preparation) or be separated by a three-week interval. There is no need for an interval between the administration of inactivated and live vaccines.

Contraindications for immunisations

- Immunisations should be postponed during an acute febrile illness, but minor infections without fever or systemic disturbance are not a contraindication.
- A clear history of a general reaction or a severe local reaction is a contraindication.
- Infants receiving prednisolone at doses of 2 mg/kg per day for ≥1 month are effectively immunosuppressed and should *not* receive live vaccines until three months after stopping therapy. Replacement corticosteroids are not a contraindication.
- Infants with impaired cell-mediated immunity commonly receive immunoglobulin preparations as part of their therapy, making most live vaccines ineffective.
- HIV-positive infants should not be given BCG (risk of dissemination of BCG). In the UK, where the risk of TB is low, withhold BCG from all infants *suspected* of being HIV-positive (such as infants of HIV-positive mothers). HIV-positive infants (with or without symptoms) may receive measles, mumps, and rubella live vaccines. IPV may be safer. They can receive the usual inactivated vaccines (diphtheria, pertussis, tetanus, *Haemophilus influenzae* type b [Hib], and hepatitis B).
- OPV should not be given to immunosuppressed infants, their siblings, or other household contacts. Instead IPV should be given.

- Stable neurological conditions (such as previous IVH or cerebral palsy) are not a contraindication to immunisation.

Schedule for primary immunisation

The immunisation schedule during the first year of life is as follows: DTwP, Hib, OPV, and meningococcal group C conjugate vaccine (Men C), three doses of all four vaccines being administered at four-weekly intervals with the first doses at two months of age. Where DTwP is contraindicated (because of a previous reaction), DTaP may be used (but with the Hib component being given in a separate site). These are followed by a single dose of the measles, mumps, and rubella vaccine (MMR), at 12–15 months of age.

Nationwide surveillance for invasive *Haemophilus* infections detected an increase in cases from 1999 to 2000, which has now been linked with the increased use of the DTaP–Hib combination. A significant trend for increasing risk of vaccine failure with each additional dose of DTaP–Hib was observed. Consequently, on 1 April 2003, the Department of Health recommended an additional dose of Hib vaccine, beginning in May 2003, for all children aged six months to four years, the cohort at risk of receipt of DTaP–Hib vaccines.

Preterm infants should be immunised according to the recommended schedule from the age of two months *irrespective* of their gestational age or birth weight. The efficacy and safety of the vaccines are similar in term and preterm infants using the recommended schedule. The magnitude of immune responses in preterm infants is directly proportional to gestational age and birth weight, with ELBW infants more likely to have decreased, although protective, immune responses when completing a primary immunisation schedule. The safety of diphtheria and tetanus toxoids and whole-cell pertussis (DTwP)/acellular pertussis (DTaP), Hib, and IPV vaccines in term infants is comparable to that in preterm and LBW infants, with no increase in vaccine adverse effects. However, some studies have reported the occurrence of apnoeas within 72 h (peak, 12–24 h) of administration of DTwP vaccine to ELBW infants (<31 weeks' gestation), but not after the administration of DTaP. It is recommended, therefore, that hospitalised ELBW infants be observed for up to 72 h after immunisation.

Additional vaccinations

BCG vaccine

BCG vaccine was introduced for general use in the UK in 1953. It has an efficacy of 70–80% in protecting against tuberculosis when given to British schoolchildren. This protection lasts 15 years. It is a live, attenuated form of *Mycobacterium bovis*, of which there are two types, one for percutaneous use (for infants only, by the multiple puncture technique), and one for intradermal injection. Neonatal immunisation policies vary widely, but, generally, they aim to target those at higher risk of tuberculosis. In the UK, this generally means the following:

- infants born to immigrants from regions with a high prevalence of tuberculosis (such as those of the Indian subcontinent and Africa) and the infants of refugees

- infants born to parents with a recent family history of tuberculosis
- newborns whose parents request BCG immunisation
- infants who will be taken on travel into countries/regions with a high prevalence of tuberculosis.

BCG vaccine should be administered strictly intradermally (0.05 ml for those aged <3 months), using a separate tuberculin syringe and needle for each subject (not by jet injectors); alternatively, the percutaneous route may be used (same site) by the multiple puncture technique (and an appropriate vaccine). Use the insertion of the deltoid muscle near the middle of left arm as the main site of injection (keloid formation is more common if higher sites are used). Alternatively, use the upper and lateral thigh (but clearly record this in the records).

Interestingly, one recent report has noted that infants with a family history of allergic rhinitis or eczema who received BCG vaccine appeared to have a lower prevalence of asthma.

Hepatitis B

This should be performed on infants born to mothers who are chronic carriers of hepatitis B virus or to mothers developing acute hepatitis B during pregnancy (see 'Hepatitis B and C').

Varicella (chickenpox)

Varicella is an acute, highly infectious disease transmitted directly by droplet spread and personal contact, and indirectly via articles (such as towels and clothing) which have been in contact with an affected individual. The disease can be life-threatening in neonates and immunosuppressed infants. Herpes zoster is a reactivation of the patient's varicella virus. Infants in the following groups are particularly at risk of developing severe disseminated or haemorrhagic varicella if exposed to varicella-zoster and should be given human varicella-zoster immunoglobulin (VZIG):

- infants with evidence of impaired cell-mediated immunity (as in severe combined immunodeficiency [SCID] or DiGeorge syndrome)
- infants and children with evidence of immunosuppression (as in immunosuppressive treatment, including those who have received corticosteroids in the previous three months at the following dose equivalents of prednisolone: 2 mg/kg daily for at least one week or 1 mg/kg daily for one month)
- infants with symptomatic HIV infection
- neonates whose mothers develop chickenpox from five days before delivery to two days after delivery
- neonates exposed to chickenpox or herpes zoster in the first 28 days of life and who are varicella-zoster antibody negative
- preterm infants born before 28 weeks' gestation or who weighed under 1000 g at birth but whose mothers have a positive history of chickenpox (inadequate transfer of maternal antibody).

VZIG, which is available from Public Health Laboratory Service, Bio Products Laboratory, or Scottish National Blood Transfusion Service (1 vial, 250 mg), is given by i.m. injection as soon as possible but within ten days after exposure. Immunocompromised infants at long-term risk should be immunised with varicella vaccine (such as Varilrix, GlaxoSmithKline). This is a live, attenuated varicella-zoster virus (Oka strain) and must not be given to individuals with primary or acquired immunodeficiency or to those receiving immunosuppressive therapy.

Respiratory syncytial virus (RSV)

RSV is a highly contagious and potentially fatal disease in high-risk infants (young infants, preterm infants, and infants with CLD and CHD). RSVIG (Synagis, Abbott Laboratories) provides passive immunity against RSV infections. It decreases the occurrence and duration of moderate to severe RSV infection in infants under 24 months of age who were born at <35 weeks' gestation, or with those with CHD and CLD. Currently, this is the only effective means of preventing severe RSV lower respiratory tract infection in high-risk preterm infants. However, prophylactic RSVIG has to be administered by i.m. injection (15 mg/kg into the anterolateral thigh) once each month, during the season for RSV at a cost of £2000–3500 per infant per season.

Influenza vaccine

Preterm and LBW infants are at increased risk of excess morbidity from influenza virus infections, with mortality rates of up to 10%. Annual influenza immunisation is recommended for all preterm infants (particularly oxygen-dependent infants with CLD), beginning at six months of age and before the onset and during the influenza season. Two doses of vaccine (given four weeks apart) are required in preterm and LBW infants receiving the vaccine for the first time. The vaccines are prepared in chick embryos and therefore contraindicated in those hypersensitive to eggs.

Pneumococcal conjugate vaccine

All LBW and preterm infants are considered at increased risk of invasive pneumococcal disease, and it is recommended that they receive full doses of the 7-valent pneumococcal polysaccharide-conjugated vaccine (Prevenar, Wyeth Pharmaceuticals), beginning at two months of age and up to the age of two years. The number of doses required for primary immunisation varies according to age. A polyvalent (23-valent) unconjugated pneumococcal polysaccharide vaccine is used for the immunisation of children over the age of two years.

Useful websites

www.VaccineAction.com
A useful website with information on vaccine developments and updates, UK and worldwide.

www.vaccineinformation.org
The Immunization Action Coalition (IAC), funded by the US CDC. This features a comprehensive selection of links, slides, and video clips.

Further reading

American Academy of Pediatrics. Immunization of preterm and low birth weight infants. *Pediatrics* (2003) **112:**193–8.

American Academy of Pediatrics, Committee on Infectious Diseases. Recommended childhood and adolescent immunization schedule–United States, 2003. *Pediatrics* (2003) **111:**212–16.

Groothuis JR, Simoes EA, Hemming VG. Respiratory syncytial virus (RSV) infection in preterm infants and the protective effects of RSV immune globulin (RSVIG). Respiratory syncytial virus immune globulin study group. *Pediatrics* (1995) **95:**463–7.

Salisbury DM, Begg NT (eds). *Immunisation Against Infectious Disease.* London: HMSO, 1996.

Slack MH, Schapira D. Severe apnoeas following immunisation in premature infants. *Archives of Disease in Childhood Fetal and Neonatal Edition* (1999) **81:**F67–8.

Tulloh R, Marsh M, Blackburn M et al. Recommendations for the use of palivizumab as prophylaxis against respiratory syncytial virus in infants with congenital cardiac disease. *Cardiology in the Young* (2003) **13:**420–3.

Vaccine Administration Taskforce. *UK Guidance on Best Practice in Vaccine Administration.* London: Shire Hall Communications, 2001.

WHO/UNICEF. Global programme on AIDS and expanded Programme on Immunisation. Joint WHO/UNICEF statement on early immunisation for HIV infected children. *Weekly Epidemiology Records* (1989) **7:**48–9.

Whitney C, Farley M, Hadler J et al. Decline in invasive pneumococcal disease after the introduction of protein–polysaccharide conjugate vaccine. *New England Journal of Medicine* (2003) **348:**1737–46.

Related topics of interest

- chronic lung disease
- discharge planning and follow-up
- hepatitis B and C
- HIV and AIDS.

Infants of diabetic mothers

The term 'infants of diabetic mothers' (IDM) is used here to describe infants of insulin-dependent diabetics. Babies born to mothers with gestational diabetes are less severely affected, particularly with regard to congenital abnormalities. Over the last 80 years since the discovery of insulin, the outcome of pregnancies complicated by diabetes mellitus has continued to improve. Currently, except for those deaths due to major malformations, perinatal mortality in the pregnancies of women with insulin-dependent diabetes mellitus who receive excellent medical care approaches that of the general population.

Problems in pregnancy

- Polyhydramnios.
- IUGR especially in mothers with a diabetic nephropathy (characterised by macro-proteinuria, hypertension, retinopathy, declining glomerular filtration, and uraemia). IUGR may be three to seven times more common in diabetic than non-diabetic pregnancy.
- Sudden unexpected foetal death in the third trimester is associated with maternal ketoacidosis, pre-eclampsia, and maternal vascular disease, but many such deaths are unexplained. It is the fear of this that results in many IDMs being delivered at 38–39 weeks. Delivery earlier than that is contraindicated because of pulmonary immaturity.

Problems for the neonate

Many of the problems are secondary to foetal hyperinsulinism. They can therefore be reduced or prevented by good diabetic control before and throughout the pregnancy. Prepregnancy counselling of the parents helps them to understand the importance of tight control.

Congenital abnormalities

These are two to eight times more common in IDMs than in other babies, though this may be reduced by tight preconceptual diabetic control. The incidence of major congenital malformations remains at 6–9%, accounting for approximately 40% of all perinatal deaths among IDMs. The caudal regression syndrome (sacral agenesis) is particularly common (600 times more common than with nondiabetic mothers). Other CNS anomalies include microcephaly, anencephaly, and other neural tube defects (3–20-fold risk of normals). Others reported include situs inversus, arthrogryposis, skeletal abnormalities, renal and genital anomalies (hydronephrosis, renal agenesis, and ureteral duplication), gastrointestinal anomalies (duplex livers, duodenal atresia, anorectal atresia, and small left colon syndrome), cardiac anomalies (VSDs, single ventricle, hypoplastic left heart syndrome, pulmonary valve stenosis and atresia, transposition of the great arteries with or without VSD, and coarctation of the aorta with or without VSD, PDA, or ASD), and single umbilical artery.

Current evidence supports the notion that hyperglycaemia and its resulting metabolic derangements are teratogenic, and that strict metabolic control in the preconceptual period may reduce the overall incidence of diabetes-related malformations.

Macrosomia

A birth weight of >90th percentile or a birth weight of ≥4000 g is secondary to foetal hyperinsulinism in the poorly controlled diabetic. The incidence of infants with birth weights of ≥4000 g is 8% in nondiabetic women and 26% in diabetic women. Insulin is a growth factor causing hypertrophy of organs and deposition of fat. Macrosomia is associated with protracted labour, birth asphyxia, shoulder dystocia, and nerve and skeletal injuries. Consequently, up to 47% of such infants are delivered by caesarean section. The macrosomic neonate is especially at risk of other complications seen in IDMs.

Hypoglycaemia

Hypoglycaemia is most common in macrosomic babies—'diabetic cherubs'—with an onset immediately after birth. Approximately 47% of macrosomic infants and 20% of nonmacrosomic IDMs become hypoglycaemic. The neonate is hyperinsulinaemic as a result of the hyperglycaemic intrauterine environment, and rapidly becomes hypoglycaemic once delivered. IDMs who develop hypoglycaemia have elevated cord C-peptide and free insulin levels at birth. Some IUGR babies will have inadequate glycogen stores and become hypoglycaemic some hours later. Maternal blood glucose control in the later part of pregnancy, including during labour and delivery, significantly influences the frequency and severity of neonatal hypoglycaemia.

Respiratory distress

This is more common in IDMs because of their delayed lung maturation. Delivery at 30–37 weeks' gestation is associated with much higher respiratory morbidity than in normal babies.

Hypocalcaemia

Hypocalcaemia is also common (seen in ~50%), possibly caused by a delay in the usual postnatal rise of parathyroid hormone. In most infants, this will resolve spontaneously within a few days, but in some it may be prolonged and require a slow infusion of intravenous 10% calcium gluconate or added vitamin D to enhance calcium absorption.

Hypomagnesaemia

Often coexists with hypocalcaemia and may present with jitteriness, irritability, apnoea, and sometimes frank seizures. Symptomatic infants with a normal serum calcium but a magnesium level of <0.7 mmol/l should receive a single i.m. injection of 0.1–0.3 ml/kg of 50% magnesium sulphate solution.

Polycythaemia

Polycythaemia is most common in IDMs who have suffered placental insufficiency. Reduced oxygen delivery secondary to elevated glycosylated haemoglobin may also contribute. Renal vein thrombosis and other complications may occur. Hyperbilirubinaemia is more common.

Myocardial dysfunction

Ventricular septal hypertrophy secondary to hyperinsulinism is common. It can cause subaortic obstruction and lead to cardiac failure. Once the insulin levels are normal, the hypertrophy resolves over 8–12 weeks. Other cardiac abnormalities may occur.

Intrapartum asphyxia

There is an increased incidence of asphyxia in pregnancies complicated by diabetic nephropathy. There may be an accompanying vasculopathy of the placental bed leading to foetal compromise. The macrosomic infant may also be more prone to delivery complications which predispose to birth trauma and asphyxia, such as failure to progress, foetal distress, and instrumental delivery.

Long-term complications

Long-term complications associated with diabetic pregnancies include childhood obesity (which correlates with maternal prepregnant weight), neuropsychological deficits, and an increased tendency (risk of up to 20-fold compared with offspring of nondiabetic mothers) to develop diabetes mellitus. Infants of gestational diabetic mothers and infants of diabetic fathers also have an increased incidence of diabetes. It remains unclear whether maternal diabetes predisposes the offspring to subtle developmental problems.

Further reading

Coetzee EJ, Levitt NS. Maternal diabetes and neonatal outcome. *Seminars in Neonatology* (2000) **5:**221–9.

Cordero L, Landon MB. Infant of the diabetic mother. *Clinics in Perinatology* (1993) **20:**635–48.

Glaser B. Hyperinsulinism of the newborn. *Seminars in Perinatology* (2000) **24:**150–63.

Harman CR, Menticoglou SM. Foetal surveillance in diabetic pregnancy. *Current Opinions in Obstetrics and Gynecology* (1997) **9:**83–90.

Kalter H. *Of Diabetic Mothers and their Babies.* London: Martin Dunitz, 2000.

Schwartz R, Teramo KA. Effects of diabetic pregnancy on the foetus and newborn. *Seminars in Perinatology* (2000) **24:**120–35.

Suevo DM. The infant of the diabetic mother. *Neonatal Networks* (1997) **16:**25–33.

Related topics of interest

- blood-glucose homeostasis
- congenital malformations and birth defects
- hypoxic-ischaemic encephalopathy
- polycythaemia
- respiratory distress.

Infection—general

Newborn infants, particularly preterm infants, are especially vulnerable to infections due to an immaturity of their host defence systems. Their impaired immunological competence is partly due to an opsonisation defect and the functional immaturity of their white blood cells. Consequently, sepsis remains a major cause of morbidity and mortality in the neonatal period.

Aetiology

Infections presenting in the neonatal period may antedate delivery by several days or weeks (congenital infections), be acquired during delivery (perinatal infections), or appear later in postnatal period (postnatal infections). Causative organisms are varied, ranging from the common bacteria and viruses, through fungi to unusual protozoa.

Clinical features

These vary from nonspecific to obvious signs of sepsis with pallor and shock.

General
- fever
- lethargy
- temperature instability
- irritable or unresponsive
- being just 'not right'
- hypothermia
- poor colour
- acute collapse.

Respiratory
- tachypnoea
- recession
- grunting
- apnoea
- cyanosis.

Cardiovascular
- poor peripheral perfusion and prolonged capillary refill time (>3s)
- tachycardia >160/min
- hypotension
- cold and clammy
- shock.

Gastrointestinal
- ileus
- vomiting

- jaundice
- poor weight gain
- abdominal distension
- hepatosplenomegaly
- periumbilical staining
- loose and/or bloody stools
- abdominal redness and induration.

Metabolic
- hyperglycaemia ($\pm$glycosuria)
- hypoglycaemia.

Haematological
- petechiae
- purpura or bleeding from puncture sites, gut, or renal tract.

Neurological
- hypotonia
- high-pitched cry
- seizures
- bulging fontanelle
- retracted head
- coma.

Musculoskeletal
- swollen and tender limb(s) or joint(s)
- pseudoparalysis and crying when moved (arthritis or osteomyelitis).

Skin
- pallor
- erythema
- septic spots
- omphalitis
- paronychia
- discharging umbilicus
- mottled skin (cutis marmorata).

Investigations

For suspected serious infection in a symptomatic infant, carry out a full septic infection screen. Lumbar puncture may be omitted in the symptomatic but, less unwell patients. The following investigations should be included:

- blood cultures
- FBC, differential and film: WBC <5 or $>20 \times 10^3/mm^3$, neutrophils <2 or $>10 \times 10^3/mm^3$, or immature leucocytes (band cells) with toxic granulation, or the immature-to-total neutrophil ratio of greater than 0.2, and thrombocytopenia suggest sepsis

- urine culture of suprapubic aspirate or clean catch specimen (on microscopy, eight organisms per high-power field suggests infection)
- surface swabs of ear, nose, throat, and umbilicus; microscopy and Gram stain, culture, and virology ($\pm$electron microscopy for virus particles)
- stools for bacteriology and virology
- CSF for microscopy and Gram stain, culture and sensitivity, virology and biochemistry (protein >1.5–2.0g/l in term infants and >3.7g/l in preterm infants, CSF glucose less than 50% of blood glucose or <1.0mmol/l, with >1 WBC per 500 red cells (traumatic samples) or >20–30 polymorphonuclear leucocytes/mm^3 (atraumatic samples), all suggest meningitis); CSF serology for group B streptococcal or *E. coli* antigen, and CSF antigen tests for group B or type-specific polysaccharide antigens in body fluid
- clotting screen (when bleeding present or serious infection suspected)
- blood gases, glucose, U and E, and C-reactive protein (CRP)
- chest radiograph(s) and abdominal radiograph(s), in the presence of abdominal signs
- abdominal ultrasound (intra-abdominal masses and sepsis, renal and urinary tract infection, and ascites).

Management

- Commence broad-spectrum IV antibiotics immediately. In general, if cultures are negative and the infant is well, antibiotics may be discontinued after 48–72 h. Where cultures are negative but a temporal improvement in the infant's condition is noted with antimicrobial therapy, therapy is continued for 5–7 days. If sepsis is confirmed by positive culture(s), therapy is continued for at least ten days and occasionally longer, depending on the focus of infection (such as brain or bone) and the pathogen isolated.
- In sick infants, commence continuous monitoring of physiological parameters, including transcutaneous oxygen saturations, by pulse oximetry.
- Commence assisted ventilation for recurrent apnoea and respiratory failure.
- Monitor arterial blood gases 4–6-hourly in infants with respiratory distress or those receiving assisted ventilation.
- Monitor BP by an indwelling arterial device or noninvasively regularly (1–4-hourly) in all ill and unstable infants; do this more frequently in the sicker infants.
- Correct hypotension with FFP or normal saline (10–15ml/kg) and add inotropes (dopamine/dobutamine at 10–20 µg/kg per min) if BP still suboptimal.
- Administer IV dextrose solutions to maintain normal blood glucose and electrolytes (check U and E).
- Monitor the core-peripheral temperature gap in sick infants as a guide to the adequacy of tissue perfusion.
- Modify drug therapy according to the evolution of the illness, taking into account reports from bacteriology (pathogens isolated and their sensitivity).
- Where response to therapy is muted or absent, consider nonbacterial infections such as herpes simplex (add aciclovir), and systemic candidiasis (add amphotericin and flucytosine).

Useful websites

www.emedicine.com/ped/neonatology.htm
Part of the largest and most current online clinical knowledge base available to health professionals.

www.neonatology.com
Neonatology on the web – an extensive resource on neonatology.

Further reading

Edwards WH. Preventing nosocomial bloodstream infection in very low birth weight infants. *Seminars in Neonatology* (2003) **7:**325–33.

Gerdes JS. Clinicopathologic approach to the diagnosis of neonatal sepsis. *Clinics in Perinatology* (1991) **18:**361–81.

Isaacs D, Moxon ER. *Handbook of Neonatal Infections: A Practical Guide.* Philadelphia: WB Saunders, 1999.

Remington JS, Klein JO (eds). *Infectious Diseases of the Fetus and Newborn Infant,* 5th edn. Philadelphia: WB Saunders, 2001.

Romero R, Espinoza J, Chaiworapongsa T, et al. Infection and prematurity and the role of preventive strategies. *Seminars in Neonatology* (2002) **7:**259–74.

Stoll B, Weisman L (eds). Infections in perinatology. *Clinics in Perinatology* (1997) **24**(1).

Related topics of interest

- acute collapse
- apnoea and bradycardia
- infection—neonatal
- infection—perinatal
- infection—prenatal
- respiratory distress
- resuscitation
- shock
- transfusion of blood and blood products.

enzyme coagulase. Organisms able to ferment mannitol and produce coagulase are called coagulase-positive organisms, such as *Staphylococcus aureus* (*S. aureus*). Organisms negative for these products are called coagulase-negative staphylococci (CNS), the most important being *S. epidermidis* and *S. saprophyticus*. Gram stain shows Gram-positive cocci. In recent years, coagulase-negative staphylococci have assumed predominance as NICU pathogens. Infants are colonised by coagulase-negative staphylococci and *S. aureus* soon after birth, mostly by staff contact. Hand washing is one of the most effective means of reducing colonisation. The virulence of *S. aureus* is related to the production of coagulase, alpha-haemolysin, and leucocidin, whereas coagulase-negative staphylococci produce a polysaccharide mucoid (slime), which facilitates their adherence to foreign bodies (such as catheters) and hinders phagocytosis.

S. aureus causes the following infections:

- impetigo
- septicaemia
- pneumonia
- septic arthritis
- osteomyelitis
- breast abscesses
- chronic recurrent furunculosis
- eye, ear, nose, and throat infections
- toxic epidermal necrolysis (staphylococcal scalded skin syndrome)
- endocarditis (rare, more likely with CNS and intravascular catheters).

Coagulase-negative staphylococci are an important cause of nosocomial infections, especially in VLBW infants, and the risk of infection is increased in the presence of indwelling medical devices (such as venous catheters or CNS shunts).

- *S. epidermidis* is the most frequent bacterial species isolated from blood.
- *S. aureus* and coagulase-negative staphylococci are now widely resistant to penicillin G due to β-lactamase production.
- In recent years, resistance to semisynthetic β-lactamase-resistant penicillins (such as methicillin) has produced problematic infections with methicillin-resistant *S. aureus* (MRSA) and methicillin-resistant coagulase-negative staphylococci.
- Once introduced into a hospital, MRSA are difficult to eliminate.

Treatment
First-line agents for methicillin-susceptible strains of *S. aureus* include flucloxacillin, oxacillin, and some 'first-generation' cephalosporins (such as cephalexin). Glycopeptide antimicrobials (such as vancomycin and teicoplanin) are the agents of choice for methicillin-resistant staphylococcal infections, and coagulase-negative staphylococci infections resistant to the common first-line drugs.

Respiratory syncytial virus (RSV)
RSV is a pneumovirus of the family Paramyxoviridae, of which two types (A and B) exist. It causes annual outbreaks of infection (bronchiolitis) during the winter months. The incubation period is 2–8 days, with viral shedding lasting 3–4 weeks. Spread is by aerosol or direct contact with infected secretions.

- Clinical features include upper respiratory tract symptoms (cough and rhinitis) followed by lower respiratory tract symptoms (tachypnoea, recessions, and cyanosis).
- Symptoms and disease severity are age dependent. The very young (<4 weeks) may present with apnoea and nonspecific signs of infection (lethargy, poor feeding, irritability, and fever). Disease is more severe in infants over 12 weeks of age, especially preterm infants with chronic lung disease, who are more likely to require assisted ventilation.
- Infants with congenital heart disease (CHD) are also at high risk of severe disease (more likely to require supplemental oxygen (83%), intensive care (30%), and assisted ventilation (19%) and to die (3.4%)).
- Diagnosis is by direct fluorescent antibody detection of virus and enzyme-linked immunosorbent assays of nasopharyngeal aspirates.
- Therapy is mainly supportive (fluids, supplemental oxygen, and antibiotics for pneumonia), with ribavirin being given early to the high-risk groups (CLD and CHD).
- The hyperimmune RSV immunoglobulin, palivizumab (Synagis, Abbott Laboratories), a humanised monoclonal antibody, is an effective prophylaxis for preterm infants (<36 weeks' gestation and age <6 months old at onset of RSV season), infants with CLD (reduces the incidence and severity of RSV infection), and children with CHD who are less than two years old. This is administered once a month (15 mg/kg i.m.) during the RSV season.

Mycoplasmas

Over 150 different species of mollicutes or mycoplasmas exist, of which *Mycoplasma hominis* and *Ureaplasma urealyticum* are of particular relevance to humans. These organisms, which are unique in lacking a cell wall, have been associated with several diseases, including septicaemia, pneumonia, meningitis, hydrocephalus, and CLD. However, most of the evidence linking mycoplasmas to disease is epidemiological, suggesting an association rather than cause and effect. Vertical transmission varies from 0–55% in full-term infants to 29–55% in preterm infants born to infected mothers, being higher in the presence of chorioamnionitis or intra-amniotic infection. *U. urealyticum* has been isolated from blood and CSF cultures, and shown to cause pneumonia (especially in infants of <1250 g). Several studies have shown an increased risk of CLD in infected infants with a birth weight <1250 g though a definite cause-and-effect relationship has not been shown.

Investigations

- Mycoplasmas may be cultured in blood, CSF, urine, pleural fluid, and tracheo-bronchial secretions. Specimens should be stored at 4 °C, not room temperature.
- PCR is faster and more sensitive.
- Detection of serotype-specific IgM and IgG is indicative of infection.

Management

Macrolides (such as erythromycin) and tetracycline (especially for CSF infection) are the drugs of choice (though resistance to both has been reported, particularly with *M. hominis*). Consider treating preterm infants with evidence of infection where bacterial cultures are consistently negative, where there is failure to respond to broad-spectrum antibiotics, or in neonates with unexplained CSF pleocytosis. In infants without CSF involvement, 10–14 days of IV erythromycin lactobionate (25–40 mg/kg per day in three to four divided doses) should suffice; in CNS infections, start with erythromycin and monitor clinical progress (repeat CSF cultures). Switch to tetracycline if there is no response or further deterioration occurs.

Useful websites

www.cdc.gov/az.do
The US Centers for Disease Control and Prevention – the largest clinical knowledge base available.

www.emedicine.com/ped/neonatology.htm
One of the largest and most current online clinical knowledge bases available to health professionals.

www.neonatology.com
Neonatology on the web – an extensive resource on neonatology.

Further reading

Isaacs D, Moxon ER. *Handbook of Neonatal Infections: A Practical Guide*. Philadelphia: WB Saunders, 1999.
Lyon AJ. Genital mycoplasmas and infection in the neonate. In: TN Hansen, N McIntosh (eds). *Current Topics in Neonatology*, No. 1. London: WB Saunders 1996: 1–20.
Phillips AGS. Perinatal infection: detection and prevention. *Seminars in Neonatology* (2002) **7**(4).
Pickering LK (ed.). *The Red Book: 2003 Report of the Committee on Infectious Diseases,* 26th edn. Elk Grove Village, IL: American Academy of Pediatrics, 2003.
Remington JS, Klein JO (eds). *Infectious Diseases of the Fetus and Newborn Infant*, 5th edn. Philadelphia: WB Saunders, 2001.
Stoll BJ, Weisman LE (eds). Infections in perinatology. *Clinics in Perinatology* (1997) **24**(1).

Related topics of interest

- infection—general
- infection—perinatal
- infection—prenatal.

Infection—perinatal

Infections presenting in the immediate postnatal period are likely to have been acquired during the delivery or in utero. Such infections often mimic respiratory distress syndrome (RDS) and if untreated may rapidly progress to fulminant and fatal illness. Therefore, where there are risk factors for sepsis, appropriate antibiotic therapy should be started immediately with recourse to full intensive care support if required. The traditional 'early-onset' infections, that is, those occurring during the first week of life, are covered in this section.

General infections

Common causative organisms

Bacterial infections
- group B streptococcus (GBS)
- *Haemophilus influenzae*
- *Escherichia coli*
- *Listeria monocytogenes*
- *Neisseria gonorrhoea.*

Viral infections
- herpes simplex
- varicella-zoster
- hepatitis B
- hepatitis C
- HIV.

Common risk factors for perinatal infections
- prolonged (>24 h) rupture of membranes
- maternal infection or intrapartum pyrexia
- cloudy or foul-smelling liquor
- instrumental delivery
- premature labour
- long labour.

Clinical features
These vary from non-specific signs to obvious signs of sepsis with pallor and shock. See 'Infection—general'.

Investigations
- FBC
- CRP
- chest radiograph
- blood culture
- GBS antigen in urine and CSF
- coagulation studies in severe sepsis

- *Chlamydia*—direct immunofluorescence test and specific IgM
- virus identification by electron microscopy in vesicle fluid, PCR, or serology.

Management
- For symptomatic infants, perform a full septic screen and commence broad-spectrum antibiotics (commonly ampicillin/penicillin and an aminoglycoside).
- For asymptomatic infants, perform a septic screen (omitting lumbar puncture) followed by broad-spectrum antibiotics.
- Discontinue antibiotics if bacteriology shows no growth at 48 h and infant is well. However, continue antibiotics for at least five days if mother received antibiotics intrapartum.

Specific infections

Group B streptococcus (GBS)
GBS disease is caused by beta-haemolytic streptococci of the Lancefield group B classification (*Streptococcus agalactiae*). In the developed nations, GBS disease is the commonest cause of fatal bacterial infection in newborns. Nine serotypes of GBS have been identified, with serotypes 1a and III being the most important cause of invasive GBS infection in the Western Hemisphere. A quarter to a third of all adults carry GBS. It is found primarily in the gastrointestinal tract, but also in the genital tract, where it is usually asymptomatic. During labour, about 20% of mothers are colonised. Fifty per cent of infants passing through a colonised birth canal become colonised, and 1–2% of colonised infants develop invasive GBS disease. Invasive disease has been categorised as early-onset GBS disease (EOGBS), occurring within the first week after birth (though most affected infants become ill within 24 h of birth), or late-onset disease (typically occurring at 3–4 weeks from birth, range day seven to three months). EOGBS is more common in preterm infants, while late-onset GBS disease affects term and preterm infants equally. The UK mortality rate is 4–6% in term infants, 18% in preterm infants, and 10.6% overall. The current incidence of EOGBS disease in the UK and Ireland is 0.5 per 1000 births, approximating to 340 infants per year (but varying from 0.21 per 1000 births in Scotland to 0.73 per 1000 births in Northern Ireland). There has been a dramatic fall in the US incidence from two per 1000 live births in the early 1990s to 0.39 per 1000 live births in 1999, following the introduction of universal maternal screening for GBS and intrapartum antibiotic prophylaxis for colonised mothers. This is estimated to have reduced the incidence of EOGBS by 86%. Adopting a similar programme in the UK would require 7000 colonised women to be given intrapartum antibiotics to prevent one neonatal death from EOGBS, which in turn would require 24000 women to be screened.

GBS predominantly invades the blood, lungs, or the CSF. Maternal colonisation (vertical transmission) is a prerequisite for EOGBS disease. Infants acquire the infection via the maternal bloodstream, from ascending infection through ruptured membranes, or through aspiration of contaminated amniotic fluid. Some 75% of cases of GBS are early-onset with septicaemia in 25–40%, pneumonia in 35–55%, and meningitis in 5–10%. Late-onset GBS commonly presents with meningitis or bacteraemia, with serotype III (the predominant cause of meningitis) being primarily involved. Horizontal transmission is the primary route of infection (from a colonised mother, human milk, or the community). Breast-feeding, however, does not increase the risk of neonatal GBS disease.

Risk factors for EOGBS disease
- maternal colonisation
- maternal chorioamnionitis
- young maternal age (<20 years)
- intrapartum pyrexia (>37.8 °C)
- GBS bacteriuria
- low serotype-specific antibody (anti-GBS IgG)
- preterm labour (<37 weeks' gestation)
- preterm premature rupture of membranes (PPROM)
- prolonged rupture of membranes (PROM, ≥18 h)
- previous birth of an infant with GBS infection
- twin with EOGBS infection.

Clinical features
- apnoea
- grunting
- respiratory distress
- acute collapse and/or shock.

Diagnosis
- isolation of GBS from blood, CSF, trachea, or body fluids (such as pleural or joint fluid)
- detection of group B or type-specific polysaccharide antigens in body fluids (mainly CSF; urine testing may yield false-positive results from contamination)
- chest radiograph clinically identical to RDS in 50% of affected infants.

Treatment
- As most infants with EOGBS disease have symptoms at or soon after birth, symptomatic infants should be treated promptly with broad-spectrum antibiotics which cover the common local pathogens, including GBS.
- Initial therapy is empirical with IV penicillin (or ampicillin) and gentamicin after performing an infection screen.
- Penicillin G alone may be used after microbial confirmation and ascertainment of sensitivity patterns (including sensitivity to erythromycin and clindamycin).
- Septicaemia requires treatment for 7–10 days.
- Uncomplicated meningitis requires treatment for 14–21 days.
- Complicated meningitis (ventriculitis or abscess) may require 21–28 days.
- Endocarditis or esteomyelitis may require 4–6 weeks' therapy.
- Duration of therapy may be guided by CRP levels returning to normal.

Most infections can be prevented by the intrapartum administration of penicillin (or, if penicillin sensitive, clindamycin, erythromycin, or vancomycin) to the high-risk group. Antibiotic prophylaxis is most beneficial when administered more than 4 h prior to delivery (reduces colonisation to 1.2%, compared to 47% in infants of untreated GBS-colonised mothers, and 2.9% when prophylaxis was 2–4 h prior to delivery). The current indications for maternal intrapartum prophylaxis are as follows:

- GBS bacteriuria
- GBS detected incidentally
- maternal chorioamnionitis
- preterm premature rupture of membranes (PPROM)
- previous birth of an infant with GBS infection.

Antibiotics (five-day course) should also be given to infants born to mothers who should have received intrapartum antibiotics but did not, infants born to mothers who received the first dose of antibiotics less than 4h prior to delivery, and preterm infants whose mothers received intrapartum antibiotics. As up to 90% of infants with EOGBS infection present in the first 12h of life, healthy term infants with a risk factor including the incidental finding of maternal GBS carriage, with or without intrapartum antibiotics, may be observed for 12h and discharged thereafter if they remain well, since the risk of disease in such infants may then be similar to that of infants with no risk factors. The incidence of EOGBS disease in term infants without antenatal risk factors in the UK is 0.2 cases/1000 births. For a mother whose previous infant had GBS disease, the infant should either be observed for 12–24h or have blood cultures taken and be started on IV penicillin until culture results are known.

Listerosis

Neonatal listerosis accounts for the largest recognisable group of infections caused by *Listeria monocytogenes*. The incidence of neonatal listerosis in Europe and the USA is 13 per 100000 live births. Early-onset listerosis has similarities to GBS with respiratory symptoms which mimic RDS. Classically, it develops within the first 48h of life. Most cases are clinically apparent at delivery, with meconium staining, cyanosis, respiratory distress, and pneumonia. A transient, pink, papular rash may be seen over the trunk. The chest radiograph may resemble RDS or aspiration pneumonitis. Disseminated disease is often fatal. Mothers acquire *Listeria* from refrigerated dairy products (soft cheeses, milk, and paté), may have a fever prelabour, and have a discoloured amniotic fluid. Diagnosis is by cultivation of *L. monocytogenes* (a Gram-positive motile bacterium) from blood and other tissues. High-dose ampicillin with an aminoglycoside is the treatment of choice. The long-term morbidity is unclear, but if meningitis is not present, outcome may be generally good.

Varicella-zoster

Severity of neonatal disease is dependent on the timing of maternal illness. Maternal rash soon after delivery or within five days before delivery greatly increases the risk of a severe perinatal infection. Varicella-zoster immunoglobulin, VZIG (one vial, 125 units), should be administered as soon as possible after birth to infants whose mothers are diagnosed with chickenpox with lesions starting from five days before to two days after delivery. VZIG will ameliorate or prevent disease. Some 50% of infants develop chickenpox. Aciclovir should be administered to symptomatic infants (10–15mg/kg eight-hourly IV, reduced in renal failure).

Herpes simplex

Herpes simplex virus (HSV) exists in two forms, types 1 and 2 (HSV-1 and HSV-2, respectively). HSV-2 accounts for 60–70% of neonatal HSV infection. The incidence of neonatal HSV infection in the UK is 0.03–0.05 per 1000 live births and 0.1–0.3 per 1000 in the USA (where the incidence is rising). Most HSV infection in neonates occurs intrapartum. The attack rate is ~33% in women with a primary infection, but only ~3% in women having a reactivation. Less commonly, HSV can be acquired in the postpartum period (mostly due to HSV-1). Skin vesicles may be diagnostic. Clinical signs may initially be mild and nonspecific but may progress to a severe illness with pneumonitis, encephalitis, or myocarditis. Note, however, that presentation may be delayed for up to eight weeks. *Diagnosis* is by virus culture (urine, stool, blood, CSF, vesicle fluid, conjunctival scrapings, and swabs of the eye, throat, and rectum), light microscopy (intranuclear inclusions) or electron microscopy of conjunctival scrapings, and PCR to detect HSV DNA (as in CSF and serum). EEG may show localising signs of high-voltage, low-frequency activity, and CT or MRI scans may show temporal lobe necrosis or haemorrhage. *Treatment* is with aciclovir (or vidarabine) with full intensive care support. Mortality is 15% with CNS involvement, and 57% with disseminated disease. Risk of death is increased in infants with DIC, seizures, HSV type 2, and in coma. If in doubt, treat and review later!

Chlamydia trachomatis

Conjunctivitis is the commonest early manifestation of an intrapartum chlamydial infection.

Chlamydiosis (including conjunctivitis) requires 1% tetracycline drops and a full course of oral erythromycin.

Parent information and support group

Group B Strep Support
P.O. Box 203
Haywards Heath
West Sussex RH16 1GF, UK
Tel: 01444 416176
www.gbss.org.uk

Useful websites

www.rcog.org.uk/resources/Public/GroupB_strep_no36.pdf
Royal College of Obstetricians and Gynaecologists guidelines on the prevention of early onset neonatal group B streptococcal disease.

www.cdc.gov/az.do
The US Centers for Disease Control and Prevention – the largest clinical knowledge base available.

www.emedicine.com/ped/neonatology.htm
One of the largest and most current clinical knowledge basis available to health professionals.

Further reading

Isaacs D, Moxon ER. *Handbook of Neonatal Infections: A Practical Guide.* Philadelphia: WB Saunders, 1999.

Phillips AGS (ed.). Perinatal infection: detection and prevention. *Seminars in Perinatology* (2002) **7**(4).

Pickering LK (ed.). *The Red Book: 2003 Report of the Committee on Infectious Diseases*, 26th edn. Elk Grove Village, IL: American Academy of Pediatrics, 2003.

Remington JS, Klein JO (eds). *Infectious Disease of the Fetus and Newborn Infant*, 5th edn. Philadelphia: WB Saunders, 2001.

Stoll BJ, Weisman LE (eds). Infections in perinatology. *Clinics in Perinatology* (1997) **24**(1).

Related topics of interest

- hepatitis B and C
- HIV and AIDS
- infection—general
- infection—neonatal
- infection—prenatal
- intrauterine growth restriction.

Infection—prenatal

TORCH infections

Several maternal infections during pregnancy may have permanent or long-lasting effects in the foetus. The outcome following such intrauterine infections may depend on the maturity of the foetus when the infection is contracted. The commonest congenital infections of significance constitute the 'TORCH' infections—namely, *Toxo*plasmosis, *O*ther (particularly syphilis), *R*ubella, *C*ytomegalovirus, and *H*erpes simplex.

Toxoplasmosis

Infection with *Toxoplasma gondii* results in toxoplasmosis, one of the commonest infections in the world, with a marked variation in prevalence from <50% to 90% (as in France). The incidence of toxoplasmosis during pregnancy varies from 3–6 per 1000 to 1–2 per 1000 in low-risk countries (such as the UK and the USA). The mother can be infected by an infected cat, or by eating raw or inadequately cooked meat or contaminated vegetables. Most individuals will have either no or minimal signs of acute infection. The risk of foetal infection increases from the first trimester to the third trimester, while the risk of serious infection in the foetus decreases from 75% in the first trimester to being negligible in the third trimester. Congenital toxoplasmosis with clinical manifestation of disease in the newborn occurs when the foetus is infected before 26 weeks' gestation. The incidence of congenital toxoplasmosis in the UK is approximately 1:10000. Approximately 60% of all infants born to infected mothers escape infection, 25% have subclinical infection without sequelae, and only 5–10% develop clinical infection. The classic tetrad of congenital toxoplasmosis comprises chorioretinitis, intracranial calcification, epilepsy, and hydrocephalus. Affected infants may also be growth restricted and present with petechiae, jaundice, and hepatosplenomegaly. Diagnosis is based on serological tests for toxoplasmosis, particularly of the CSF. Antenatal diagnosis is possible. Treatment with spiramycin, pyrimethamine, and sulphonamides may improve foetal outcome for mothers who seroconvert during pregnancy. Infected neonates receive a year's therapy with spiramycin, sulphadiazine, and pyrimethamine. Prognosis for mild or subclinical cases is good, but 25% of those with neonatal symptoms die. Infection in the first 20 weeks of pregnancy may be an indication for termination.

Rubella

Congenital rubella is rare in the UK with ≤10 cases reported each year. Rubella was made notifiable in the UK in 1988, the same year the MMR vaccine was introduced. In 1995, there were only eight confirmed rubella infections in pregnant women reported to the Communicable Disease Surveillance Centre. Currently, about five cases of the congenital rubella syndrome (CRS) are reported annually to the National Congenital Rubella Surveillance Programme. The risk of foetal infection decreases with advancing gestation. In 90% of cases, maternal rubella infection in the first 8–10 weeks of pregnancy results in serious foetal infection and damage, whereas by 16 weeks the risk declines to 10–20%, and thereafter foetal damage is rare. The clinical features of extended CRS include petechiae, jaundice, hepatosplenomegaly, eye and bone anomalies, a murmur, and, in 33%, birth weight below the third percentile. Multiple foetal defects are common: eyes (cataract, glaucoma, and microphthalmia), CNS (microcephaly, mental retardation, and cerebral palsy), deafness (bilateral and sensorineural), cardiovascular (PDA and peripheral pulmonary artery stenosis), liver (hepatitis and prolonged jaundice), bone (osteitis), and haematological (anaemia and thrombocytopenia). Diagnosis is by culturing the virus from a throat swab or urine and demonstrating rubella-specific IgM in the infant's blood. Antiviral treatment is not available, and infants remain very infectious during the first months of life (hazard to female staff). Glaucoma and cataracts require ophthalmological intervention, and hearing should be formally assessed.

Cytomegalovirus (CMV)
Occurring with an incidence of 0.2–2.5% of all live births (UK 0.3–0.4%, USA ~1%), congenital CMV is the commonest disease of newborns with a significant morbidity. Both primary and recurrent maternal infections during pregnancy can result in foetal infection, but the rate of foetal transmission is higher (24–75%) with a primary maternal infection than with a reactivation of infection (<1%). Approximately 90% of congenitally infected infants born to mothers who had their primary infection during pregnancy are asymptomatic at birth, but they are more likely to develop adverse sequelae than those infants born to mothers with reactivation of infection. The characteristic features include petechiae, hepatosplenomegaly, sensorineural hearing impairment, microcephaly, intracranial calcification, chorioretinitis, jaundice, growth restriction, and thrombocytopenia. The standard diagnostic test is viral culture (the most sensitive and specific test) of urine, saliva, or other bodily secretions/tissues obtained within the first three weeks of life, so as to distinguish congenital from perinatal and postnatal infection. Other tests include serology for CMV-specific IgM antibody, detection of CMV DNA by PCR, and urine electron microscopy for viral particles. These infants shed the virus for long periods (hazard to female staff). Therapy with ganciclovir and CMV immunoglobulin should be considered in severe disease, though efficacy has not been proven. Prognosis is generally good, with most infants developing normally. Approximately 10% of asymptomatic neonates develop deafness in later life. Of those with CNS signs in the neonatal period, 73% develop long-term sequelae, while 30% will have neurological sequelae in the absence of signs in the neonatal period.

Herpes simplex virus (HSV)
HSV exists in two forms, types 1 and 2 (HSV-1 and HSV-2, respectively). HSV-2 causes about 85% of genital herpes, while HSV-1 causes mainly ophthalmic, orolabial, and CNS disease. HSV-2 accounts for 60–70% of neonatal HSV infection. The incidence of neonatal HSV infection in the UK is 0.03–0.05 per 1000 live births and 0.1–0.3 per 1000 in the USA (where the incidence is rising). Most HSV infection in neonates occurs intrapartum, but true congenital infection occurs in about 5% of cases as a result of both primary infection and (rarely) recurrent maternal infection. Congenital HSV is defined as the presence of vesicles or scarring at birth, abnormal brain CT scan within the first week of life, microcephaly, microphthalmia, or chorioretinitis. Congenital HSV has a different presentation from intrapartum HSV. The

major clinical findings are cutaneous lesions (94%), CNS lesions (79%) (microcephaly, hydranencephaly, cerebral atrophy, and intracranial calcification), prematurity (59%), ocular lesions (42%) (chorioretinitis and microphthalmia), and organomegaly (hepatitis). HSV-2 causes >90% of congenital infection. The congenitally infected infant may be mildly affected with eye involvement only, or severely affected with skin lesions, chorioretinitis, and microcephaly (or hydranencephaly). *Diagnosis* is by virus culture (urine, stool, blood, CSF, vesicle fluid, conjunctival scrapings, and swabs of the eye, throat, and rectum), light microscopy (intranuclear inclusions) or electron microscopy of conjunctival scrapings, and PCR to detect HSV DNA (as in CSF and serum). EEG may show localising signs of high-voltage, low-frequency activity, and CT or MRI scans may show temporal lobe necrosis or haemorrhage. *Treatment* is with aciclovir (30–60 mg/kg per day IV) with full intensive care support. Mortality is 15% with CNS involvement, and 57% with disseminated disease. Rarely, infants with congenital HSV develop normally.

Other infections

Syphilis

Infected newborn infants may appear normal or be severely affected with extensive skin eruptions through to marked hydrops fetalis. All pregnant mothers should be screened (VDRL, TPHA, or ELISA test) for syphilis. False-positives may occur after *Treponema pertenue* infection (yaws). Maternal infection leads to intrauterine infection in up to half of all pregnancies, with increased foetal loss from abortions or stillbirths.

Clinical features
- infant initially appearing normal, with signs only appearing weeks to months later
- extensive mucocutaneous lesions in the absence of systemic disturbance but with hepatosplenomegaly and lymphadenopathy
- severe systemic disturbance but without the typical skin rashes
- cutaneous manifestations (maculopapular rash with circinate lesions involving palms and soles of feet)
- rhinitis followed by mucopurulent, blood-stained nasal discharge
- destruction of nasal cartilage and bone producing flattened nasal bridge and saddle nose
- fissures and bleeding from lesions at mucocutaneous junctions
- rhagades
- condylomata around anus and female genitalia
- osteochondritis, especially wrists, elbows, and knees
- periostitis, especially in limb bones and skull
- meningitis and hydrocephalus.

Investigations
- FBC
- liver function tests
- syphilis serology (VDRL, TPHA, or ELISA test with rising or persistently high titres)
- dark-field microscopy of fluid from skin lesions and nasal discharge

- radiography of long bones (periostitis and osteochondritis)
- CSF examination (lymphocytosis, raised protein, normal glucose level, and syphilis serology positive).

Management
Take precautions as skin lesions are infectious. Procaine penicillin 30 mg/kg per day i.m. for ten days or single i.m. injection of long-acting benzathine penicillin 60 mg/kg. Treat mother and partner(s)!

Varicella-zoster
Varicella-zoster virus (VZV) infection during pregnancy (incidence ~0.7 in 1000), particularly during the first 20 weeks, may result in foetal loss or the congenital varicella-zoster syndrome with cutaneous lesions (scars) (70%), ocular abnormalities (chorioretinitis, microphthalmia, cataracts, and Horner's syndrome), CNS lesions (50%) (cortical atrophy, calcifications, and mental retardation), and abnormal limb development (hypoplasia, and abnormal or absent digits). Administration of varicella-zoster immune globulin (VZIG) after exposure may prevent foetal infection, and aciclovir therapy during pregnancy may be safe.

Parvovirus B19
Parvovirus B19, the causative agent of erythema infectiosum (fifth disease), has a predilection for bone-marrow erythroid precursors. Lysis of the erythroid precursors is responsible for the decreased red cell production. The incidence of B19 infection is reported as 3.7%, with a vertical transmission of 16% during the first 20 weeks and 35% after 20 weeks' gestation. Infection-related foetal loss is low at 0.6 per 1000 women. The commonest symptomatic presentation of prenatal infection is nonimmune hydrops secondary to severe foetal anaemia, but this only occurs in about 1% of infected infants. Most infants with prenatal B19 infection are normal. No studies support a correlation between maternal infection and an increased risk of birth defects. Diagnosis is by electron microscopy of virions in tissue specimens, detection of viral DNA by PCR, or serology (IgM and IgG antibodies). Negative IgM assay at birth does not rule out congenital infection.

HIV infection
From 8% to 24–50% of the total HIV vertical transmission is estimated to occur in utero. Vertical transmission is reduced by prenatal, perinatal, and early neonatal antiretroviral therapy. No HIV-associated dysmorphic syndrome exists. (see 'HIV and AIDS' chapter.)

Useful websites

www.cdc.gov/az.do
The US Centers for Disease Control and Prevention. The largest clinical knowledge base available.

www.emedicine.com/ped
One of the largest and must current online clinical knowledge bases available to health professionals.

www.neonatology.com
Neonatology on the web – an extensive resource on neonatology.

Further reading

Greenough A, Osborne J, Sutherland S (eds). *Congenital, Perinatal and Neonatal Infections.* Edinburgh: Churchill Livingstone, 1992.

Isaacs D, Moxon ER. *Handbook of Neonatal Infections: A Practical Guide.* Philadelphia: WB Saunders, 1999.

Pickering LK (ed.). *The Red Book: 2003 Report of the Committee on Infectious Diseases*, 26th edn. Elk Grove Village, IL: American Academy of Pediatrics, 2003.

Remington JS, Klein JO (eds). *Infectious Diseases of the Fetus and Newborn Infant*, 5th edn. Philadelphia: WB Saunders, 2001.

Stoll BJ, Weisman LE (eds). Infections in perinatology. *Clinics in Perinatology* (1997) **24**(1).

Related topics of interest

- infection—general
- infection—neonatal
- infection—perinatal
- intrauterine growth restriction.

Inherited metabolic disease—investigation and management

As over a hundred inherited metabolic diseases (IMDs) can present in newborn infants, it would be impractical to cover these disorders in any detail in a brief synopsis of IMDs. A summary of an approach to the investigation and management of IMDs may be more useful. The diagnosis of IMD has implications for future pregnancies, as prenatal diagnosis is now possible for many of these conditions. Though IMDs may present in myriad ways, certain details offer important clues to the possibility of IMD, namely, unexplained neonatal deaths, a previously affected sibling or close relative, and consanguinity. A history of sudden illness in a previously well infant (particularly when vomiting, acidosis, and circulatory disturbance are followed by depressed consciousness and convulsions or neurological features out of proportion to the perceived insult) is also highly suggestive of IMD.

For simplicity, IMDs may be divided into three groups.

Group 1

These disorders lead to toxicity from accumulation of compounds proximal to the metabolic block; for example, aminoacidopathies, organic acidurias, urea cycle defects, and sugar intolerances. There is a symptom-free period followed by signs of acute intoxication (such as vomiting, lethargy, and coma). Metabolic disturbances are common (such as hypoglycaemia, ketosis, acidosis, and hyperammonaemia). Diagnosis relies on the assay of urine and plasma amino acids and organic acids. Therapy entails removal of toxic compounds by extrarenal procedures or special diets.

Group 2

These disorders arise partly from a defect in utilisation or production of energy due to a metabolic defect in the liver, muscle, myocardium, or brain; for example, glycogenosis types I and III, congenital lactic acidaemia, fatty acid oxidation defects, and mitochondrial respiratory chain defects. Symptoms include hypoglycaemia, hyperlacticacidaemia, severe hypotonia, myopathy, cardiomyopathy, cardiac failure, and sudden infant death syndrome. These disorders may arise antenatally.

Group 3

These disorders disturb the synthesis or catabolism of complex molecules. Symptoms are permanent, progressive, and not related to food intake, as in lysosomal disorders, peroxisomal disorders, α_1-antitrypsin deficiency, and carbohydrate-deficient glycoprotein (CDG) syndrome. As therapies are not available for most of these conditions, ascertaining the correct diagnosis is important.

Presentation of IMD in the neonatal period

For simplicity, three presentations may be described: neurological, hepatodigestive, and cardiac.

Neurological presentations
This may present primarily as hypotonia, seizures, or neurological dysfunction.

Neurological dysfunction
In group 1 (toxicity) disorders, there is often a normal pregnancy and delivery, and an initial normal and symptom-free postnatal period followed by unprovoked progressive deterioration unresponsive to symptomatic therapy. Typically, the affected infant feeds poorly and then progresses into a coma with apnoea, bradycardia, hiccups and involuntary movements (tremors and myoclonic jerks), axial hypotonia, and limb hypertonia.

In group 2 (energy-deficiency) disorders, there is no intervening symptom-free postnatal period. Commonly, there are generalised hypotonia, rapidly progressive neurological deterioration, hypertrophic cardiomyopathy, occasional malformations, and dysmorphic features.

Seizures
Seizures occur as early signs of IMD in pyridoxine dependency, sulphite oxidase deficiency, nonketotic hyperglycinaemia (NKH), and peroxisomal disorders. Of note, seizures rarely occur in organic acidurias or urea cycle defects unless the affected infant is comatose, hypoglycaemic, or in a pre-existing stupor.

Hypotonia
Predominant or isolated hypotonia is seen in only a few IMDs (such as peroxisomal disorders, NKH, respiratory chain disorders, sulphite oxidase deficiency, and urea cycle defects).

Hepatodigestive presentations
Hepatomegaly with hypoglycaemia and seizures suggests glycogenosis types I and III, fructose diphosphatase deficiency, or hyperinsulinism.

Liver failure syndrome (jaundice, haemorrhagic disease, hepatocellular necrosis with raised transaminases, ascites, and hypoglycaemia) suggests galactosaemia, fructosaemia, tyrosinosis type I (after 2–3 weeks), neonatal haemochromatosis, and respiratory chain disorders.

Cholestatic jaundice with failure to thrive is primarily observed in α_1-antitrypsin deficiency, bile acid metabolic defects, peroxisomal disorders, Niemann–Pick type C disease, CDG syndrome, and Byler disease. Hepatic presentations of fatty acid oxidation defects or urea cycle defects include fatty degeneration or Reye-like syndrome with slightly prolonged prothrombin time, raised transaminases, and normal bilirubin levels, but not true liver failure.

Cardiac presentations
Cardiac failure with cardiomyopathy (dilated hypertrophic), and hypotonia, muscle weakness, and failure to thrive, suggests Pompe's disease, respiratory chain disorders, fatty acid oxidation defects, or CDG syndrome. Long-chain fatty acid oxidation

defects may present with conduction defects (A–V block, bundle branch blocks, and ventricular tachycardia).

Investigations

Investigations must proceed alongside supportive therapy. Certain findings may be especially significant in suspected IMD, namely, metabolic acidosis with large anion gap (organic acidurias), acetonuria (always abnormal in newborn), and raised lactate concentration with ketosis (especially in the absence of hypoxic insult, infection, and circulatory collapse). Hyperammonaemia often suggests a urea cycle defect (with associated respiratory alkalosis), organic acidaemia (with ketoacidosis), or transient hyperammonaemia in preterm infants. Leucopenia, thrombocytopenia, and even sepsis may also be present, especially in organic acidurias. Obtain adequate amounts of plasma, urine, and CSF for immediate analysis and storage. Expert metabolic advice is essential.

Urine
- note smell and colour
- reducing substances (Clinitest, Ames)
- pH (pH Stix, Merck)
- acetone (Acetest, Ames)
- keto acids (dinitrophenylhydrazine [DNPH])
- sulphitest (Merck)
- uric acid
- electrolytes
- organic acid chromatography.

Each fresh urine sample should be collected separately and either frozen ($-20\,°C$) for storage or refrigerated if not being assayed immediately.

Blood
- FBC
- blood gases
- blood glucose
- ammonia
- liver function tests (including transaminases)
- coagulation screen
- amino acid chromatography
- electrolytes (check anion gap) and calcium
- lactate and pyruvate
- uric acid
- free fatty acids
- acetoacetate and 3-hydroxybutyrate.

For storage, obtain 5 ml of heparinised plasma and freeze ($-20\,°C$), and whole blood (10 ml in EDTA tube) and freeze for DNA studies. In addition, obtain blood on filter paper (Guthrie test cards). For white and red cells, spin blood sample, separate plasma, and store frozen ($-20\,°C$), keeping infranatant (red and white cells) at $+4\,°C$ (for up to two days).

Other investigations

- lumbar puncture (CSF biochemistry, store some CSF at $-20\,^{\circ}$C)
- skin biopsy (fibroblast culture)—place in culture medium or normal saline and store at $+4\,^{\circ}$C
- liver and muscle biopsies (before or after death). Freeze the liver biopsy tissue immediately on dry ice or in liquid nitrogen
- cerebral ultrasound and EEG
- echocardiography and ECG
- chest radiograph
- postmortem.

Management

General

The primary goal is to correct the biochemical derangement(s) while ensuring adequate nutrition. The production of toxic metabolites should be suppressed while encouraging their elimination by extrarenal and alternate pathways.

Supportive cure is required, and this includes mechanical ventilation, circulatory support, maintenance of good hydration, and diuresis with correction of electrolytes, correction of severe acidosis (pH <7.15), and treatment of sepsis.

Specific therapies

Peritoneal dialysis, haemodialysis, and exchange transfusion (with fresh blood) may be useful in some IMDs where the accumulation of toxic metabolites is detrimental (organic acidurias and urea cycle defects). Adequate nutrition suppresses endogenous tissue breakdown. At the earliest opportunity, enteral or total parenteral nutrition should be commenced with appropriate glucose, lipid, and amino acids and mixtures built up to provide the recommended dietary allowance (RDA).

- Insulin infusion (0.2–0.3 units/kg per h) when combined with high glucose concentration (such as 1 unit insulin per 4 g of glucose), may suppress catabolism.
- Sodium benzoate (250–500 mg/kg per day) and sodium phenylbutyrate (250–650 mg/kg per day) may be useful in urea cycle defects by enhancing nitrogen excretion as hippurate and phenylacetylglutamine, respectively.
- Arginine becomes an essential amino acid in urea cycle defects and therefore requires supplementation (at doses of 100–150 mg/kg per day) to maintain plasma concentrations of 50–200 µmol/l. Alternatively, substitute citrulline (up to 700 mg/kg per day) for arginine.
- L-Carnitine (100 mg/kg per day), orally or intravenously, is useful in organic acidaemias (propionic, isovaleric, and methylmalonic acidaemias, and 3-methylcrotonyl glycinuria), as it enhances specific acylcarnitine excretion.
- Dichloroacetate (DCA), a potent inhibitor of pyruvate dehydrogenase kinase, is useful in congenital lactic acidosis unresponsive to other therapies. All severe hyperlacticacidaemias (primary or secondary) are responsive to DCA (50 mg/kg per day).

Long-term outcome

Despite several advances in the diagnostic techniques for these disorders, the long-term outlook remains largely poor. Most patients with urea cycle defects and hyperammonaemia have a very poor outcome, most survivors being handicapped. Those known to be affected prenatally may initially do better if treated expectantly, but a favourable long-term outlook may be secured only by liver transplantation. The organic acidaemias generally have a poor outcome, and affected infants may benefit significantly only from liver transplantation or futuristic gene therapy. Isovaleric acidaemia has a better outlook than the other acidaemias, with neurodevelopmental outcome depending on early diagnosis and compliance with treatment. With early diagnosis and meticulous therapy, infants with maple syrup urine disease (MSUD) can be expected to survive long term with at times satisfactory neurodevelopmental outcomes. The excellence of long-term metabolic control and length of time after birth for which the plasma leucine levels were above 1 mmol/l directly influence intellectual outcome.

Useful website

www.ssiem.org.uk/bimdg.html
British Inherited Metabolic Disease Group and Society for the Study of Inborn Errors of Metabolism (includes the UK directory of laboratories diagnosing inborn errors of metabolism).

Further reading

Burton BK. Inborn errors of metabolism in infancy: a guide to diagnosis. *Pediatrics* (1998) **102:**E69.

Chaves-Caballo E. Detection of inherited neurometabolic disorders: a practical clinical approach. *Pediatric Clinics of North America* (1992) **39:**801.

Greene CL, Goodman SI. Inborn errors of metabolism. In: WW Hay, JR Groothuis, AR Hayward et al (eds). *Current Pediatric Diagnosis and Treatment*, 13th edn. Stamford, CT: Appleton & Lange, 1997: 864.

Hoffman GF, Nyhan WL, Zschocke J et al. *Inherited Metabolic Diseases*. Philadelphia: Lippincott, Williams & Wilkins, 2001.

Ogier de Baulny H, Saudubray JM. Emergency treatments. In: J Fernandes, JM Saudubray, G Van den Berghe (eds). *Inborn Metabolic Disease: Diagnosis and Treatment*, 2nd edn. New York: Springer-Verlag, 1995: 47–55.

Saudubray JM, Narcy C, Lyonnet L et al. Clinical approach to inherited metabolic disorders in neonates. *Biology of the Neonate* (1990) **58:**44.

Saudubray JM (ed.). Inborn errors of metabolism. *Seminars in Neonatology* (2002) **7**(1).

Related topics of interest

- acute collapse
- death of an infant
- inherited metabolic disease—recognisable patterns
- prenatal diagnosis.

Inherited metabolic disease—recognisable patterns

Several clinical signs and laboratory findings are especially valuable in diagnosing inherited metabolic diseases (IMDs). The following patterns may be recognised.

Altered neurological status

Toxic type with hypertonia and abnormal movements
Principal investigations
Urine and plasma amino acid chromatography.

Findings
Urine DNPH strongly positive, no acidosis, and minor or no acetonuria. Normal lactate, glucose, and calcium. Ammonia normal or raised.

Usual diagnoses
Maple syrup urine disease (characteristic smell).

Toxic type with dehydration
Principal investigations
Urine and plasma organic acid chromatography, plasma and urine carnitine esters, and plasma carnitine.

Findings
Moderate acetonuria and acidosis. Urine DNPH slightly positive or negative. Ammonia raised. Lactate normal or raised; glucose and calcium normal or raised. Leucopenia and thrombocytopenia.

Usual diagnosis
Ketolytic defects, organic acidurias (isovaleric acidaemia, propionic acidaemia, and methylmalonic acidaemia).

Energy-deficiency type with liver or cardiac symptoms
Principal investigations
Plasma and urine organic acids, plasma carnitine, loading or fasting test, and fatty acid oxidation studies on lymphocytes or fibroblasts.

Findings
Acidosis without acetonuria and urine DNPH negative. Lactate and ammonia raised with low/normal calcium or glucose, and normal blood count.

Usual diagnoses
Fatty acid oxidation and ketogenesis defects.

Energy-deficiency type, hypotonia, and tachypnoea
Principal investigations
Lactate/pyruvate ratios, hydroxybutyrate/acetoacetate ratio, urine organic acids, and enzyme assays (muscle, fibroblast, or lymphocytes).

Findings
Marked acidosis, acetonuria, and lacticacidaemia. Ammonia normal or raised. Normal calcium and glucose.

Usual diagnoses
Multiple carboxylase deficiency and congenital lactic acidosis (pyruvate carboxylase, pyruvate dehydrogenase, Krebs cycle, and respiratory chain).

Toxic type, hypotonia, seizures, coma, and moderate hepatocellular disturbances
Principal investigations
Plasma and urine amino acids, urine organic acids, and liver or intestinal enzyme studies (such as ornithine carbamyl transferase and carbamyl phosphate synthetase).

Findings
Alkalosis without acetonuria and DNPH negative. Ammonia raised, lactate normal or raised with normal blood glucose, calcium, and blood count.

Usual diagnoses
Urea cycle defects and fatty acid oxidation defects (glutaric aciduria type II, carnitine palmitoyltransferase II, long-chain acyl-CoA dehydrogenase, and 3-hydroxy long-chain acyl-CoA dehydrogenase).

Severe hypotonia, myoclonic jerks, and seizures
Principal investigations
Amino acid chromatography, CSF amino acids, plasma phytanic acid, and plasma very long chain fatty acids.

Findings
No acidosis, and acetonuria and DNPH negative. Ammonia, lactate, glucose, and blood count all normal.

Usual diagnoses
NKH, sulphite oxidase, xanthine oxidase, peroxisomal disorders, pyridoxine dependency, and trifunctional enzyme.

Hepatomegaly with deranged liver function

Hepatomegaly and hypoglycaemia
Principal investigations
Fasting and loading tests. Liver, fibroblast, and lymphocyte enzyme studies.

Findings
Acetonuria with acidosis. Ammonia normal, lactate raised, moderate hypoglycaemia, and normal blood count.

Typical diagnoses
Fructose diphosphatase deficiency, glycogenosis type I (Acetest negative), and glycogenosis type III (moderate acetonuria).

Hepatomegaly, jaundice, liver failure, and hepatocellular necrosis

Principal investigations

Enzyme studies to exclude galactosaemia, fructosaemia, and tyrosinaemia. Urinary organic acids.

Findings

Slight acidosis and acetonuria. Ammonia normal or raised, lactate significantly raised, and glucose normal or decreased.

Typical diagnoses

Galactosaemia, fructosaemia, tyrosinosis type I, neonatal haemochromatosis, and respiratory chain disorders.

Hepatomegaly, cholestatic jaundice, chronic diarrhoea, and failure to thrive

Principal investigations

Plasma and urine organic acids, protein electrophoresis, phytanic acid, very long-chain fatty acids, pipecolic acid, and phytanic acid.

Findings

Acidosis and ketosis are absent with normal glucose, lactate, and ammonia.

Typical diagnoses

α_1-Antitrypsin deficiency, peroxisomal disorders, and inborn errors of bile acid metabolism.

Hepatosplenomegaly, storage signs, chronic diarrhoea, and failure to thrive

Principal investigations

Enzyme studies, mucopolysaccharides, sialic acid, and oligosaccharides.

Findings

Acidosis and ketosis absent. Ammonia and glucose normal with normal or raised lactate.

Typical diagnoses

Storage disorders, gangliozide I, gangliosidosis, infantile sialic acid storage disease (sialidosis II), I-cell disease, mucopolysaccharidosis type VII, and galactosialidosis.

Useful websites

www.ssiem.org.uk/bimdg.html
British Inherited Metabolic Disease Group and Society for the Study of Inborn Errors of Metabolism (includes the UK directory of laboratories diagnosing inborn errors of metabolism).

www.emedicine.com/emerg/topic768.htm
eMedicine topic on inborn errors of metabolism. eMedicine is one of the largest and most current online clinical knowledge bases available to health professionals.

www.neonatology.com
Neonatology on the web – an extensive resource on neonatology.

Further reading

Clarke JTR. *A Clinical Guide to Inherited Metabolic Diseases*, 2dn edn. Cambridge: Cambridge University Press, 2003.

Lyon G, Adams RD, Kolodny EH. *Neurology of Hereditary Metabolic Diseases of Children*, 2nd edn. New York: McGraw-Hill, 1996.

Saudubray JM, Ogier H, Charpentier C. Clinical approach to inherited metabolic diseases. In: J Fernandes, J-M Saudubray, G Van den Berghe (eds). *Inborn Metabolic Disease: Diagnosis and Treatment*, 2nd edn. New York: Springer-Verlag, 1995: 3–39.

Saudubray JM (ed.). Inborn errors of metabolism. *Seminars in Neonatology* (2002) **7**(1).

Scriver CR, Beaudet AL, Sly WS et al (eds). *The Metabolic and Molecular Basis of Inherited Disease*, 7th edn. New York: McGraw-Hill, 1995.

Wraith JE. Inborn errors of metabolism in the neonate. In: JM Rennie, NRC Roberton (eds). *Textbook of Neonatology*, 3rd edn. Edinburgh: Churchill Livingstone, 1999: 986–1002.

Related topics of interest

- acute collapse
- death of an infant
- inherited metabolic disease—investigation and management
- prenatal diagnosis.

Intrauterine growth restriction

The provision of adequate nutrition for the growing foetus is essential for its normal development and has implications for future health and well-being during childhood and adulthood. Intrauterine growth restriction (IUGR) is largely a consequence of foetal malnutrition. It is well known that the lighter a newborn infant is at birth, the more likely it is to become ill or die. Recently, convincing evidence has accumulated linking foetal malnutrition with increased morbidity and mortality from cardiovascular disease in adulthood.

Pathophysiology

Most foetuses, including those in multiple gestations, follow similar growth curves during the first 20 weeks of pregnancy, with any slowing of growth usually occurring only in the second half of pregnancy. Where the cause is physiological (such as multiple pregnancy or inherited genetic factors), slow growth is confined to the third trimester. The more severe the pathology, the earlier foetal growth restriction becomes evident. The earliest slowing of growth (during second trimester) occurs when the foetus is inherently abnormal (as in congenital or chromosomal anomaly) or has sustained significant first trimester insult (as from intrauterine infection or drug exposure).

Recent studies have given considerable insight into the pathophysiology of IUGR. At the start of gestation, growth appears to be controlled by nutritional input and growth factors acting locally by autocrine and paracrine mechanisms. Among these, the insulin-like growth factors (IGFs, especially IGF-I) and their binding proteins (IGFBPs) appear to have a central regulatory role. Foetuses showing IUGR have low IGF-I and IGFBP-3 levels but elevated growth hormone (GH) levels. Following birth and renutrition, a rapid increase in IGF-I and a decrease in GH levels are observed. Thus, GH, though playing a role in foetal and infantile growth, appears not to be the key hormone for foetal growth. On the other hand, insulin appears to play a major role in the regulation of foetal growth, perhaps by increasing IGF-I production.

Definition

Newborn infants may be described, according to their birth weight for gestation, as appropriate for gestational age (AGA), small for gestational age (SGA), or large for gestational age (LGA). The definition of SGA varies from a birth weight below the 10th percentile to one of less than the 3rd percentile. In the UK, just over 2% of all babies may be SGA, whereas in some developing nations up to one in three newborns may be SGA and every other infant may be of low birth weight (LBW) (weighing <2.5 kg). Although the terms 'IUGR' and 'SGA' are often used interchangeably, IUGR is not strictly synonymous with SGA. Whereas SGA indicates an atypical growth pattern, IUGR implies either inhibition or restriction of a normal growth potential. Thus, healthy SGA infants whose smallness is genetically predetermined are not IUGR.

Causes of IUGR and SGA

Physiological
Foetal
- multiple pregnancy
- inherited genetic factors.

Maternal
- small stature
- young or elderly mothers.

Pathological
Foetal
- intrauterine infection
- chromosomal anomalies (2% of SGA infants)
- congenital malformation (up to 15% of SGA infants).

Maternal
- smoking
- irradiation
- undernutrition
- socioeconomic status
- uteroplacental vascular insufficiency
- drugs—therapeutic and addictive (such as cocaine)
- pregnancy-induced hypertension, pre-eclampsia, diabetes mellitus, collagen disorders, and renal disease.

SGA infants may be symmetrically or asymmetrically growth restricted. Symmetrical growth restriction suggests early onset of intrauterine growth restriction (as in chromosomal anomaly, intrauterine infection, or constitutionally small babies) producing equal reduction in brain and body size. Asymmetrically growth-restricted infants (majority of SGA infants) have relative sparing of head size and length but marked reduction in weight, with onset of growth restriction in the last few weeks of pregnancy (as in placental insufficiency, pre-eclampsia, and maternal smoking). Symmetric IUGR is associated with a less favourable prognosis than asymmetric IUGR, affecting only the weight.

Clinical correlates of SGA infants

Hypoglycaemia
Reduced glycogen liver stores, impaired gluconeogenesis, relative hyperinsulinaemia, and deficient catecholamine secretion predispose to hypoglycaemia (symptomatic and asymptomatic).

Hypothermia
SGA infants have relatively large surface area to weight ratios and less subcutaneous fat, making them more vulnerable to cold stress.

Birth asphyxia
Foetal distress is twice as common in SGA infants due to the inability to maintain anaerobic metabolism. There may be a greater risk of meconium aspiration.

Polycythaemia
Risk is increased due to the relatively hypoxic intrauterine environment of SGA infants. A haematocrit of ≥ 0.65 may be found in 50% of SGA infants. Treatment is by partial exchange transfusion with human albumin or normal saline.

Respiratory problems
Recurrent apnoea, pulmonary haemorrhage, and persistent pulmonary hypertension of the newborn may be more common. RDS is less common.

Infection
Immunity is impaired with defective cell-mediated (decreased T lymphocytes) and humoral responses (deficient IgG). Furthermore, polymorphs have reduced chemotactic mobility and bactericidal capacity.

Neurobehavioural problems
SGA infants are less active and responsive, have poor muscle tone, are jittery, and show variable feeding and sleeping patterns.

Detection of intrauterine growth restriction

Up to 90% of SGA infants may be detected by serial ultrasound measurements of the biparietal diameter (BPD), abdominal circumference (AC), and femoral lengths (FL), and by comparing ratio of BPD to AC or FL to AC.

Management of intrauterine growth restriction

Prenatal
- Advise cessation of smoking.
- Treat hypertension and pre-eclampsia.
- Obtain foetal blood samples for karyotype and acid–base status in severe IUGR.

Serial umbilical artery Doppler wave forms discriminate between foetuses at high or low risk of intrauterine/perinatal death. Absent end-diastolic flow (EDF) is associated with hypoxaemia, acidosis, and unfavourable outcome. Reversed EDF is a more ominous sign.

Postnatal
- Start feeds early and screen for asymptomatic hypoglycaemia (check four-hourly capillary glucose).
- Avoid hypothermia, monitor temperature, and provide a heated mattress if necessary.
- Treat polycythaemia with partial exchange transfusion.
- Avoid rapid increments of feeds, and use breast milk in preference (high risk of NEC).

- If oral feeds are not tolerated, provide parenteral nutrition and gradually reintroduce enteral feeds.
- Thrombocytopenia and leucocytopenia are common. Treat suspected infection early.

Long-term outcome

The postnatal growth of infants born with IUGR is characterised by a rate of growth superior to that seen in the normal infant ('catch-up growth'). This affects first the weight and then the length, and by the end of the second year, the majority have attained a normal size, while approximately 13% have not. The severity and duration of antenatal growth restriction affect later growth potential. Infants who experience prolonged antenatal growth restriction will remain small, whereas infants who experience short periods of foetal growth restriction show catch-up growth. However, approximately 8% of IUGR infants whose birth weight or length are below the 3rd percentile will have a final adult height below the 3rd percentile. Of all the possible causes of small stature at the end of adolescence, 20% are due to IUGR. Recent therapeutic trials with GH (Genotropin, Pharmacia and Upjohn) have, however, been encouraging, suggesting that a satisfactory final adult height might be achieved with GH therapy.

Severely growth-restricted infants also have an excess of serious neuromotor impairments and deficits of cognitive function (such as cerebral palsy) compared to AGA infants. For the less severely affected infants, long-term outcomes in terms of physical growth, neurodevelopmental outcome, or school performance may not differ significantly from matched peer groups, morbidity being largely determined by gestation. However, some recent UK epidemiologic studies have suggested an increased risk of death from cardiovascular disease in adult life and an adverse effect on adult cognitive performance. These studies have shown that low birth weight is a risk factor for syndrome X, also known as insulin-resistance syndrome, which includes glucose intolerance (non-insulin-dependent diabetes mellitus), hypertension, and dyslipidaemia, all risk factors for cardiovascular and cerebrovascular diseases. Although the mechanisms of these illnesses are not known, they illustrate the complex effects of foetal malnutrition on the 'programming' of illnesses in later life.

Further reading

Barker DIP. *Mothers, Babies and Health in Later Life*, 2nd edn. London: BMJ Publishing, 1998.

Barker DIP, Gluckman PD, Godfrey KM et al. Fetal nutrition and cardiovascular disease in adult life. *Lancet* (1993) **341:**938–41.

Boguszewski M, Albertsson-Wikland K, Aronsson S et al. Growth hormone treatment of short children born small-for-gestational age: the Nordic Multicentre Trial. *Acta Paediatrica* (1998) **87:**257–63.

Cowett RM, Stern L. The intrauterine growth retarded infant: etiology, prenatal diagnosis, neonatal management and long term follow-up. In: F Lifshetz (ed.). *Pediatric Endocrinology*, New York: Marcel Dekker, 1990: 93–110.

Czernichow P. Pathophysiology and consequences of intrauterine growth retardation. In: CJH Kelnar (ed.). *Baillière's Clinical Paediatrics*, Vol. 4/No. 2, *Paediatric Endocrinology*. London: Baillière Tindall, 1996: 245–57.

Eyal FG. The small-for-gestational-age preterm infant. In: FR Witter, LG Keith (eds). *Textbook of Prematurity: Antecedents, Treatment, and Outcome*. Boston: Little, Brown, 1993: 361–9.

Rodeck CH, Whittle M (eds). *Foetal Medicine: Basic Science and Clinical Practice*. Edinburgh: Churchill Livingstone, 1999.

Sorensen HT, Sabroe S, Olsen J et al. Birth weight and cognitive function in young adult life: historical cohort study. *British Medical Journal* (1997) **315**:401–3.

Related topics of interest

- blood-glucose homeostasis
- necrotising enterocolitis
- prenatal diagnosis
- polycythaemia.

Intubation

Infants are most frequently intubated in the perinatal period, the primary indication being respiratory failure secondary to prematurity. Other infants requiring intubation have either failed to respond to the other means of resuscitation, including bag and mask ventilation, or are electively intubated for other reasons. Thus, the procedure is done either electively or as an immediate and urgent response to the clinical condition of the infant. It is desirable for the procedure to be done calmly, a condition which is aided by the assurance of assistance being readily available from a senior colleague if required. Practitioners who are new to the discipline should be supervised by senior colleagues until they have acquired sufficient skills and confidence to undertake the procedure independently.

Indications

- prematurity ($\leq$28 weeks' gestation)
- failure to respond to bag and mask or T-piece ventilation
- respiratory distress with abnormal blood gases and an oxygen requirement (F_iO_2 $\geq$0.60)
- poor respiratory drive with recurrent apnoea (and bradycardia) and/or respiratory arrest
- planned elective intubation as for surgery.

Premedication

For nonurgent intubations such as elective intubation for surgery, it is appropriate and desirable to provide analgesia (such as morphine 100 µg/kg) and/or muscle relaxation (such as suxamethonium 2 mg/kg IV with atropine 15 µg/kg i.m./IV) just prior to intubation. This reduces the infant's stress response to the procedure and may make the procedure easier, as the infant will not be struggling. It is not necessary to paralyse the infant first; this is risky if intubation fails.

Procedure

Use a laryngoscope with a short blade, especially for the small preterm infant. Suction the oropharynx to clear the view. Partially extend the neck. Introduce the laryngoscope from the right side of the mouth and gradually tilt and lift the blade anteriorly but *without* resting the blade on the lower gum (that traumatises the lower gum). Gently withdraw the laryngoscope until the epiglottis flips into view. The vocal cords then immediately come into view just below the epiglottis; this may be aided by light cricoid pressure. Introduce the endotracheal (ET) tube through the open cords (without forcing) and then adjust the position of the tube (depth of insertion down the trachea) by checking that air entry is equal on both sides. Secure the ET if artificial ventilation is to be maintained.

Common problems

Infant not responsive to artificial ventilation

- ET tube may have been misplaced or dislodged.
- Lung inflation pressure may be too low—increase by 5–10 cm of water.
- Gas flow (or oxygen) is turned off!
- A tension pneumothorax may be present (unilateral or bilateral). Transilluminate and, if necessary, needle the chest.

Partial improvement followed by rapid deterioration

- ET tube is blocked (as by meconium, blood, and thick secretions)—replace ET tube.
- Acute pneumothorax—transilluminate and aspirate affected side.
- ET tube is dislodged.

Failed intubation

Do not persist unnecessarily long if the initial intubation is unsuccessful! Discontinue the attempt if still unsuccessful after 2 min. Reoxygenate the infant by bag and mask or T-piece ventilation. If still unsuccessful after two further attempts, let someone else try (do not be too proud to ask for help). Note, however, that infants can be effectively ventilated by bag and mask (or T-piece) for prolonged periods of time until assistance arrives. However, infants may be traumatised and subjected to repeated hypoxic insults by repeated failed intubation attempts.

Common causes of failed intubation

- inexperience
- neck overextension
- ET tube inappropriately large
- inadequate visualisation of airway—notwithstanding your experience, most 'blind' intubations fail!
- rarely—unusual anatomy or congenital malformations.

Complications

- pulmonary haemorrhage
- pharyngeal tears from laryngoscope
- tracheal, laryngeal, and mediastinal perforating injuries
- penetrating injuries of the brain from attempted nasal intubation
- pneumothorax, especially right-sided (selective intubation of right main bronchus)
- trauma to alveolar margin by laryngoscope (resting and rotating laryngoscope on gum)
- vocal cord trauma (forcing ET tube plus introducer through closed cords or using inappropriately large ET tube)
- marked abdominal distension from excessive mask bagging and/or oesophageal intubation.

Further reading

Angelos GM, Smith DR, Jorgenson R et al. Oral complications associated with neonatal oral tracheal intubation: a critical review. *Paediatric Dentistry* (1989) **11:**133–40.

Black AE, Hatch DE, Nauth-Misir N. Complications of nasotracheal intubation in neonates, infants and children: a review of 4 years experience in a children's hospital. *British Journal of Anaesthesia* (1990) **65:**461–7.

Cameron D, Lupton BA. Inadvertent brain penetration during neonatal nasotracheal intubation. *Archives of Disease in Childhood* (1993) **69:**79–80.

Macdonald M, Ramsethu J. *Atlas of Procedures in Neonatology*, 3rd edn. Philadelphia: Lippincott, Williams & Wilkins, 2002.

Rawlings DJ, Lawrence S, Goldstein JD. Acquired tracheoesophageal fistula in a premature infant. *American Journal of Perinatology* (1993) **10:**164–7.

Shukla HK, Hendricks-Munoz KD, Atakent Y et al. Rapid estimation of insertional length of endotracheal intubation in newborn infants. *Journal of Pediatrics* (1997) **131:**561–4.

Sutherland PD, Quinn M. Nellcor Stat Cap differentiates oesophageal from tracheal intubation. *Archives of Disease in Childhood Fetal and Neonatal Edition* (1995) **73:**F184–6.

Ziegler JW, Todres ID. Intubation of newborns. *American Journal of Diseases in Childhood* (1992) **146:**147–9.

Related topics of interest

- acute collapse
- complications of mechanical ventilation
- mechanical ventilation
- respiratory distress
- resuscitation.

Jaundice

All neonates have a transient rise in bilirubin, and some 30–50% become visibly jaundiced. Preterm and term infants become jaundiced for similar reasons as follows:

- increased bilirubin load on the liver due to a high red cell mass, the shorter survival of the neonatal erythrocyte, and the increased intestinal reabsorption of bilirubin (the enterohepatic circulation)
- decreased hepatic uptake of bilirubin from the circulation
- impaired bilirubin conjugation.

The bilirubin excretory pathway is therefore both overloaded and operationally inefficient, leading to a transient unconjugated hyperbilirubinaemia that peaks around day three, fades rapidly over the next three days, and clears by days 10–14. Hyperbilirubinaemia is more pronounced and almost universal in preterm infants, as a result of hepatic and gastrointestinal immaturity. The delayed initiation of enteral feeds in sick preterm infants (which further enhances the enterohepatic circulation) and the slower maturation of hepatic bilirubin uptake and conjugation contribute to the greater magnitude and duration of jaundice in these infants.

Jaundice in neonates is considered as either physiological or pathological. *Physiological* jaundice is the consequence of transient immaturity and the inefficiency of the bilirubin conjugation and excretory pathways. Prematurity, bruising, polycythaemia, breast-feeding, and other factors can increase physiological jaundice (sometimes to the point of needing treatment). Jaundice is *pathological* and important if:

- It is in the first 24 h of life—haemolysis until proven otherwise.
- It is associated with another illness.
- The bilirubin concentration is above the normal range.
- It has become prolonged (>10 days at term; >14 days in preterm infants).

Term infants

The 97th percentile for bilirubin concentration in the first few days of life in the well, breast-fed term baby is approximately 250 μmol/l, and it is 210 μmol/l in the formula-fed baby. These thresholds of concentration and time may therefore be taken as levels above which jaundice should be investigated for potentially pathological causes. They are not thresholds for initiating treatment, nor are they thresholds below which pathological causes for jaundice are absent. Vigilance is always needed.

Investigations

In the well term infant who clinically looks jaundiced enough to need treatment, the following are required:

- serum bilirubin concentration
- blood group and Coombs' test.

Further tests are not indicated unless the need for treatment is confirmed by a high bilirubin concentration without evidence of haemolytic disease. Tests on treated infants should include:

- urine culture
- urine reducing sugars (to exclude galactosuria, which tests positive on Clinitest, but negative on Clinistix)
- further estimates of total bilirubin concentration
- liver-function tests and conjugated/unconjugated bilirubin assays that may be needed to exclude cholestasis, especially if the jaundice is prolonged.

Some specific hepatic causes of jaundice are discussed under 'Liver disorders'. World-wide, glucose-6-phosphate dehydrogenase (G6PD) deficiency is the most important cause of jaundice, especially in Southeast Asian and African countries. In the UK, it is justifiable to screen jaundiced male infants who are of an ethnic origin that has a high prevalence of G6PD deficiency.

Management

The literature on bilirubin-induced brain injury in both term and preterm infants is both complex and voluminous, suggesting that no simple relationship exists between peak serum bilirubin levels and later adverse neurodevelopmental outcome. However, there is unequivocal evidence of the neuropathological damage (kernicterus) that severe hyperbilirubinaemia can cause. Kernicterus is a pathological diagnosis characterised by macroscopic yellow staining of specific subcortical nuclei and brainstem cranial nuclei, with microscopic evidence of neuronal damage in those nuclei. The long-term neuro-logical sequelae of this include deafness and choreoathetoid CP. The aim of treating hyperbilirubinaemia is therefore to prevent bilirubin-related neurodevelopmental hand-icap while avoiding harm. The cornerstones of hyperbilirubinaemia management are phototherapy and exchange transfusion. Experts differ on what constitutes 'appropriate guidelines' for these two interventions, and no 'evidence-based guidelines' exist.

Generally, if the baby is well and is feeding well, and the concentration of bilirubin is below the treatment level, no further action should be taken unless the jaundice deepens or becomes prolonged. If the bilirubin concentration is above the treatment threshold and likely to rise to a point where kernicterus is a risk, phototherapy is needed (see Table 1). Untreated severe hyperbilirubinaemia can cause fits, opisthotonos, and, indeed, death in the neonate.

There is continuing debate about the threshold above which kernicterus is likely to occur. Recent work suggests that in well term infants without haemolytic disease (including G6PD deficiency) it is higher than originally thought. The term 'vigintipho-bia' (fear of the figure 20) was coined to reflect paediatricians' fear of the total biliru-bin concentration rising above 20 mg/dl (340 μmol/l) lest kernicterus should ensue. Now, a gentler approach to jaundice is used, and kernicterus is considered to be a significant risk only above a bilirubin concentration of 450 μmol/l in this group of infants. The setting of this value also sets the level (450 μmol/l) at which exchange transfusion to prevent kernicterus is mandatory. In turn, phototherapy is started when the bilirubin concentration is 100 μmol/l below this exchange line. In well term infants, therefore, phototherapy is started at bilirubin concentrations as low as 80 μmol/l on day one, rising to 350 μmol/l on day three and later.

Neither phototherapy nor exchange transfusion is harmless, and they should be initiated only if necessary. There is, however, a greater risk of kernicterus at lower concentrations of bilirubin if the baby is preterm, has haemolytic disease, G6PD deficiency, hypoalbuminaemia, or acidosis, or is receiving any drugs that may displace bilirubin from the albumin-binding sites. The thresholds for action have therefore to be reduced accordingly.

Preterm infants

There are insufficient coherent data on jaundice in preterm infants below 35 weeks' gestation to develop scientific evidence-based guidelines about phototherapy. Table 1 contains some published recommendations and some extrapolations from them. A few observations should be noted. Despite the near universal finding of clinical jaundice in VLBW infants, kernicterus has virtually disappeared in this group of infants. It has been suggested that this might be as a consequence of the general improvements in neonatal intensive care or the increased readiness to use phototherapy. However, a report (published in 2001) of kernicterus in two infants at 31 weeks' (serum bilirubin 224 μmol/l) and 34 weeks' gestation (serum bilirubin 251 μmol/l), neither of whom was ill, have once more raised concerns about what levels of bilirubin are safe in preterm infants.

Phototherapy

From its introduction by Cremer and colleagues (Rochford General Hospital in Essex, UK, 1958), phototherapy has evolved into a widely accepted and highly effective medical therapy for jaundice to such a degree that even senior trainees in neonatology are now increasingly unsure as to how to perform an exchange transfusion safely. The greatest impact of phototherapy has been in VLBW infants, where it has made exchange transfusions virtually obsolete. There have been several recent developments in phototherapy technology. Some fibre-optic phototherapy systems ('bili-blankets') are now as effective as conventional phototherapy, and infants need not have their eyes covered (when the bili-blanket is wrapped around the baby). The efficacy of phototherapy is related to the surface area of the infant exposed to the phototherapy lights. This may readily be increased by placing an infant on a fibre-optic pad with a bank of conventional free-standing phototherapy units above and around the infant. The spectral radiance may be greatly increased by reducing the distance

Table 1 Guidelines for initiating phototherapy for jaundice.

	Postnatal age and bilirubin level (μmol/l) for phototherapy			
Gestation	<1 day	1–2 days	2–3 days	>3 days
≤27 weeks or <1000 g	85	100	100–150	150–175
28–32 weeks	85–120	100–150	125–175	175
32–35 weeks	100–150	150–200	220	220
≥37 weeks	85–170	170–260	260–350	>350

between the light source and the infant (but not too close to cause burns!). Lining the sides of the incubator with reflecting aluminium foil may further enhance the efficacy of phototherapy and avoid the need for an exchange transfusion. The most effective light source currently available is provided by special blue fluorescent tubes, which provide light mainly in the blue-green spectrum (which best penetrates the skin and is maximally absorbed by bilirubin). These should be used when bilirubin levels are approaching exchange levels. However, provided the bilirubin level is controlled by phototherapy, it is reasonable for phototherapy to be interrupted for feeds and parental visits. Finally, the bilirubin isomer, lumirubin, is excreted in bile and urine, so adequate hydration is important. It is not essential, however, to provide additional 'phototherapy fluids' as long as the infant is not subjected to heat stress and the skin temperature is kept constant (by servo-control).

Complications of phototherapy
- purpuric bullous eruptions (rare)
- diarrhoea from a decreased gut transit time
- hypothermia (naked infant in a cool environment)
- heat stress (increased fluid loss) and skin burns
- bronze baby syndrome (with conjugated hyperbilirubinaemia).

Exchange transfusion

When hyperbilirubinaemia cannot be controlled by phototherapy alone, an exchange transfusion is required in order to protect the infant from the permanent neurodevelopmental sequelae which characterise kernicterus. This is the only option available for an infant requiring an urgent reduction in serum bilirubin that is at toxic levels. It is the preferred therapy in severe haemolytic anaemia, as it corrects the anaemia and removes the excess bilirubin. Commonly, a double volume exchange is undertaken; that is, a calculated blood volume equal to twice the infant's blood volume is exchanged. This volume is calculated quite simply as: volume = infant's weight (kg) × 85 ml × 2 (or 170 ml/kg). When performing an exchange transfusion in sick (especially preterm) infants, fresh CMV-negative blood (<48 h old), cross-matched against the mother should be used. Older blood is less appropriate, as it is hyperosmolar, hypernatraemic, hypocalcaemic, and more acidic. It also has lower 2:3 diphosphoglycerate levels.

Exchange procedure
- Small aliquots of blood (5–10 ml or smaller still in the ill/preterm infant) may be gradually withdrawn (over 5 min) through a large central vein (such as the umbilical vein) and replaced (over 3–5 min) with equal amounts of fresh blood until the required volume has been exchanged.
- Alternatively, blood may be continuously removed from a large artery (or the umbilical vein) and replaced by a continuous infusion of fresh blood into a secure peripheral vein (to avoid the damaging consequences of blood extravasation into the surrounding tissues).
- Commence by withdrawing a blood sample for FBC, U and E, calcium, glucose, bilirubin, and blood gas, and repeat these investigations at the end of the procedure.

- Accurately record the blood volumes removed and replaced; the procedure should not be rushed, taking 2–4 h overall.
- Observe the infant closely while monitoring BP, gases, and the ECG continuously.

Complications of exchange transfusion
- NEC
- infection
- acidaemia
- hypoglycaemia
- cardiac arrhythmias
- hypocalcaemia (due to citrate in banked blood)—monitor ECG continuously
- hyperkalaemia (potassium rises by 0.5 mmol/day in CPDA preserved blood)
- catheter related complications (thromboembolic events, haemorrhage, and thrombocytopenia)
- haemodynamic complications (rapid shifts in blood volume may produce cardio-respiratory instability)
- death.

Prolonged jaundice

Jaundice is prolonged if it lasts over ten days in the term infant and over 14 days in the preterm. The most common cause for this is breast-milk jaundice in a well and thriving infant who has unconjugated hyperbilirubinaemia secondary to increased enterohepatic circulation. Unfortunately, there is no specific 'test' for this, and it is always a diagnosis of exclusion after other, more sinister diagnoses, including biliary atresia, are ruled out.

Investigations
Investigation starts with the question: is the hyperbilirubinaemia unconjugated or conjugated? If it is *unconjugated*, first check:

- liver function
- thyroid function
- urine culture
- haemoglobin and red cell morphology.

If these are negative and the baby is well, thriving, and breast-fed, it is safe to watch for a further 2–3 weeks, during which time the jaundice should fade and the baby remain well. If this does not happen, then more extensive investigations into the causes of haemolysis, repeat liver-function tests, and specific conditions such as Gilbert's syndrome and the Crigler–Najjar syndrome should be performed.

If the hyperbilirubinaemia is *conjugated*, it is pathological. There is then a need for prompt diagnosis, and referral to a specialist hepatology centre at the outset is often the best way to achieve this. The necessary investigations and the important diagnoses to be considered are covered in the topic 'Liver disorders'.

Further reading

Ives NK. Neonatal jaundice. In: JM Rennie, NRC Roberton (eds). *Textbook of Neonatology*, 3rd edn. Edinburgh: Churchill Livingstone, 1999: 715–32.

Maisels MJ, Newman TB. Jaundice in full-term and near-term infants who leave the hospital within 36 hours: the pediatrician's nemesis. *Clinics in Perinatology* (1998) **25:**295–302.

Maisels MJ, Watchko JF (eds). *Neonatal Jaundice*. London: Harwood, 2000.

Maisels MJ, Watchko JF. Treatment of jaundice in low birthweight infants. *Archives of Disease in Childhood Fetal and Neonatal Edition* (2003) **88:**F459–63.

Modi N. Jaundice. In: D Harvey, RWI Cooke, GA Levitt (eds). *The Baby Under 1000 g*. London: Reed, 1999: 101–12.

Seidman DS, Gale R, Stevenson DK. What should we do about jaundice? In: TN Hansen, N McIntosh (eds). *Current Topics in Neonatology*, No. 2. London: WB Saunders, 1997: 125–41.

Volpe JJ. Bilirubin and brain injury. In: *Neurology of the Newborn*, 3rd edn. Philadelphia: WB Saunders, 1995: 490–513.

Watchko JF, Oski FA. Bilirubin = 20 mg/dl = vigintiphobia. *Pediatrics* 1983: **71:**660–3.

Related topics of interest

- breast-feeding
- infants of diabetic mothers
- liver disorders
- polycythaemia
- postnatal examination.

Jitteriness

Jitteriness is a fine rhythmic 5–6-Hz tremor of the arms and legs. It is the most common involuntary movement in newborn babies. In the majority of jittery babies, there is no associated pathology.

Aetiology

- idiopathic
- prematurity
- hypoglycaemia
- hypocalcaemia
- drug withdrawal
- infants of diabetic mothers
- intrauterine growth restriction.

Differential diagnosis

The challenge is to distinguish 'jitters' from fits. The main feature is that jitteriness stops when the limb is held or gently restrained, whereas fits continue. Moreover, there are no abnormal eye movements, and 'jitters' can be provoked by stretching and then releasing a limb, in contrast to the spontaneous onset of fits.

Management

Hypoglycaemia and hypocalcaemia must be excluded or treated if necessary. While hypocalcaemia is benign, the jitteriness of hypoglycaemia may be the herald of a more profound hypoglycaemia with more severe symptoms. Jitteriness as part of a drug-withdrawal syndrome in a neonate occurs after marijuana, caffeine, and opiate drug withdrawal, and has also been reported in infants of mothers on selective serotonin reuptake inhibitors. In these situations, the overall state of the baby determines therapy, rather than any one sign. Jitteriness in other babies is thought to be due to an immaturity of the nervous system, probably a lack of myelination. Up to 44% of well term babies were observed to be jittery in one series. For these babies, no treatment is needed. Jitteriness can continue into infancy, and again is benign.

Further reading

Avery GB, Fletcher MA, MacDonald M. *Neonatology: Pathophysiology and Management of the Newborn*, 5th edn. Philadelphia: Lippincott Williams & Wilkins, 1999.

Fanaroff AA, Martin RJ (eds). *Neonatal-Perinatal Medicine: Disease of the Fetus and Infant,* 7th edn. St Louis, MO: Mosby, 2002.

Parker S, Zuckerman B, Baucher H et al. Jitteriness in full-term neonates: prevalence and correlates. Pediatrics (1990) **85:**17–23.

Polin RA, Fox WW, Abman SH (eds). *Fetal and Neonatal Physiology*, 3rd edn. Philadelphia: WB Saunders, 2004.

Related topics of interest

- intrauterine growth restriction
- maternal drug abuse
- postnatal examination
- seizures.

Liver disorders

Liver disorders commonly present with jaundice, abnormal liver function tests, hepatomegaly, or coagulopathy; less commonly, they present as part of a metabolic disorder or are discovered in the context of other investigations. While the individual disorders may be quite rare, as a group, these disorders are fairly common. However, the complete evaluation of some of these disorders can be technically difficult, and early referral to a specialist paediatric liver hepatology centre is desirable when the diagnosis remains uncertain after a detailed history and examination complemented by the appropriate laboratory investigations.

Neonatal hepatitis syndrome (NHS)

Any infant with conjugated hyperbilirubinaemia has NHS, which is defined as a state in the newborn period where, as a result of decreased bile flow, there is accumulation of substances in the liver, blood, and extrahepatic tissues that would normally be excreted in bile. The terms 'neonatal hepatitis' and 'neonatal cholestasis' are less accurate. Conjugated hyperbilirubinaemia, dark urine, and pale stools are pathognomic of NHS and require a methodological and comprehensive diagnostic investigation. There is a broad spectrum of causative disease processes, with the most important differential diagnosis being biliary atresia (BA), which ideally requires surgery to be performed before the infant is 60 days old.

Causes of NHS

Infection
- TORCH infections
- human herpesvirus-6, varicella-zoster
- HIV, hepatitis B
- enteric viral sepsis (echovirus, adenovirus, and coxsackie virus)
- parvovirus B19
- bacterial infection (extrahepatic), including listerosis and tuberculosis.

Structural
- BA
- gallstones
- Caroli's disease
- Alagille's syndrome
- choledochal cyst
- neonatal sclerosing cholangitis
- spontaneous biliary perforation.

Metabolic
- galactosaemia
- cystic fibrosis
- tyrosinaemia
- hypopituitarism
- hypothyroidism

- Gaucher's disease
- Wolman's disease
- Rotor's syndrome
- Dubin–Johnson syndrome
- α-1-antitrypsin deficiency
- neonatal haemochromatosis
- peroxisomal disorders (such as Zellweger syndrome)
- progressive familial intrahepatic cholestasis (types 1, 2, and 3).

Genetic
- trisomies 13, 18, and 21
- Turner's syndrome
- cat-eye syndrome.

Toxic
- drug-induced
- TPN-associated
- foetal alcohol syndrome.

Immune
- insipated bile syndrome
- neonatal lupus erythematosus.

Vascular
- neonatal asphyxia
- Budd–Chiari syndrome
- congestive heart failure.

Neoplasia
- neuroblastoma
- hepatoblastoma
- erythrophagocytic lymphohistiocytosis.

Miscellaneous/idiopathic
ARC syndrome (arthrogryposis, renal tubular dysfunction, and cholestasis).

Investigations in NHS
First-line
- FBC
- plasma glucose, and U and E
- thyroid function tests
- urine culture and reducing substances
- liver function tests (including total and unconjugated bilirubin, AST, ALT, and γGT)
- prothrombin time (if abnormal, give 1 mg vitamin K IV; if not corrected by 6 h, liver failure may be involved—discuss with liver unit).

Second-line
- cortisol
- iron and ferritin

- immunoreactive trypsin
- cholesterol and triglycerides
- α-1-antitrypsin level and phenotype
- galactose-1-phosphate uridyl transferase
- fasting glucose, lactate, and amino acids
- urinary amino acids, organic acids, and protein/creatinine ratio
- karyotype (with dysmorphic features)
- abdominal ultrasound (after 4-h fast)
- hepatobiliary scan (pretreatment with phenobarbital 5 mg/kg per day for three days improves resolution)
- liver biopsy (plus immunostaining, histochemistry, electron microscopy, and biochemical assays).

General management of NHS

This should aim to provide definitive treatment and, where that is not possible, supportive therapy.

- Some inborn errors of carbohydrate and amino acid metabolism require special diets (such as galactose-free diet in galactosaemia).
- Aggressive nutritional support may be required to provide 120–150% of the estimated average requirements, with a higher proportion of fat as medium chain triglyceride (MCT).
- Large doses of oral fat-soluble vitamins (A, D, E, and K) are required on a daily basis.
- Ursodeoxycholic acid (UDCA) improves pruritis and biochemical measures of cholestasis.
- Severe pruritis may be treated with rifampicin, colestyramine, or UDCA.
- Where a structural cause is evident, surgery is required to relieve the obstruction (such as choledochal cyst or BA).
- Orthotopic liver transplantation may be the final option for progressive severe infantile liver disease.

Specific disorders

Biliary atresia

In BA, all or part of the extrahepatic biliary ducts are obliterated, leading to complete biliary obstruction. BA occurs worldwide with the highest incidence in French Polynesia. The incidence in the UK and Ireland is 1:16 700 live births. The cause of BA is unknown, but two forms are recognised: an 'early' or syndromic type (10–20% of all cases) and a 'late' or nonsyndromic type. Infants with early BA have additional abnormalities (such as cardiac defects). In 'late' BA, the biliary system is normal but appears to have become involved in a fibrosing process towards the end of pregnancy or shortly after birth. Children are usually born after a normal pregnancy and show normal early growth. Pigmented stools may be passed during the first week of life before stools become acholic. Hepatomegaly is present. BA should be recognised and treated before the age of 60 days. No single preoperative investigation is completely reliable. Investigations show conjugated hyperbilirubinaemia, raised γGT, and normal clotting (unless vitamin K malabsorption is present), and ultrasound after a

4-h fast shows a small or absent gall bladder with an irregular wall (normal gall bladder does not exclude BA). Percutaneous needle liver biopsy is vital, as is radionuclide hepatobiliary imaging using technetium-99m iminodiacetic acid (IDA), which fails to show bile excretion into the bowel in BA. Pretreatment with phenobarbital (5 mg/kg per day) and a 24-h scan enhance the accuracy of the test. Magnetic resonance cholangiography, endoscopic retrograde cholangiography, and laparoscopy or minilaparotomy and cholangiography may all be required to exclude BA. α-1-Antitrypsin deficiency must be excluded before surgery. The definitive treatment is the Kasai portoenterostomy (after Morio Kasai, a Japanese surgeon), in which the obliterated extrahepatic tissue is removed and a Roux loop of jejunum anastomosed to the hepatic hilum. Outcome is related to centre experience, and age at surgery is not important until 60–80 days, when the likelihood of success falls with time especially after 100 days. In the UK, after a successful Kasai, 74% of children are alive with their native liver after seven years. Liver transplantation is required when end-stage liver disease develops. The five-year survival for the combination of Kasai portoenterostomy and liver transplantation is 90%.

α-1-Antitrypsin deficiency

α-1-Antitrypsin deficiency (A1ATD) is the commonest inherited (autosomal recessive) cause of NHS. The protease inhibitor α-1-antitrypsin produced mainly in the liver inactivates leucocyte elastase, thereby inhibiting destructive proteases. A1ATD is caused by mutations in the α-1-antitrypsin genes on chromosome 14. The normal phenotype is the so-called PIMM, which is present in 95% of the northern European population. The Z mutation is present in 2–3% of individuals, and only 1:2000–3000 are born with PIZZ associated with neonatal liver disease and adult emphysema. However, only 15% of PIZZ infants ever develop liver disease (mostly NHS), though some present with late haemorrhagic disease of the newborn. Cholestasis may be severe, with acholic stools, and a nondraining hepatobiliary scan, thus mimicking BA. In most, the liver disease eventually resolves. Clinical diagnosis depends on finding low serum levels of α-1-antitrypsin (which may not be found due to hepatic inflammation), identifying the allelic variant of α-1-antitrypsin (by isoelectric focusing), or identifying a specific gene defect by PCR. The prognosis is usually good, especially in infants in whom jaundice resolves by the age of six months, but those with prolonged jaundice have progressive liver disease. Overall, half do well; of these, half (that is, 25% of the total) are entirely normal, and the other half have mildly deranged liver-function tests, no jaundice, and hepato- or splenomegaly. The other half develop chronic liver disease with cirrhosis or die in the first year of life unless liver transplantation is carried out. Medical therapy entails aggressive nutritional support.

Galactosaemia

The incidence of galactosaemia is 1:50 000, and clinical features include vomiting, diarrhoea, jaundice, malnutrition, and poor weight gain. 'Oil-drop' cataracts are typical, and some present with septicaemia. Diagnosis is confirmed by measuring erythrocyte galactose-1-phosphate uridyl transferase (before infant receives blood transfusions). Testing urine (Clinitest) may be misleading (reducing substances may be present in other severe liver disorders). When galactosaemia is suspected, stop all feeds and commence IV glucose. If confirmed, galactose should be excluded from the diet for life. Liver disease improves, but neurodevelopmental problems may develop despite adherence to a special diet.

Multifactorial cholestasis in premature infants
Although BA may occur in preterm infants, NHS is more commonly due to other liver disorders in preterm infants whose enteral feeds have been interrupted and replaced with TPN, and who have been exposed to sepsis, hypoxia, and multiple drug therapy. Initial investigations for cholestasis should aim to exclude metabolic and other conditions contributing to NHS. Liver biopsy is deferred until the infants are term and weigh over 2 kg unless stools are acholic, there is biliary dilation, there is a nonexcreting hepatobiliary scan, or NHS persists beyond the corrected age of three months. Infants on TPN should receive some trophic enteral feeds, and TPN should be discontinued at the earliest opportunity. UDCA and fat-soluble vitamins (A, D, E, and K) should be used until jaundice resolves.

Specific disorders of bile metabolism

Two steps in the conversion of unconjugated bilirubin to a conjugated, water-soluble form involve uridine diphosphate glucuronyl transferase (UDPGT), which converts bilirubin to bilirubin monoglucuronide and is also capable of converting that to the diglucuronide. Bilirubin monoglucuronide dismutase catalyses the conversion to the diglucuronide.

Syndromes with UDPGT deficiency
Crigler–Najjar syndrome (type 1)
- autosomal recessive
- complete absence of hepatic glucuronyl transferase
- persistent unconjugated hyperbilirubinaemia, usually >340 µmol/l
- kernicterus in infancy
- death in infancy, some surviving to adulthood then developing kernicterus
- treatment—phototherapy
- transplantation—prior to neurological complications
- phenobarbital without effect.

Crigler–Najjar syndrome (type 2)
- autosomal recessive/dominant with variable penetrance
- less severe, persistent unconjugated hyperbilirubinaemia
- treatment with enzyme-inducing phenobarbital and phototherapy reduces bilirubin levels
- neurological problems unusual.

Gilbert's syndrome
- autosomal dominant
- affects 5% of the population
- benign, mild, chronic unconjugated hyperbilirubinaemia
- bilirubin clearance about one-third of normal
- impaired UDPGT activity and impaired hepatic uptake
- 50% of cases have reduced red cell survival

- bilirubin rises with fasting, exercise, and intercurrent illnesses
- rarely recognised before puberty
- phenobarbital reduces jaundice.

Dubin–Johnson syndrome
- autosomal recessive
- caused by mutation in MRP2 gene which encodes bile canalicular membrane transporter for anion conjugates
- chronic conjugated hyperbilirubinaemia
- jaundice may be seen after birth, but may not appear until fourth decade
- diagnosis is by exclusion of other causes of conjugated hyperbilirubinaemia and by typical liver biopsy appearance of deposition of melanin-like pigment
- no treatment necessary.

Rotor's syndrome
- autosomal recessive
- predominantly conjugated hyperbilirubinaemia
- benign.

Useful website

www.childliverdisease.org
Children's Liver Disease Foundation.

Further reading

Kelly DA (ed.). *Diseases of the Liver and Biliary System in Children*. Oxford: Blackwell Science, 1999.
McKiernan PJ. Neonatal cholestasis. *Seminars in Neonatology* (2002) **7:**153–65.
Mowat AP. *Liver Disorders in Childhood*. Oxford: Butterworth-Heinemann, 1998.
Roberts EA. Neonatal hepatitis syndrome. *Seminars in Neonatology* (2003) **8:**357–74.
Stringer MD. Disorders of the neonatal liver and bile ducts. *Seminars in Neonatology* (2003) **8**(5).

Related topics of interest

- jaundice
- hepatitis B and C
- inherited metabolic disease—investigation and management.

Maternal drug abuse

Drug addiction during pregnancy has deleterious effects on the mother, her foetus, her immediate family, and the rest of society. A high proportion of drug-abusing women are in relationships with men who also abuse drugs, with up to two-thirds having been subjected to physical and sexual abuse. Mental health problems are frequent among drug-abusing individuals. Self-care and diet therefore tend to be neglected, with consequential foetal compromise.

Drug abuse is on the increase, particularly in the developed nations, though prevalence rates vary widely, being highest (up to 15%) in inner-city areas. It is not confined only to women of low socioeconomic status but occurs in all social groups regardless of income level or ethnic/racial identity. Mood-altering drugs are often used along with alcohol, with a tendency for the younger age group (under 30s) to use two or more drugs. Of the infants diagnosed as having AIDS in the UK in 1996, outside London, approximately three-quarters of the mothers or their partners contracted HIV infection through intravenous drug abuse.

Indicators of possible drug abuse in pregnancy

Medical
- self-admission of use
- stillbirth or birth of infant with anomalies
- sporadic or no prenatal care before delivery
- preterm labour and delivery or abruptio placentae.

Social
- imprisonment
- family violence
- past drug or alcohol abuse
- a disruptive or dysfunctional lifestyle
- removal of other children from the home
- frequent changes of residence or employment.

Commonly abused drugs

- heroin
- codeine
- cannabis
- marijuana
- barbiturates
- amphetamines
- benzodiazepines
- alcohol (foetal alcohol syndrome)
- cocaine (microcephaly and cardiac malformations).

Management during pregnancy

Encourage mother to enter an alcohol and drug treatment programme, often in conjunction with a psychiatrist specialising in drug and substance abuse. Mothers addicted to narcotics may be switched to methadone (for decreased risk of infection and better antenatal care), from which they can be gradually weaned. Methadone, however, has more prolonged and severe withdrawal effects.

Mothers should be screened for possible hepatitis B, hepatitis C, and HIV infection after appropriate counselling. Social Services should be involved with the appointment of a key worker with arrangements for long-term follow-up.

Neonatal presentation of maternal drug abuse

Most infants will present with symptoms of drug withdrawal, the neonatal abstinence syndrome (NAS). These are not drug specific, but the timing of withdrawal symptoms is characteristic of some drugs. Opiate withdrawal (such as heroin) has a rapid onset (maximum intensity on days 2–4 and fading by days 10–14), whereas methadone withdrawal persists over weeks or months. NAS symptoms may resolve within a few days or persist for several weeks, while the growth impairment and neurobehavioural effects may last for several months. Between 30% and 80% of infants exposed to opiates in utero require treatment for NAS.

Symptoms of NAS

Central nervous system
- irritability
- restlessness
- tremulousness
- high-pitched cry
- hyperactivity (with rub marks)
- photophobia
- hyperacusis
- hypertonus
- yawning
- seizures.

Respiratory system
- sneezing
- tachypnoea
- hiccups
- stuffy nose
- apnoea
- rhinorrhoea
- respiratory distress.

Gastrointestinal system
- vomiting
- diarrhoea
- salivation
- poor feeding (especially after methadone and diazepam)
- poor weight gain.

Management of the infant

Acute
Nurse in quiet environment.

- Aim to promote normal sleep patterns.
- Firm wrapping reduces irritability and hyperactivity.
- Monitor blood glucose, especially in low-birth-weight infants with feeding difficulties.
- For severe irritability with feeding difficulties, give chlopromazine (1–3 mg/kg per day at 3–6-hourly intervals) or phenobarbital (equally effective), titrating against symptoms. Prophylactic therapy is not appropriate—only treat if symptomatic.
- Treat seizures with opioids (morphine, methadone, or diamorphine), phenobarbital, phenytoin, clonazepam, or paraldehyde.
- Opioids are the most effective treatment in controlling acute neonatal opiate withdrawal. The oral doses are morphine 0.5–0.75 mg/kg per dose six-hourly (wean by 0.5 mg/dose every two days), methadone 0.1 mg/kg per dose six-hourly (increasing by 0.05 mg/kg per dose if symptoms are not controlled, and decreasing the dose slowly by 10–20% daily once control is achieved).
- Many infants with NAS have been exposed to multiple drugs in utero, and these may be treated with phenobarbital, although a combination of agents (such as phenobarbital with diluted tincture of opium) may be more effective.
- Taper drug therapy gradually (over weeks to months).
- The use of 'score charts', comprising a record of withdrawal signs and symptoms against time, provides an objective assessment of the infant's clinical status and can guide treatment.
- Breast-feeding is discouraged, as it may complicate management (such as future placement in foster care) and prolong the withdrawal phase. It should certainly be avoided in mothers with HIV infection.

Long term
Assess social circumstances with Social Services to decide whether the child can be allowed home and decide on long-term follow-up. Infants with foetal alcohol syndrome require appropriate neurodevelopmental follow-up. Neurodevelopmental outcome may be suboptimal, particularly in infants born to mothers abusing alcohol and cocaine, and those brought up in families with disruptive or dysfunctional lifestyles. Further studies are required to determine treatment regimens with the best short- and long-term outcomes.

Useful website

www.nta.nhs.uk
National UK treatment agency for substance misuse (UK).

Further reading

Chasnoff IJ (ed.). Chemical dependency and pregnancy. *Clinics in Perinatology* (1991) **18:**1–191.
Chasnoff IJ, Scholl SH. Consequences of cocaine and other drug use in pregnancy. In: A Washton, MS Gold (eds). *Cocaine: A Clinician's Handbook*. New York: Guilford, 1987: 241.
Durand DJ, Espinoza AM, Nickerson BG. Association between prenatal cocaine exposure and sudden infant death syndrome. *Journal of Pediatrics* (1990) **117:**909.
Fetters L, Tronick EZ. Neuromotor development of cocaine-exposed and control infants from birth through 15 months: poor and poorer performance. *Pediatrics* (1996) **98:**938–43.
Finnegan LP. Perinatal substance abuse: comments and perspectives. *Seminars in Perinatology* (1991) **15:**331.
Johnson K, Gerada C, Greenough A. Treatment of neonatal abstinence syndrome. *Archives of Disease in Childhood Fetal and Neonatal Edition* (2003) **88:**F2–5.
Lester B (ed.). Prenatal drug exposure and child outcome. *Clinics in Perinatology* (1999) **26**(1).
Nicoll A, McGarrigle C, Brady T et al. Epidemiology and detection of HIV-1 among pregnant women in the United Kingdom: results from national surveillance 1988–1996. *British Medical Journal* (1998) **316:**253–8.
Shaw NJ, McIvor L. Neonatal abstinence syndrome after maternal methadone treatment. *Archives of Disease in Childhood Fetal and Neonatal Edition* (1994) **71:**F203–5.

Related topics of interest

- HIV/AIDS
- infection—perinatal
- intrauterine growth restriction
- seizures.

Mechanical ventilation

Mechanical ventilation using positive airway pressure is indicated for babies with respiratory failure secondary to lung or cardiac disease, for some with recurrent apnoea or fits, and during deep sedation or anaesthesia. The ventilators used are conventionally time-cycled, pressure-limited ventilators; that is, the time of the inspiratory and expiratory phases is set, and the ventilator delivers certain preset pressures. During the last 20 years, there have been several advances in ventilator technology, and several new modes of ventilation have become available. These new ways of ventilation have been assimilated into clinical practice on the basis of physiological studies which suggested the advantages of the new modalities over 'conventional' ventilation. Thus, newer ventilators have been adapted for patient-triggered ventilation (PTV), pressure support ventilation (PSV), proportional assist ventilation (PAV), volume guarantee (VG), volume-controlled ventilation (VCV), and high-frequency oscillatory ventilation (HFOV). In severe respiratory failure with ventilation-perfusion mismatch, nitric oxide (NO) may be introduced into the inspiratory gases to dilate the pulmonary vasculature and improve ventilation-perfusion matching. Liquid ventilation, though still experimental, has also been used. Finally, extracorporeal membrane oxygenation (ECMO), which is, in essence, not a mode of ventilation, but modified cardiac bypass support, may be used in near-term infants with severe respiratory failure who cannot be successfully supported on any of the above ventilation modalities.

Continuous positive airway pressure (CPAP)

CPAP is an attempt to mimic the positive end expiratory pressure a baby generates by grunting during expiration against a closed glottis. The generated positive pressure reduces atelectasis. CPAP can be administered by face mask, endotracheal tube or nasal prongs. Increasingly, it is applied by short, soft nasal prongs on the end of a CPAP driver circuit. These devices sense airway pressure changes secondary to the baby's spontaneous respiratory effort and alter gas flows to maintain a near-constant airway pressure. This may reduce the work of breathing. A comparison of neonatal outcomes in American units showed that the unit using early CPAP and tolerating slightly higher $PaCO_2$, had the lowest incidence of chronic lung disease. At the same time, studies from Scandinavia using similar techniques suggested benefits of early CPAP, and this modality of treatment is currently being re-explored.

Preterm babies extubated during recovery from respiratory distress onto nasal CPAP are less likely to need reintubation than those extubated into a headbox. CPAP is also an important treatment of obstructive and mixed apnoea, in which the soft structures of the upper airway may collapse inward during the baby's negative pressure inspirations. CPAP 'splints' open the airway. More recently, additional 'positive pressure breaths' have been added to some CPAP delivery systems. Such newer systems are thought to offer advantages over traditional CPAP, but formal studies demonstrating their superiority are awaited. Randomised trials comparing nasal IPPV and nasal CPAP for apnoea of prematurity have produced conflicting results.

Intermittent positive pressure ventilation (IPPV)

In IPPV, the inspiratory and expiratory pressures, the inspired oxygen fraction (FiO_2), inspiratory time (T_I), expiratory time (T_E), and hence the rate (bpm) and the T_I/T_E ratio can all be controlled. During volume-cycled ventilation (VCV), a constant volume of gas is delivered regardless of the infant's lung function. VCV is yet to be tested against 'standard IPPV', with both modes being delivered by appropriate ventilators.

Target ranges for blood gases
- pH—arterial pH should preferably be ≥ 7.25 (≥ 7.3 in the first week of life).
- PaO_2—the recommended range is 6–10 kPa.
- $PaCO_2$—this should be >5 kPa. If the pH is >7.25, there may be an advantage in letting the pCO_2 rise towards 8 kPa in the hope of avoiding baro- and volutrauma. There is increasing evidence linking early hypocapnia with an increased incidence of CLD and PVL.
- SaO_2—a range of 85–92% may be optimal in the newborn preterm infant, but arterial gases are needed to confirm adequate oxygenation and pH.

Arterial oxygenation (PaO_2)
This can be controlled by:

- changing the FiO_2
- changing the mean airway pressure by:
  —changing the peak inspiratory pressure (PIP)
  —changing the PEEP
  —changing the T_I/T_E ratio
  —lengthening the inspiratory plateau (increasing inspiratory gas flows).

As PaO_2 varies directly with mean airway pressure (MAP) between 5 and 15cmH$_2$O, increasing MAP will improve oxygenation. Most modern ventilators will automatically indicate the MAP for any given ventilator settings. Alternatively, MAP may be calculated as follows: $MAP = ([PIP - PEEP] \times [T_I/T_I + T_E]) + PEEP$

Arterial CO$_2$ tension ($PaCO_2$)
This varies inversely with minute volume, the product of rate and stroke (tidal) volume, which is 5–8ml/kg in conventionally ventilated babies. Thus, $PaCO_2$ can be controlled by:

- changing the rate
- changing the tidal volume by:
  —changing the PIP
  —changing the PEEP (likely to have the greater effect for the same degree of change).

Remember that CO$_2$ retention can be caused by inadvertent PEEP (PEEP higher than set) during high-rate ventilation with short expiratory times. Acute unexpected rises in $PaCO_2$ often indicate an endotracheal tube blockage or pneumothorax.

Synchrony between the baby and the ventilator

In IPPV, the ventilator and the baby may breathe independently of one another, causing inefficient ventilation, variable tidal volumes, and high intrapulmonary pressures that result in an increased incidence of pneumothoraces. The ventilator–baby interaction should be studied to ensure that the baby is breathing synchronously. This is achieved by:

Capturing the baby's respiration

This is done by increasing the ventilator rate to just above the baby's spontaneous rate (often 80 bpm or more in babies of <1250 g), at which point the baby tends to synchronise with the ventilator.

Sedation

The baby should be sedated to the point where the baby's own respiratory drive is depressed but not abolished.

Paralysis

This guarantees 'synchrony', but has several disadvantages, including the loss of the baby's own considerable respiratory effort.

Patient-triggered ventilation (PTV)

Here the baby's own breath initiates a ventilator breath. The most efficient systems detect early inspiratory gas flow with an anemometer, or early inspiratory pressure changes with a pneumotachygraph in the circuit. To achieve synchrony, there must be minimal delay between the baby's starting the breath and the ventilator's response; Ti must be set between 0.25 and 0.3 s as a baby's spontaneous Ti is of that order.

In synchronised intermittent positive pressure ventilation (SIPPV) or assist/control mode, the ventilator can be triggered by every breath, provided that the change in pressure, flow, etc., exceeds the critical trigger level, whereas, in synchronised intermittent mandatory ventilation (SIMV), only the preset number of breaths can be triggered regardless of the number of the infant's spontaneous breaths. A backup rate is set so that the ventilator takes over in an 'IPPV' mode if the baby becomes apnoeic. Babies probably benefit from being on caffeine to stimulate their respiration during trigger ventilation and to aid early weaning. With minor variations, control of PaO_2 and $PaCO_2$ is as above. Although physiological studies in preterm infants with RDS showed that, when compared with SIMV, PTV was associated with better synchrony, blood gases, higher tidal volumes, reduced work of breathing, and fluctuations in blood pressure, randomised trials have shown only a reduction in the duration of ventilation as the positive advantage of PTV. The international, randomised, controlled trial of PTV versus conventional ventilation in over 900 preterm infants (<32 weeks' gestation) with RDS showed no significant difference in outcomes. In fact, a greater proportion of those supported by PTV compared with IPPV developed air leaks. SIPPV has not been compared with SIMV in acute RDS. SIMV allows more flexible weaning than SIPPV, as pressure, rate, or both can be reduced. However, in preterm infants recovering from RDS, SIPPV may be superior to SIMV, although in infants with vigorous respiratory effort, SIMV is more efficacious, as it avoids hypocarbia. It should be noted, though, that oxygen consumption is increased at low ventilator rates: at least 20 breaths need to be supported to overcome the work of breathing imposed by the endotracheal tube.

Pressure support ventilation (PSV)

In PSV, the patient triggers a pressure-supported breath at a preset level. Outside the neonatal period, PSV has been shown to reduce the work of breathing during weaning. Randomised trials are required to define the role of this modality in neonatal ventilation.

Proportional assist ventilation (PAV)

During PAV, the pressure applied is servocontrolled throughout each spontaneous breath. The frequency, timing, and amplitude of lung inflation are controlled by the patient. The applied pressure increases in proportion to the tidal volume and inspiratory flow generated by the patient and thus enhances the effects of the respiratory muscles on ventilation. Large leaks around the endotracheal tube cause problems, and a backup rate is required in case of poor respiratory effort by the infant. Formal studies on PAV in neonates are, however, still awaited.

Volume guarantee (VG) ventilation

In the VG or volume-controlled ventilation (VCV) mode, PIP is servocontrolled, so that the preset volume is delivered during PSV, SIMV, or SIPPV. The expiratory tidal volume is measured and compared with the desired volume, and a new pressure plateau is calculated for the next breath. The desired volume will not be delivered, however, if the preset peak pressure is too low or there is no positive pressure plateau (airflow is too low or the inflation time is too short). VG allows adequate ventilation to be achieved at lower airway pressures. VG might reduce chronic lung disease if that is caused by (or partly by) volutrauma as opposed to barotrauma. In time-cycled pressure limited ventilation, the tidal volume varies from breath to breath, and overdistension with some breaths may be traumatic. The constant tidal volumes of VG may induce less damage, even if occasional high airway pressures have to be used. Limited experience with babies of >1200 g has been reported, and it is uncertain also whether the technique can be applied to the more difficult population of babies of <750 g.

High-frequency oscillatory ventilation (HFOV)

In HFOV, the inspiratory gases are oscillated around a mean airway pressure by a piston or diaphragm cycling at 10–15 Hz (600–900 cycles/min). Reducing the frequency below 10 Hz can improve CO_2 elimination, because the delivered volume increases when the rate is decreased. Tidal breaths such as those seen in spontaneous breathing, IPPV, or trigger ventilation are not generated. Gas dispersion occurs primarily through diffusion and convection, but also by pendelluft, asymmetric velocity profiles, and turbulence in the small airways, and tidal ventilation of very short-path alveoli. Pendelluft is the generation of local oscillating currents between neighbouring respiratory units of different physical properties and time constants. HFOV can be delivered alone or added to either or both of the inspiratory and expiratory phases of IPPV (though this may predispose to volutrauma). Recruitment of alveoli is important: the MAP is increased until the baby is in a FiO_2 of 0.3–0.4 and/or nine posterior ribs are seen above the diaphragm on the chest radiograph. Babies with the most severe lung disease will still be in a high FiO_2 even with the lungs radiologically expanded, but many will have diminished their oxygen demand as additional alveoli were recruited. Oxygenation is controlled by changes in FiO_2 and MAP. CO_2 elimination varies with the amplitude of the oscillation and with the frequency (see above).

Earlier studies used HFOV with a low-volume strategy (minimising pressures with the hope of preventing further trauma to the lungs). However, animal studies showed that a high-volume strategy in which lung recruitment is employed results in less lung injury than either low-volume HFOV strategy or IPPV. Meta-analysis of the early randomised trials suggested that HFOV, especially when a high-volume strategy is used, was associated with a reduction in CLD. While no major differences were noted between HFOV and 'conventional' ventilation, there have been consistent reports of an increased incidence of intracerebral haemorrhage in infants supported by HFOV. The most recent and largest randomised trial (UK Oscillation Study, 2002), which recruited 800 infants within 1 h of birth, compared HFOV and 'conventional' ventilation in newborns of 28 weeks' gestation or less. No significant differences were noted in the primary outcomes (death or CLD), or a range of other secondary outcomes, including air leaks and serious brain injury. The results of long-term effects, however, are awaited. One earlier trial (reported in 1994) comparing HFOV and IPPV in infants born at or near term with severe respiratory failure, and who were candidates for ECMO, similarly showed no differences between the two groups.

Thus, on the basis of current evidence, the host of new ventilation modalities complementing 'conventional ventilation techniques' have not been proven to be superior to 'standard' IPPV. Likewise HFOV, in spite of its earlier promise based on physiological studies, has not been shown by randomised trials to be superior to 'conventional' ventilation.

Useful websites

www.emedicine.com/ped/topic2770.htm
eMedicine article on Assisted Ventilation of the Newborn.

www.neonatology.com
Neonatology on the web – an extensive resource on neonatology.

Further reading

Avery ME, Tooley WH, Keller JB et al. Is chronic lung disease in low birth weight infants preventable? A survey of eight centers. *Pediatrics* (1987) **79:**26–35.
Baumer JH. International randomised controlled trial of patient triggered ventilation in neonatal respiratory distress syndrome. *Archives of Disease in Childhood Fetal and Neonatal Edition* (2000) **82:**F5–10.

Goldsmith JP, Karotkin EH (eds). *Assisted Ventilation of the Neonate*, 4th edn. Philadelphia: WB Saunders, 2003.

Goldsmith JP, Spitzer AR (eds). Controversies in neonatal pulmonary care. *Clinics in Perinatology* (1998) **25**(1).

Greenough A. Update on modalities of mechanical ventilators. *Archives of Disease in Childhood Fetal and Neonatal Edition* (2002) **87**:F3–6.

Henderson-Smart DI, Bhuta T, Cools F, et al. Elective high frequency oscillatory ventilation versus conventional ventilation for acute pulmonary dysfunction in preterm infants (Cochrane Review). In: The Cochrane Library, Issue 2, 2004. Chichester: John Wiley & Sons.

Johnson AH, Peacock JL, Greenough A et al (United Kingdom Oscillation Study Group). High-frequency oscillatory ventilation for the prevention of chronic lung disease of prematurity. *New England Journal of Medicine* (2002) **347**:633–42.

Related topics of interest

- complications of mechanical ventilation
- intubation
- pulmonary air leaks
- respiratory distress syndrome
- sedation and analgesia on the NICU.

Meconium aspiration syndrome

This life-threatening condition occurs with increasing frequency as gestation advances. The incidence of meconium aspiration syndrome (MAS) varies in different parts of the world, ranging from one to five per 1000 births. Higher rates are reported from North America and the Middle East than Europe. Though up to 15% of all deliveries may be complicated by meconium staining of amniotic fluid, only 5–10% of babies born through meconium-stained liquor develop pulmonary disease. In utero passage of meconium is uncommon because of the good anal sphincter tone, lack of strong intestinal peristalsis, and the meconium sludge normally plugging the rectum. Acidosis, asphyxia, and compression of the foetal head all stimulate relaxation of the anal sphincter and intestinal peristalsis. Foetal hypercarbia and hypoxia stimulate gasping, which can lead to meconium aspiration. Passage of meconium before 34 weeks is rare, but consider listerosis (causes liquefaction of meconium) if it occurs.

Pathogenesis

Aspirated meconium reaches the peripheral airways causing partial or complete obstruction. Partial obstruction causes gas trapping and lung overdistention (a 'ball-valve' effect). Complete obstruction leads to atelectasis and ventilation-perfusion mismatch. Meconium inhibits surfactant action, the normal bacteriostatic qualities of amniotic fluid, and also produces chemical pneumonitis. Furthermore, hypoxia, acidosis, and hypercarbia produce pulmonary vasoconstriction, leading to pulmonary hypertension, right-to-left shunting, and worsening gas exchange.

Clinical features

- post-term delivery and/or IUGR
- foetal distress during labour
- meconium staining of the skin, nails, and umbilical cord
- hypoglycaemia
- metabolic acidosis
- cyanosis and hypoxaemia
- tachypnoea or gasping respiration
- pneumothorax (30% with severe MAS)
- postasphyxial signs (CNS, renal, or cardiovascular)
- PPHN.

Diagnosis

Diagnosis is based on presence of meconium-stained liquor, meconium below the cords, or chest radiological appearances (lung overinflation, widespread, coarse, fluffy opacities, pneumothorax, and pneumomediastinum).

Management

Admit all infants with meconium below the cords for observation. Symptomatic infants should have pulse oximetry, supplemental oxygen (as required), blood-gas analysis, and a chest radiograph. Commence broad-spectrum antibiotics after blood cultures. Respiratory failure and severe hypoxaemia require intubation and mechanical ventilation. Surfactant administration, fast rates and low PEEP, and high-frequency ventilation may improve gas exchange. Inhaled nitric oxide (a selective pulmonary vasodilator) may further improve oxygen when used in conjunction with conventional or high-frequency ventilation. Refractory hypoxaemia (with an oxygenation index of $\geq$25–30) unresponsive to the above measures is an indication for ECMO. Neonates with severe MAS are ideal candidates for ECMO support. ECMO ensures adequate oxygenation and provides time for the pulmonary vasculature and parenchyma to recover while avoiding the damaging effects of high pressure ventilation. Ventilation parameters can be dramatically reduced, and the meconium cleared by intensive chest physiotherapy. The Extracorporeal Life Support Organisation reports a worldwide survival rate of 94% for this group of infants. Asphyxiated infants with MAS may have multisystem involvement (as in renal failure, seizures, and hypotension) requiring specific therapy.

Prevention

Identify foetuses at risk of asphyxia (IUGR, post-term, and oligohydramniotic) and monitor carefully during labour.

A skilled neonatal resuscitator should attend deliveries complicated by meconium staining of liquor. Clear the mouth and pharynx when the head is delivered and view the larynx; if meconium is present, aspirate carefully. If thick meconium is present or meconium is seen below the cords, aspirate the trachea with a large-bore suction catheter, or carefully intubate and then repeatedly aspirate the trachea.

Endotracheal tube adapters or other mechanical aspirators should be used to prevent the resuscitator from being contaminated with any infectious agents (such as HIV) present in the amniotic and vaginal fluids. Although up to half of all meconium-stained infants may have meconium in their trachea, and one in ten may have meconium below the cords although it is absent from the mouth or pharynx, intubation of all meconium-stained infants is associated with a greater morbidity.

Prognosis

Mild disease not requiring mechanical ventilation has an excellent prognosis of recovery within a few days. Recently, mortality from severe MAS has declined from almost 50% to 4–18%. Most deaths are due to air leaks, PPHN, respiratory failure, or associated perinatal asphyxia. There is an increased risk of asthma and exercise-induced bronchial reactivity in survivors. The use of hyperventilation-induced hypocapnia ($PaCO_2$ <25 mmHg or <3.5 kPa) in treating PPHN is associated with adverse neurodevelopmental outcome (such as sensorineural hearing loss and low psychomotor developmental test scores). Perinatal asphyxia is associated with a mortality and neurodevelopmental morbidity related to the severity of the asphyxial insult.

Further reading

Cleary GM, Wiswell TE. Meconium-stained amniotic fluid and the meconium aspiration syndrome: an update. *Pediatric Clinics of North America* (1998) **45:**511–29.

Cunningham AS, Lawson EE, Martin RJ et al. Tracheal suction and meconium: a proposed standard of care. *Journal of Pediatrics* (1990) **138:**153.

Greenough A, Milner AD (eds). *Neonatal Respiratory Disorders*, 2nd edn. London: Arnold, 2003.

Halahakoon CN, Halliday HL. Other acute lung disorders. In: VYH Yu (ed.). *Baillière's Clinical Paediatrics*, Vol. 3/No. 1. *Pulmonary Problems in the Perinatal Period and their Sequelae.* London: Baillière Tindall, 1995: 87–114.

Kirkpatrick BV, Mueller DG. Respiratory disorders in the newborn. In: V Chernick, T Boat (eds). *Kendig's Disorders of the Respiratory Tract in Children*, 6th edn. Philadelphia: WB Saunders, 1998: 328–64.

Taeusch HW, Ballard RA, Gleason CA (eds). *Avery's Diseases of the Newborn*, 8th edn. Philadelphia: WB Saunders, 2005.

Wiswell TE. Handling the meconium-stained infant. *Seminars in Neonatology* (2001) **6:**225–31.

Wiswell TE, Gannon CM, Jacob J et al. Delivery room management of the apparently vigorous meconium-stained neonate: results of the multicenter international collaborative trial. *Pediatrics* (2000) **105:**1–7.

Related topics of interest

- chronic lung disease
- extracorporeal membrane oxygenation
- intubation
- intrauterine growth restriction
- hypoxic-ischaemic encephalopathy
- mechanical ventilation
- persistent pulmonary hypertension of the newborn
- respiratory distress.

Metabolic acidosis

Normal cellular function requires that the hydrogen ion concentration (or pH) be kept within a narrow range. In order to maintain a normal pH, intracellular and extra-cellular proteins, inorganic phosphate and the bicarbonate buffer hydrogen ions. Bicarbonate is the most important buffer in the body (accounting for over 60% of blood buffering capacity) and is central to all the other important homeostatic mechanisms for dealing with hydrogen ions. Metabolic acidosis arises from the excessive production or inadequate excretion of hydrogen ions, or the increased loss of bicarbonate.

The Henderson–Hasselbalch equation for the bicarbonate system is expressed thus:

$$pH = 6.1 + \log[HCO_3^-]\backslash[CO_2]$$

In metabolic acidosis, the excess hydrogen ions combine with bicarbonate, thus reducing its concentration ($[HCO_3^-]$), and thereby reducing the ratio $[HCO_3^-]:[CO_2]$; this causes a fall in pH. The bicarbonate may be lost in the urine or gastrointestinal tract, may fail to be generated, or may be utilised in buffering H^+. The base deficit and $[HCO_3]$ are calculated automatically from the pH and the PCO_2 measurements. The normal range of base excess for preterm babies on the first day of life is from -2 to -6. As their renal function improves and the clearance of H^+ increases with age, so the base excess rises to 0, and then by three or four weeks of age it may be $+2$ to $+4$, and more in babies with compensated CLD.

The commonest cause of metabolic acidosis in neonatal intensive care is tissue hypoxia, which causes lactic acidosis. However, as several other disorders may produce similar biochemical changes, a systematic approach to metabolic acidosis is required in order to identify correctly its aetiology and therefore the appropriate management. Recognised causes of metabolic acidosis include the following:

Systemic

- hypoxia
- sepsis
- shock
- cold stress
- birth asphyxia
- maternal acidosis
- amino acid intolerance during parenteral nutrition
- drug therapy (such as acetazolamide therapy for glaucoma—inhibits carbonic anhydrase)
- neonatal diabetes.

Central nervous system

- prolonged seizures
- intracranial haemorrhage
- arteriovenous malformations.

Pulmonary system (mixed metabolic and respiratory acidosis more likely)

- pneumothorax
- congenital lung malformations
- large pleural effusions
- pulmonary haemorrhage.

Cardiovascular system

- congenital heart disease (such as TGA, HLHS, and coarctation of aorta)
- myocardial dysfunction (as in myocardial ischaemia)
- hypotension and/or hypovolaemia
- cardiac failure.

Gastrointestinal system

- excessive loss of HCO_3^- in intestinal secretions (as in via fistulae or severe diarrhoea)
- gut ischaemia (as in NEC, volvulus, and mesenteric occlusion/infarction).

Renal system

- renal glomerular failure
- renal tubular failure (as in renal tubular acidosis or renal Fanconi's syndrome)
- renal immaturity in preterm infants (inappropriate urinary HCO_3^- loss)
- polycystic kidneys
- obstructive uropathies.

Inborn errors of metabolism

Consider an inborn error of metabolism especially in term infants, particularly where there is a family history of unexplained neonatal illnesses and/or deaths and consanguinity. Typically, after being initially well, the infant becomes ill with unexplained severe or persistent acidosis with a large anion gap. The main group of inborn errors of metabolism presenting with severe metabolic acidosis are as follows:

- defects of gluconeogenesis (such as glucose-6-phosphatase deficiency, and fructose-1,6-biphosphatase deficiency)
- organic acidaemia (such as propionic, methylmalonic, and isovaleric acidaemia)
- defects of pyruvate metabolism and electron transport chain (as in pyruvate carboxylase deficiency—these infants may be dysmorphic).

Hyperlacticacidaemia is most commonly due to tissue hypoxia, and this resolves with adequate cardiac and tissue perfusion. In contrast, the acidosis in congenital lactic acidaemias persists in spite of an adequate cardiac output and tissue perfusion. It may be present from birth, with a large anion gap, a blood lactate of $\geq 5\,mmol/l$, and ketosis.

Summary of findings in metabolic acidosis

- $[HCO_3^-]$ always low
- PCO_2 usually low (compensatory change)
- pH low (uncompensated or partially compensated) or normal (fully compensated)
- Chloride concentration usually normal; raised in renal tubular acidosis (RTA) or with administration of acetazolamide or ammonium chloride.

Deleterious effects of metabolic acidosis

Metabolic acidosis, particularly when the pH is <7.2, causes a failure of intracellular metabolism, resulting in further metabolic acidosis and end-organ failure. Acidosis is associated with impaired cerebral blood flow, increased peripheral vascular resistance, decreased myocardial function, and IVH. Additionally, a falling cardiac output and poor tissue perfusion may increase tissue hypoxia, further worsening the acidosis. Preterm infants are more prone to disorders that cause metabolic acidosis (such as RDS and cold stress) and have a reduced capacity to prevent and correct acidosis. The ability to compensate for a metabolic acidosis by increasing the excretion of carbon dioxide is further diminished in infants with respiratory disease.

Investigations

Laboratory
First-line
- blood gases (tracking changes in pH and HCO_3^-)
- urea and electrolytes (renal function)
- liver function tests
- blood glucose (hypoglycaemia in gluconeogenic disorders and neonatal diabetes)
- FBC (anaemia and sepsis)
- blood culture (sepsis)
- CRP (sepsis)
- urinalysis (failure to acidify urine in RTA, haematuria in acute renal failure, renal vein thrombosis, ketones, and reducing sugars).

Second-line
- anion gap (sum of sodium and potassium, less sum of chloride and bicarbonate [normal value: 6–14 mmol/l]—large anion gap suggests possible inborn error of metabolism)
- plasma chloride (high Cl^- with normal 'anion gap' suggests RTA; in acidosis due to most other causes, Cl^- is normal and 'anion gap' increased)
- metabolic tests—plasma lactate, ammonia, serum amino acids, urine amino acids and organic acids, ketones, and urine-reducing substances.

Imaging as clinically appropriate
- chest radiograph (pneumothorax and effusions)
- abdominal radiograph (NEC with or without perforation and volvulus)
- cranial ultrasonography (intracranial haemorrhage and vascular malformations)

- echocardiography (myocardial dysfunction and congenital heart disease)
- abdominal ultrasound (renal arterial or venous thrombosis, and bladder outlet obstruction).

Management

Interventions should be aimed to correct the underlying abnormality.

- Treat hypothermia.
- Treat hypoxia by administering oxygen (head box, CPAP, or mechanical ventilation).
- Transfuse with blood if anaemic, or administer colloid/crystalloid if hypovolaemic.
- Commence appropriate first- or second-line antibiotics for suspected sepsis.
- Treat hypotension with volume replacement and/or inotropes.
- Reduce or discontinue drug therapy (such as acetazolamide) or parenteral nutrition if it is contributing to the acidosis.
- Treat bowel ischaemia/NEC by withholding oral feeds and commencing parenteral nutrition and antibiotics. Administer colloid (FFP or blood) and augment the blood pressure with inotropes, where appropriate. For suspected volvulus, intestinal perforation, and bowel infarction, refer for surgery.
- Treat RTA with alkali (oral bicarbonate or citrate) (1–2 mmol/kg per day for distal RTA and 2–5 mmol/kg per day for proximal RTA).
- In the absence of a specific contraindication (such as irreversible glomerular failure when the administration of sodium bicarbonate to a patient with impaired sodium excretion is inappropriate), correct base deficit by administering 4.2% bicarbonate or THAM (1/2 correction) intermittently or as a constant infusion for persistent acidosis.
- Perform echocardiography to rule out congenital heart disease or myocardial dysfunction.
- In suspected inherited metabolic disease, protein catabolism may be reduced by commencing a glucose infusion at rates of up to 10 mg/kg per min with insulin, starting at 0.01 U/kg per h while monitoring blood-glucose concentration. Specific cofactors may be administered in pharmacological amounts to correct partially or wholly a few inborn errors of metabolism (such as biotin in holocarboxylase synthase deficiency, glycine [250–500 mg/kg per day] in isovaleric acidaemia, and L-carnitine [up to 50 mg/kg per h] in organic acidaemias).

Further reading

Arnon S, Litmanovits I, Regev R et al. Dichloroacetate treatment for severe refractory metabolic acidosis during neonatal sepsis. *Pediatric Infectious Disease Journal* (2001) **20**:218–19.
Modi N. Renal function, fluid and electrolyte balance and neonatal renal disease. In: JM Rennie, NRC Roberton (eds). *Textbook of Neonatology*, 3rd edn. Edinburgh: Churchill Livingstone, 1999: 1009–37.
Walter JH. Metabolic acidosis in newborn infants. *Archives of Disease in Childhood* (1992) **67**:767–9.
Wyckoff MH, Perlman J, Niermeyer S. Medications during resuscitation—what is the evidence? *Seminars in Neonatology* (2001) **6**:251–9.

Related topics of interest

- acid–base balance
- blood pressure
- inherited metabolic disease—investigation and management
- mechanical ventilation
- necrotising enterocolitis
- renal and urinary tract disorders—nephrology.

Multiple pregnancy

Multiple pregnancy rates vary worldwide. For instance, the prevalence of twin births varies from 6.7 per 1000 deliveries in Japan to 40 per 1000 deliveries in Nigeria. This is due largely to variations in dizygotic twinning, as the prevalence of monozygotic twinning is relatively constant worldwide at 3.5 per 1000 births. Dizygotic twins arise when two ova are released and fertilised in one menstrual cycle; monozygotic twins arise when one ovum is fertilised and the resulting zygote divides into two. Over the last two decades, the incidence of twins and higher-order births has been rising, partly due to the more widespread use of assisted-reproductive techniques. However, multiple pregnancy is associated with greater risks for both mothers and foetuses than with a singleton pregnancy. This is because every complication of pregnancy occurs more commonly. The most important complication of multiple pregnancy is preterm delivery, with its concomitant increased perinatal morbidity and mortality. Thus, twins account for only 2% of births, but 9% of all perinatal deaths due to their prematurity and low birth weight. The perinatal mortality rate among higher-order births is directly related to the number of foetuses. The average length of twin pregnancy is 20 days shorter than a singleton one. The mean duration of pregnancy decreases as the number of foetuses in utero increases. Approximately 25% of twins are born preterm. The mean gestational age at delivery for triplets is 33 weeks (with 85–90% delivering before 37 weeks and 20–30% before 32 weeks). Almost all quadruplets experience preterm delivery (half before 32 weeks' gestation).

Maternal risks associated with multiple pregnancy

- increased symptoms of early pregnancy (such as nausea and vomiting)
- increased risk of miscarriage
- the vanishing twin syndrome
- preterm labour and delivery
- hypertension (pre-eclampsia and eclampsia)
- antepartum haemorrhage
- hydramnios (in up to 12% of multiple pregnancies)
- possible need for prenatal hospitalisation for prolonged periods
- antepartum foetal death (risk of DIC in up to 25%)
- risk of operative delivery (increased risk of trauma and infection)
- increased likelihood of caesarean delivery
- post-partum haemorrhage
- postnatal problems (such as increased risk of depression).

Foetal risks associated with multiple pregnancy

- Congenital abnormalities (twice as common as with singletons)
- IUGR (25–33% have birth weight <10th percentile)
- preterm labour and delivery (rates of 30–50%)
- twin-to-twin transfusion
- death of a cotwin

- hydramnios (malpresentation)
- operative vaginal delivery
- cord accidents (carry perinatal mortality of up to 50%)
- risk of asphyxia (mortality risk from asphyxia for twins is four to five times that of a singleton)
- stillbirth or neonatal death (perinatal mortality rate of twins is up to ten times that of singletons)
- the 'stuck' twin phenomenon (occurs in 8% of twin pregnancies but mortality is over 80% for both twins)
- twin entrapment (rare, typically occurring in monoamniotic twins; incidence of one in 800, and high risk of foetal death).

Specific problems associated with multiple pregnancy

Determining zygosity
This is of importance, as monozygotic pregnancies have increased morbidity and mortality. Twins of different sex are obviously dizygotic. Monozygosity can be proven on the basis of a monochorionic placenta. However, monozygotic twins with dichorionic placentas may be distinguished reliably from like-sex dizygotic twins only by blood grouping, red cell and tissue enzymes, serum proteins, or minisatellite DNA probe tests.

Foetal nutrition and growth
Of necessity, multiple foetuses compete for nutrition. Foetal growth in twins is usually similar to that of singletons until approximately 24 weeks' gestation. Thereafter, body weight falls disproportionately more than head growth. The average birth weight of a newborn twin is 500 g less than a singleton. Dichorionic twins are heavier than monochorionic twins.

Twin–twin transfusion syndrome
Placental arteriovenous vascular anastomoses can result in the twin–twin transfusion syndrome, usually in monozygotic monochorionic twins. A cord-blood haemoglobin difference of at least 5 g/dl is noted between the twins. An incidence of 5–15% of all twin pregnancies has been reported, and the acute severe twin–twin transfusion syndrome occurs in 1% of monochorionic gestations. The donor twin becomes anaemic, hypovolaemic, oligohydramniotic, and growth restricted. The recipient twin becomes polycythaemic, hypervolaemic, and polyhydramniotic, and may develop cardiac failure, ascites, and pleural and pericardial effusions. Hydrops fetalis may develop in both. Antenatal treatment includes laser ablation of anastomoses, repeated amniocentesis, transfusion of donor, and exsanguination of recipient. Mortality may be high (80–100%) for twins presenting acutely at 18–26 weeks' gestation.

'Stuck' twin phenomenon
One foetus in a diamniotic pregnancy lies in a severely oligohydramniotic sac, while the co-twin lies in a severely polyhydramniotic sac. Mortality is high (>80%). Most result from twin–twin transfusion syndrome.

Congenital anomalies

Major anomalies are twice as common in multiple pregnancies than in singleton. Cardiac anomalies, bowel atresia, neural tube defects, and chromosomal abnormalities are more common in multiple pregnancies. Certain malformations uniquely occur in monozygotic twins (namely, conjoined twins) (one in 50 000 pregnancies), the commonest form being thoracopagus and acardia (one in 30 000–35 000 deliveries).

Death of a cotwin

Foetal demise of one twin occurs in 0.5–6.8% of twin pregnancies after the first trimester. The emboli and debris from the dead foetus may enter the circulation of the surviving (monochorionic) twin, producing multiple brain, gastrointestinal, and renal lesions. In contrast, surviving dichorionic twins have a good prognosis. Regardless of zygosity, males fare less well than females, and male–male pairs have the highest perinatal mortality rates. In male–female pairs, female infants fare better. The second-born twin may be at greater risk of death and morbidity.

Further reading

Foley MR, Strong TH (eds). *Obstetric Intensive Care: A Practical Manual.* Philadelphia: WB Saunders, 1997.

Fowler MG, Kleinman JC, Kiely JL et al. Double jeopardy: twin infant mortality in the United States 1983 and 1984. *American Journal of Obstetrics and Gynecology* (1991) **165:**15–22.

Fusi L, McParland P, Fisk N et al. Acute twin–twin transfusion: a possible mechanism for brain-damaged survivors after intrauterine death of a monochorionic twin. *Obstetrics and Gynecology* (1991) **78:**517–20.

Hawrylyshyn PA, Barkin M, Bernstein A et al. Twin pregnancies—a continuing perinatal challenge. *Obstetrics and Gynecology* (1982) **59:**463–6.

Keith LG, Papiernik E, Keith DM et al (eds). *Multiple Pregnancy. Epidemiology, Gestation and Perinatal Outcome.* London: Parthenon, 1995.

Little J, Bryan E. Congenital anomalies. In: I MacGillivary, DM Campbell, B Thompson (eds). *Twinning and Twins.* Chichester: Wiley, 1988: 207–40.

Seng YC, Rajadurai VS. Twin–twin transfusion syndrome: a five year review. *Archives of Disease in Childhood Fetal and Neonatal Edition* (2000) **83:**F168–70.

Related topics of interest

- complications of pregnancy
- congenital malformations and birth defects
- intrauterine growth restriction
- prenatal diagnosis.

Necrotising enterocolitis

The first reported cases of necrotising enterocolitis (NEC) appeared over 150 years ago, although the term 'NEC' was first used in the 1950s. NEC is a maladaptive response of the immature gastrointestinal tract to perinatal/postnatal injury. Damage to the intestinal mucosa in the presence of intraluminal feeds and microbial infection are important aetiological factors. Intestinal ischaemia, from any cause, rapid oral feeds, non-human-milk formula, and bacterial infection are thought to be particularly important. Abnormal prenatal umbilical wave forms (absent and reversed end diastolic flow) and marked intrauterine growth restriction are particularly associated with NEC. Approximately 90% of cases occur in premature infants, with the incidence varying with gestational age from 0.1 per 1000 live births in term infants to almost 8% in the very low-birth-weight infants. It is most frequently seen within the first two weeks of life, though it may occur in infants who are several weeks old. Approximately 300 cases occur annually in the UK with 70–100 deaths.

Although the caecum, ascending colon, and terminal ileum are the most commonly affected sites, any part of the gastrointestinal tract may be involved. The affected segment of gut may show only small perforations or be severely affected and necrotic.

Clinical features

These vary, from the nonspecific signs of hypotonia, lethargy, and apnoea with temperature instability, to the signs of septic shock with hypotension, bradycardia, pallor with abdominal distension, bloody stools, bilious aspirates, and DIC. A silent tender abdomen with a red and indurated abdominal wall suggests a perforation.

Investigations

Radiology

Plain abdominal radiography shows thickened dilated loops of bowel (which may be fixed) occasionally with fluid levels. In the acute phase of the disease, daily radiographs should be performed. A lateral abdominal film (right side up for better air–liver contrast) is important in the acute stage of the disease, as perforations may be difficult to detect otherwise. Typical radiographs show intramural gas (pneumatosis intestinalis); in later stages, air may also be seen in the liver, along with ascites. Intra-abdominal abscesses and ascites may be more readily recognised with ultrasound.

Haematology
- FBC
- coagulation screen.

Biochemistry
- U and E
- blood gases.

Microbiology
Perform a full septic screen (omit LP if diagnosis is clear).

Management

Stop oral feeds to rest the gut and commence parenteral nutrition for at least ten days. Deflate the abdomen with a nasogastric tube on free drainage. Administer FFP in the acute phase of the disease at 10–20 ml/kg, depending on clinical state (wide core–peripheral temperature gap, poor capillary refill, and hypotension). Transfuse with packed red cells if anaemic. Support the blood pressure (keep mean arterial blood pressure at ≥35 mmHg) with colloids and inotropes (dopamine 10–20 μg/kg per min or dobutamine 10–30 μg/kg per min). Monitor arterial blood gases, correct acidosis, and commence ventilation if patient is hypoxic and retaining carbon dioxide and/or in the presence of apnoea. Carefully monitor electrolytes and hydration with 6–12-hourly electrolytes in the acute phase of the disease, and then less frequently later when more stable. Control infection with intravenous broad-spectrum antibiotics including metronidazole. Correct DIC and transfuse platelets if marked thrombocytopenia is present (platelet count $<20 \times 10^3/mm^3$). Provide adequate analgesia by infusing opiates (10–40 μg morphine/kg per h). Treat intercurrent problems, such as electrolyte imbalance and hypoglycaemia, promptly.

Surgery is required when a perforation has occurred or when there is continuing deterioration (with persistent acidosis) despite adequate medical treatment. In the unstable sick VLBW infant, simple drainage of the peritoneal cavity under local anaesthetic may be a useful interim measure until the infant is fit for surgery.

Enteral feeds (preferably expressed breast milk or a simplified formula, such as Prejestimil, Mead Johnson) may be recommenced slowly in the well infant after 10–14 days (or longer if surgery was required). Relapses may occur in up to 10% of cases after reintroduction of enteral feeds. Complications include stricture formation with intestinal obstruction and short bowel syndrome following bowel resection.

Prevention

- Antenatal steriods are protective.
- Breast milk has a protective effect against NEC.
- Promptly correct shock, hypotension, hypoxia, and acidosis.
- Withhold feeds early in the presence of large gastric aspirates, bilious aspirates, or abdominal distension.
- Delay oral feeds for 5–7 days if reversed end-diastolic flow was demonstrated in the umbilical artery prenatally, or previous perinatal ischaemic events.
- Small-volume, nonnutritive feeds ('gut priming') soon after birth minimises mucosal atrophy, improve intestinal motility, and may prevent NEC or lessen its severity.
- Avoid aggressive feeding with cautious incremental volumes (maximum enteral incremental rate ~20 ml/kg per day).

Further reading

Clark DA, Miller MJS. What causes neonatal necrotizing enterocolitis and how can it be prevented? In: TN Hansen, N McIntosh (eds). *Current Topics in Neonatology*, 1. London: WB Saunders, 1996: 160–76.

Faix RG, Nelson M. Neonatal necrotizing enterocolitis: progress, problems, and prospects. In: TJ David (ed.). *Recent Advances in Paediatrics*, No. 16. Edinburgh: Churchill Livingstone, 1998: 1–24.

Lee JS, Polin RA. Treatment and prevention of necrotising enterocolitis. *Seminars in Neonatology* (2003) **8:**449–59.

Malcolm G, Ellwood D, Devonald K et al. Absent or reversed end diastolic flow velocity in the umbilical artery and necrotizing enterocolitis. *Archives of Disease in Childhood* (1991) **66:**805–7.

Pierro A, Hall N. Surgical treatment of infants with necrotizing enterocolitis. *Seminars in Neonatology* (2003) **8:**223–32.

Reber KM, Nankervis CA. Necrotizing enterocolitis: prevention strategies. *Clinics in Perinatology* (2004) **31:**157–67.

Related topics of interest

- abdominal distension
- acute collapse
- neonatal surgery
- shock
- surgical emergencies
- vomiting.

Neonatal screening for inherited disease

Mass screening for newborns for metabolic disorders was introduced by Bob Guthrie (Guthrie test for phenylketonuria [PKU]) some four decades ago. Conditions which merit screening occur frequently, have gradual onset (allowing time for detection before the onset of symptoms), and can be detected by inexpensive and accurate assays. Early treatment should produce a good outcome. This is ideal for PKU.

Phenylketonuria (PKU)

PKU has an incidence of one in 12000 births and in the classic form is due to phenylalanine hydroxylase deficiency. However, tetrahydrobiopterin cofactor defects may also produce PKU. The PKU screening test identifies all infants with elevated serum phenylalanine. An amino acid chromatogram is performed on a heel prick spot of blood collected onto filter paper. Other disorders can also now be detected from this same blood sample, including tyrosinaemia, MSUD, and some genetic disorders (from DNA analysis).

Infants with serum phenylalanine values persistently above 1.0 mmol/l (18 mg/dl) need treatment. Infants with phenylalanine levels of 0.2–0.6 mmol/l (4–10 mg/dl) on the first test should have a repeat test. Levels of ≥0.6 mmol/l (10 mg/dl) need further assessment and may need treatment. Infants should be tested when on full feeds (commonly days 6–10) and off intravenous fluids.

Treatment should be carried out by those expert in this area. In essence, most of the amino acid requirements are provided in synthetic form, and natural proteins are only used in sufficient amounts to supply the phenylalanine requirements for growth, leaving no excess to be broken down to tyrosine.

Hypothyroidism

Hypothyroidism has an incidence of one in 3500 births. Most screening programmes use a single blood sample taken at days 5–10 (when relative stability has returned to the thyroid axis after the abrupt changes at birth). A heel prick spot of blood is collected onto filter paper at the same time and onto the same paper as the PKU test. Thyroxine screening alone is inadequate because of the overlap between normal and hypothyroid values. Thyroid-stimulating hormone (TSH) assay is the primary test performed, though this may miss the rarer cases of secondary hypothyroidism (pituitary or hypothalamic hypothyroidism with an incidence of one in 60–100000 births).

Normal TSH levels are <25 mU/l. Levels of 25–80 mU/l are equivocal and the infant should be retested. Levels of >80 mU/l are abnormal and the infant should be recalled urgently for full thyroid function tests. Treatment should be started as soon as possible (without waiting for results) with thyroxine 8–10 µg/kg per day (once-daily dose).

The commonest cause of congenital primary hypothyroidism is thyroid dysgenesis (dysplasia), which is associated with trisomy 21, with females affected twice as often as males and with an incidence of one in 3500. The second commonest cause is thyroid dyshormonogenesis (autosomal recessive biochemical defects of iodothyronine synthesis), which has a frequency of one in 30000–50000 and equal sex incidence; it accounts for 10–15% of infants detected by screening.

Galactosaemia

Galactosaemia has a prevalence of one in 44000 births and screening detects 60–70% while they are still asymptomatic. The effect of screening at 4–6 days upon final outcome is still uncertain. Routine screening is not practised in the UK.

Hereditary tyrosinaemia

Screening for this uncommon disorder is routine only in certain parts of the world, such as Norway, Sweden, and Quebec, Canada. There is a defect in fumaryl aceto-acetate, and excretion of succinylacetone in urine is diagnostic. Treatment is with low tyrosine and phenylalanine milk. If the disorder is undetected, there is progressive liver dysfunction, hypoglycaemia, renal tubular defects, and eventually cirrhosis. However, transient tyrosinaemia is common in preterm infants (responds to 50 mg vitamin C daily for one week).

Cystic fibrosis

DNA analysis now affords a useful screening tool for CF, especially where there is a strong family history of the disorder or one parent is known to be affected. Routinely, the commonest mutations are screened for, namely, ΔF508, 621 + 1G > T, G542X, G551D, and R553X. Absence of the above mutations gives an 80% certainty of excluding CF as a diagnosis in the indigenous UK population. An optimal screening programme should screen for most common mutations in a given population, as these vary in different ethnic groups and geographic locations. Meconium ileus in the neonatal period is associated with CF. Fifteen per cent of infants with CF present with bowel obstruction caused by meconium ileus, but only 75% of infants with meconium ileus have CF. The blood immunoreactive trypsin (IRT) level should be assayed. Elevated IRT (normal values are $<70 \mu g/l$) suggests CF. Similarly, low tryptic activity (normal faecal chymotrypsin $120 \mu g/g$) in the stool suggests CF.

Haemoglobinopathies

The two most important haemoglobinopathies, numerically and clinically, are sickle cell disease (SCD) and thalassaemia major (homozygous β-thalassaemia). Both are β-globin chain defects and therefore rarely cause problems before 3–6 months of age, when the β-chain of adult haemoglobin (HbA; $\alpha_2\beta_2$) normally becomes predominant as foetal haemoglobin (HbF; $\alpha_2\gamma^2$) disappears. The thalassaemia syndromes are the commonest inherited single-gene defects in the world. The main 'at-risk' groups are individuals from the Mediterranean region and the Middle East, Asians, Afro-Caribbeans, and Orientals.

Sickle haemoglobin can be identified by alkaline cellulose acetate electrophoresis backed by acid citrate-agarose electrophoresis of a haemolysate of packed red cells.

Thalassaemia can be diagnosed by analysis of globin chain synthesis and gene mapping. α-Thalassaemia (homozygous α-thalassaemia) presents as hydrops fetalis and is incompatible with survival.

Further reading

Evans MI (ed.). Metabolic and genetic screening. *Clinics in Perinatology* (2001) **28**(2).

Gaston M. Why we should screen newborns for sickle cell disease. *Contemporary Pediatrics* (1989) **1:**175.

Griffiths P, Mann JR, Darbyshire PJ et al. Evaluation of eight and a half years of neonatal screening for haemoglobinopathies in Birmingham. *British Medical Journal* (1988) **296:**1583–5.

Hall DMB, Michel JM. Screening in infancy. *Archives of Disease in Childhood* (1995) **72:**93–6.

Laird L, Dezateux C, Anionwu EN. Neonatal screening for sickle cell disorders: what about the carrier infants? *British Medical Journal* (1996) **313:**407–11.

Murray J, Cuckle H, Taylor G, et al. Screening for cystic fibrosis. *Health Technology Assessment* (1999) **3:**8.

Scriver CR, Beaudet AL, Sly WS et al (eds). *The Metabolic and Molecular Basis of Inherited Disease*, 7th edn. New York: McGraw-Hill, 1995.

Seymour CA, Thomason MJ, Chalmers RA et al. Newborn screening for inborn errors of metabolism: a systematic review. *Health Technology Assessment* (1997) **1:**1.

Van Vliet G, Czernichow P. Screening for neonatal endocrinopathies: rationale, methods and results. *Seminars in Neonatology* (2004) **9:**75–85.

Wald N, Leck I. *Antenatal and Neonatal Screening*, 2nd edn. Oxford: Oxford University Press.

Wonke B, Modell B. Impact and future of screening for haemoglobin disorders. *Current Paediatrics* (1998) **8:**55–61.

Related topics of interest

- inherited metabolic disease—investigation and management
- inherited metabolic disease—recognisable patterns
- prenatal diagnosis.

Neonatal surgery

Several medical conditions presenting in the neonatal period require surgical intervention. Such surgery is best performed in a dedicated surgical unit where anaesthetists experienced in neonatal anaesthesia are available along with designated paediatric surgeons. The need for surgery may arise unexpectedly or have been previously anticipated and therefore planned.

Preoperative preparations

- Obtain parental consent in good time.
- Cross-match an appropriate amount of blood if perioperative blood loss is likely. A maternal blood sample is required for this in the newborn period.
- Obtain a baseline FBC and electrolytes, especially if the infant is several days old.
- Secure adequate venous and arterial access for the preoperative administration of colloid and crystalloid and continuous perioperative monitoring of blood pressure and blood gases for infants who are ready for surgery.
- In the immediate preoperative period, it may be necessary to intubate and ventilate infants requiring general anaesthesia for their surgical procedures. Check endotracheal tube placement radiographically and adjust ventilation if necessary after some baseline blood gases.

Intraoperative medical management

During surgery, several parameters should be monitored to maintain the infant in an optimal physical and metabolic status.

- Monitor temperature and provide additional heating to prevent excessive cooling.
- Monitor blood pressure (invasively where possible).
- Monitor blood gases and blood glucose during prolonged surgical procedures.
- Maintain an intravenous infusion of a dextrose solution (newborns) or dextrose/electrolyte solution (older infants), administering colloid (such as blood or 4.5% human albumin) should blood losses become significant (falling BP or rising pulse).
- Where necessary, administer antibiotics with induction of anaesthesia.

Postoperative management

This is determined partly by the surgical procedure previously performed, especially whether it was major or minor, and the general condition of the infant (that is, whether well or critically ill). Following minor surgery (such as uncomplicated hernia repair), the infant may be otherwise well and require only minimal analgesia, which may be administered orally. Oral or intravenous feeds may be commenced soon after the infant has recovered from anaesthesia. Following major surgery, however, intensive care monitoring is usually necessary with particular reference to the following:

- Monitor urine output, aiming to maintain a urine flow rate of ≥1 ml/kg per h; patients with renal failure should be closely monitored to avoid hyperkalaemia, fluid overload, acid–base disturbance, and drug toxicity (as from aminoglycosides).
- Monitor BP and support if necessary with colloid (blood, 4.5% albumin, or FFP) and inotropes (dopamine/dobutamine 10–30 µg/kg per min).
- Monitor adequacy of peripheral circulation/perfusion by monitoring core–peripheral temperature gap (maintain at <2 °C) and/or capillary refill time (normal is <3 s); administer colloid if above parameters are unsatisfactory.
- Continue infusion(s) of analgesia in appropriate amounts (such as morphine 40 µg/kg per h or fentanyl 1–2 µg/kg per h) following an appropriate loading dose, and, if necessary, an intravenous sedative (such as midazolam 50–100 µg/kg per h).
- Restrict crystalloids after major surgery because of inappropriate ADH secretion, as fluid overload may otherwise develop.
- Monitor U and E, FBC, blood glucose, and, if still ventilated, arterial blood gases.
- Commence total parenteral nutrition (via central venous line if possible) if full enteral nutrition is likely to be delayed (as after repair of abdominal wall defects).
- Ongoing losses (such as that secondary to nasogastric suctioning or drainage through stoma fistula or dressing) should be replaced every 2–4 hours with normal saline to avoid dehydration.
- Monitor wound healing; if wound appears infected, swab and commence antibiotics empirically. Review choice of antibiotics with culture results.

The place for surgery

In most neonatal centres, surgery is performed in the operating theatre, not in the intensive care unit, on the assumption that the neonatal intensive care unit (NICU) does not provide a sufficiently clean area, and so predisposes the infant to a higher risk of infection. However, when the patient undergoing surgery is an unstable, extremely low-birth-weight infant, the need for transportation (at times to an off-site centre), the extra handling, and the change of ventilator equipment all increase the risk of disrupting vascular lines or chest tubes, accidentally dislodging the endotracheal tube, and hypothermia, which may all further compromise the ill preoperative infant. With good planning and organisation, an area of the NICU can easily be set aside for the surgery of critically ill preterm or more mature infants who would be too unwell to transfer to a dedicated operating theatre. The surgical team, anaesthetists, operating theatre staff, and the NICU staff can work quite harmoniously on the NICU, allowing continuity of care for the infant (and the continued use of 'neonatal' technologies such as high-frequency ventilation), while avoiding transportation of the infant and its associated complications. With good organisation, both minor operations and some major procedures may be performed on the unit without placing the infant at disadvantage.

Further reading

Gavilanes AWD, Heineman E, Herpers MJHM et al. Use of neonatal intensive unit as a safe place for neonatal surgery. *Archives of Disease in Childhood Fetal and Neonatal Edition* (1997) **76:**F51–3.

Puri P (ed.). *Newborn Surgery*, 2nd edn. London: Arnold, 2003.

Reyes HM, Vidyasagar D (eds). Neonatal surgery. *Clinics in Perinatology* (1989) **16**(1).

Rowe MI, Lloyd D. Pre-operative and post-operative management. In: L Spitz, HH Nixon (eds). *Rob and Smith's Operative Surgery: Paediatric Surgery*, 4th edn. London: Butterworths, 1988: 4–10.

Spitz L, Steiner GM, Zachary RB. *A Colour Atlas of Paediatric Surgical Diagnosis*. London: Wolfe Medical, 1981.

Stringer MD, Oldham KT, Mouriquand PDE et al (eds). *Pediatric Surgery and Urology: Long Term Outcomes*. Philadelphia: WB Saunders, 1998.

Wetzel RC. Pediatric anesthesia. *Pediatric Clinics of North America* (1994) **41**(1).

Related topics of interest

- analgesia and anaesthesia
- abdominal distension
- abdominal wall defects
- congenital malformations and birth defects
- necrotising enterocolitis
- Hirschsprung's disease
- surgical emergencies.

Neural tube defects

In the human embryo, the developing CNS becomes recognisable by day 19 as the neural plate. This differentiates into the neural tube, the forerunner of all the major structures of the brain, and the spinal cord. Defects in the early organogenesis of the neural tube lead to the host of developmental defects manifest as brain and spinal cord malformations, often accompanied by unfavourable neurodevelopmental outcome.

In recent years, there has been a consistent steady decline in the incidence of congenital CNS malformations. Neural tube defects (NTDs) occur less frequently in the higher social classes. Maternal serum alpha-fetoprotein (AFP) is raised in pregnancies with NTDs. Folic acid (4 mg daily) appears effective in preventing the first occurrence as well as the risk of recurrent NTDs if administered periconceptually. Detailed antenatal ultrasound examination will detect most foetuses with severe NTDs.

Anencephaly

Here, the posterior skull fails to develop, exposing a rudimentary brain with absent cerebral hemispheres, associated with polyhydramnios and spina bifida. It is incompatible with life. There is increased risk of NTDs in future pregnancies.

Spina bifida occulta

This may affect approximately one in every 20 individuals. It has an excellent prognosis. Defects are often detected only by chance on spinal radiographs, but few have outward sign (hairy patch, dimple, and naevus). There is no increased risk of NTDs in future pregnancies.

Meningocele

This is a relatively benign condition in which the spinous process is absent and a CSF-containing sac protrudes through the gap. It may be sited anywhere from the cervical spine to the sacral region. Hydrocephalus may develop (10%) but is less severe and may resolve spontaneously. Operative closure is advised and prognosis is excellent. Antenatally, AFP is not raised, and unless detailed spinal ultrasound views are obtained, the diagnosis may be missed antenatally.

Myelomeningocele

This is usually thoracolumbar (worst prognosis) but may be lumbar, sacral, or lumbosacral. Defects often span several segments of spinal cord with various vertebral anomalies (wedge-shaped or hemivertebrae, fusion or absence of some ribs, and splayed out spinal laminae) and spinal scoliosis. Occasionally, defects of the skull membranous bones are present (craniolacunia) with characteristic radiologic appearance. The site and size of exposed abnormal neural elements (the 'neural plaque') partly determine the outcome.

Common clinical findings
- flaccid paralysis and analgesia, affecting lower limbs. Cervical/upper thoracic lesions may affect upper limbs similarly
- lower limb deformities: due to imbalanced paralysis of muscle groups (commonly with flexed and abducted hips, hyperextension of knees, talipes, and calcaneovalgus—lesion below L3)
- paralysed sphincters and urinary tract anomalies: dribbling incontinence, paralysed rectal sphincters, and patulous anus, with associated retention of urine, bladder trabeculation, hydronephrosis, and/or ureteric reflux. Other renal defects (pelvic kidney, duplex collecting system, and horseshoe kidney) are also more common
- hydrocephalus: present at birth in 90% (head shape and size may be normal).

Investigations
- spinal radiographs (to determine extent of skeletal anomalies)
- cranial ultrasound scan (to assess severity of hydrocephalus)
- renal ultrasound scan
- micturating cystourethrogram (bladder anomalies and ureteric reflux)
- electrolytes (excessive sodium loss with CSF leak).

Management
Treatment is now selective. Infants with serious defects and a projected poor outcome receive palliative care (with parents' agreement). Determine the neurologic deficits—assess the sensory and motor levels of the lesions. Orthopaedic assessment is required (fixed anomalies of spine and limbs and hip anomalies).

Indications for palliative care
- .paralysis below L3
- gross hydrocephalus
- marked kyphosis and scoliosis
- associated major congenital malformations
- thoracolumbar or thoracolumbosacral lesion.

If the outcome is favourable, active treatment may be undertaken, ideally in a specialised unit, beginning with closure of the lesion. Mild to moderate hydrocephalus may be treated medically and then surgically if this fails (see 'Hydrocephalus').

Cranial meningocele

Skull bone is deficient and a cystic swelling (containing CSF only) projects through the defect (usually occipital). It has a good outcome.

Encephalocele

Abnormal brain tissue is in a sac protruding from the occipital, parietal, or frontal areas or into the upper nasal cavity. Microcephaly and hydrocephaly are common. Associated anomalies include myelomeningocele and Klippel–Feil syndrome. Small encephaloceles may be treated surgically, but large lesions have a poor prognosis (cortical blindness or partial sight, spastic quadriplegia, epilepsy, and death). The worst prognosis is associated with large lesions and microcephaly.

Agenesis of the corpus callosum

Whole or part of the corpus callosum is missing, so the third ventricle extends between the hemispheres to the skull. This is associated with hypertelorism and megalencephaly. Cranial ultrasound or CT scan will reveal the absent corpus callosum.

Holoprosencephaly

This is a rare condition with absent olfactory bulbs and tracts and failure of cleavage of the forebrain. A large, single, dilated ventricle is present, and the corpus callosum may be absent. It is associated with other major malformations, including chromosomal defects (such as trisomy 13), and has a high mortality, as no treatment is available. Genetic counselling is required, as recurrence is common.

Megalencephaly

This is usually a benign familial trait, presenting with a large head, but without the signs of hydrocephalus, and growth at the normal rate. Measure siblings' and parents' head circumference, which should also be large.

Hydranencephaly

Hydranencephaly is a rare condition in which the cerebral hemispheres have been destroyed or failed to develop. The infant's head freely transilluminates (distinguish from extreme hydrocephalus), and prognosis is poor with high mortality despite surgical treatment (shunt insertion).

Microcephaly

Microcephaly is very common. It has multiple aetiologies, ranging from infection (as in CMV, rubella, and toxoplasmosis) and syndromic origin (as in foetal alcohol, and Roberts and Seckel syndromes) through chromosomal defects (such as autosomal recessive familial type). Head circumference is below 2nd percentile in relation to birth weight, with a sloping forehead. Prognosis is poor with neurodevelopmental delay, spasticity, and seizures.

Family support group and information

Association for Spina Bifida and Hydrocephalus
42 Park Road
Peterborough PE1 2UQ, UK
Tel: 01733 555988
www.asbah.org/

Further reading

Czeizel AE, Dudas I. Prevention of the first occurrence of neural-tube defects by periconceptional vitamin supplementation. *New England Journal of Medicine* (1992) **317:**1832–5.

Kaufman BA. Neural tube defects. *Pediatric Clinics of North America* (2004) **51:**389–419.

Levene MI, Chervenak FA, Whittle M (eds). *Fetal and Neonatal Neurology and Neurosurgery.* Edinburgh: Churchill Livingstone, 2001.

MRC Vitamin Study Research Group: Prevention of Neural Tube Defects. Results of the Medical Research Council Vitamin Study. *Lancet* (1991) **338:**131–7.

Volpe JJ. *Neurology of the Newborn*, 4th edn. Philadelphia: WB Saunders, 2001.

Related topics of interest

- congenital malformations and birth defects
- hydrocephalus
- prenatal diagnosis.

Neurological evaluation

History

Often overlooked, the history is an important part of neonatal assessment. It includes:

- family history
- outcome of previous pregnancies
- current pregnancy and mode of delivery
- evidence of foetal distress, Apgar scores, and cord-blood pH
- behaviour prior to examination, especially fits, jitteriness, and feeding difficulties.

Clinical examination

This assesses four main areas:

- tone
- behaviour
- 'automatic' or 'primitive' responses
- conventional signs as elicited in older children.

Tone

This is the resistance of muscles to stretch. It is generally lower when the baby is asleep. Passive tone is reflected in the posture of a baby. Active tone is elicited by manoeuvres such as pulling to sit from a supine position (head-lag), and in the resistance to stretching of a flexed limb. Healthy, full-term neonates lie in a flexed posture, with the hips flexed and adducted, and and the knees flexed so that the legs are drawn up under the body. The shoulders are adducted, and the elbows flexed. This posture persists for a week or so after birth before flexor tone diminishes. Preterm babies have lower tone, so the tight flexion is not seen: the very preterm baby lies with arms and legs abducted and extended.

The normal active tone of an alert term baby will enable him briefly to hold his head in line with the body during 'pull to sit' and ventral suspension manoeuvres. The degree of recoil when a limb is extended is also a useful sign of tone. As tone varies with gestational age, it is used in gestational age assessment. Conversely, it is important to know the gestation of a baby in order to assess the appropriateness of a baby's tone when neurologic compromise is suspected.

Primitive reflexes

These are complex responses present in newborns, but then diminishing and disappearing. Persistence beyond the normal age suggests that the higher cortical centres are not gaining control of tone and movement as expected, and can, for example, be an early sign of cerebral palsy.

- The Moro (startle) reflex is elicited by gently dropping the head of a baby from one hand into the palm of the other some 5 cm below. The full reflex shows abduction and extension of the arms with hand opening followed by adduction and extension of the arms over the chest with hand closure. It wanes rapidly after 1–2 months and is abnormal if it persists at all beyond six months. The Moro reflex is often absent in preterm babies.

- Primitive walking is elicited by holding an alert baby vertically with the feet firmly in contact with a flat surface and leaning him slightly forwards. It has usually disappeared by 4–6 weeks. It can also be started through a 'placing reaction' in which the dorsum of the baby's foot is brought up against the underside of a tabletop. The baby then raises the foot and places it on the table, and may then begin primitive walking.
- The asymmetric tonic neck reflex is most marked at 2–4 months and may not be easily elicited in the newborn. The head is turned to one side to elicit extension of the arm on that side with some extension of the ipsilateral leg. It has usually disappeared by 6–7 months.
- The palmar grasp disappears by eight weeks, to be replaced by voluntary grasp 6–8 weeks later, as cortical control develops.
- Rooting persists until 3–4 months, after which visual cues predominate in the normal baby, who will recognise the breast or the bottle and move towards them, but no longer root and suck on a finger placed at the corner of the mouth.

Conventional signs

These include:

- Maximum head circumference and examination of the head shape, sutures, and fontanelles.
- Eye examination that must include eliciting a 'red reflex'. The light of an ophthalmoscope reflected from the red retina is absent in congenital cataracts and retinoblastomas. This examination may also detect colobomata of the iris. Corneal haziness can be caused by oedema in congenital glaucoma (buphthalmos), which needs immediate referral to an ophthalmologist. In the very preterm baby, the lens remains vascularised up to 32 weeks, and this may initially prevent the red reflex. In any case, such a baby should be seen by an ophthalmologist for retinopathy screening. Given time, sophisticated assessment of a baby's eyes and visual behaviour can be achieved, but at routine neonatal examination the one thing that *must* be checked is the red reflex. Missed cataracts can lead to permanent reductions of visual acuity if they are removed too late.
- Gross movements of the limb should be noted during examination. Knee and biceps jerks are easily elicited; the others less so. Isolated sustained clonus at the ankles can occur in jittery babies. Plantar reflexes are variable. Responses should be symmetrical. Asymmetry may indicate a unilateral peripheral nerve palsy or unilateral brain damage, though the signs of the latter can be very subtle in a newborn baby.

Behaviour

This is important, and not just during examination. These responses have been quantified by a number of workers, including Brazelton, who produced a Neonatal Behavioural Assessment Scale, which includes the arousal sequence described below. Use of these scales requires training, experience, and patience on the part of the neonatologist. If approached when asleep the normal term infant may progress through the following steps:

1. being deeply asleep with eyes closed, regular breathing, and no movements, to
2. light sleep with rapid eye movements, some random movements, and irregular breathing, onto
3. a drowsy state with eyes open and small movements, to
4. being alert, looking bright, and having minimal movements, and then to
5. grosser movements with fussing, and finally into
6. crying.

At the correct state of arousal and with some patience on the part of the examiner, a term baby will fix and follow an interesting object, such as a face or a brightly coloured ball, though following up to eight weeks postterm does not depend on an intact visual cortex. Babies will also respond to sound. Abnormal neurological signs can be elicited in babies with HIE, PVL, and IVHs. These detailed and sometimes subtle signs again require particular expertise to elicit, and tend not to be used regularly by clinicians, particularly for PVL and IVH, which can be more readily detected by ultrasound scanning.

In addition to history and clinical examination, a number of techniques can contribute to the neurological evaluation of a newborn baby:

- ultrasound scanning of the brain
- computerised tomography (CT scan)
- MRI, including diffusion-weighted and perfusion MR imaging
- magnetic resonance spectroscopy (^{31}P- and ^{1}H-MR spectroscopy)
- EEG
- auditory evoked brainstem responses
- visual evoked responses.

Further reading

Brazelton TB. *Neonatal Behavioural Assessment Scale*, 2nd edn. London: Spastics International Medical Publications, 1962.

Dubowitz LMS. *The Neurological Assessment of the Preterm and Full-term Infant*, 2nd edn. Clinics in Developmental Medicine, No. 148, Cambridge: Cambridge University Press, 1998.

Levene MI, Chervenak FA, Whittle M (eds). *Fetal and Neonatal Neurology and Neurosurgery*. Edinburgh: Churchill Livingstone, 2001.

Paneth N, Rudelli R, Kazam E et al (eds). *Brain Damage in the Preterm Infant*. Clinics in Developmental Medicine, No. 131. London: MacKeith Press, 1994.

Volpe JJ. *Neurology of the Newborn*, 4th edn. Philadelphia: WB Saunders, 2001.

Related topics of interest

- childbirth complications and foetal outcome
- germinal matrix-intraventricular haemorrhage
- hypotonia
- hypoxic-ischaemic encephalopathy
- neuromuscular disorders—muscular
- neuromuscular disorders—neurological
- periventricular leucomalacia
- postnatal examination
- seizures.

Neuromuscular disorders—muscular

Congenital muscular dystrophy (CMD)

Congenital muscular dystrophies (CMDs) are autosomal recessive muscle disorders, which may be classified into two major groups depending on the association with structural brain anomalies. CMDs without structural CNS anomalies (the 'classic' or 'occidental' CMDs) form a heterogeneous group of disorders. In those with associated structural CNS anomalies, eye involvement and neurological abnormalities are common. In CMDs, the muscle biopsy is abnormal, though no unique identifying features exist.

CMDs without structural CNS anomalies

- These can now be subclassified on the basis of merosin (laminin α_2-chain) staining. The merosin gene maps to chromosome 6q22.
- The merosin-negative subgroup is more severely affected clinically, with peripheral nerve involvement, associated hypomyelination of brain white matter on cranial MRI scans, and relatively high serum CPKs. Most patients will be unable to walk, in contrast to merosin-positive patients, most of whom will walk.
- Both subgroups can present in the neonatal period with weakness, hypotonia, raised CPK, and joint contractures.
- Diagnosis is made from EMG, nerve conduction studies, elevated CPK, muscle biopsy and merosin staining, and cranial CT or MRI.

CMDs with structural CNS anomalies

Fukuyama muscular dystrophy
- The most common form of the CMDs with brain anomalies, mainly found in Japan.
- Inheritance is autosomal recessive, and the gene locus is on chromosome 9q31–33.
- At birth, there is hypotonia, generalised weakness, joint contractures, depressed deep tendon reflexes, microcephaly with neurodevelopmental delay, convulsions (50%), and raised CPK.
- Death occurs by age ten years.

Walker–Warburg syndrome
- This is predominantly inherited as an autosomal recessive trait.
- There is weakness, hypotonia, macrocephaly, hydrocephaly, and eye abnormalities.
- CNS malformations include lissencephaly, cerebellar hypoplasia, Dandy–Walker malformation, hydrocephalus, absent corpus callosum, and heterotopia.
- Most patients die in early infancy.

Muscle-eye-brain disease
- Inheritance is autosomal recessive.
- The disorder is similar to Walker–Warburg syndrome, though the phenotype is milder.
- The symptoms include early hypotonia, delayed development, seizures, hydrocephalus, and eye involvement (optic atrophy, retinal dysplasia, and progressive visual failure).
- Death occurs between six and 16 years.

Congenital myotonic dystrophy

This autosomal-dominant, multisystem disorder is the most prevalent form (five per 100000) of muscular dystrophy that is inherited almost exclusively from mothers.

- Severe neonatal disease is associated with polyhydramnios, poor foetal movements, and premature delivery.
- The clinical features include hypotonia, talipes, poor respiratory function, impaired sucking and swallowing, 'tented upper lip', facial weakness, ptosis, dilation of cerebral ventricles, and moderate intellectual impairment.
- Mortality is high (up to 50%).
- The milder form is nonlethal and so can occur in all age groups, and initial hypotonia resolves.
- Management is supportive; prolonged ventilation may be required.
- Always examine mothers for myotonia or weakness of distal muscles and neck flexors.
- Diagnosis is by DNA assay for a trinucleotide CTG repeat located in the 3′ untranslated region of a gene coding for myotonin protein kinase on chromosome 19q13.3. Disease severity is related to the length of the expansion, with normals having up to 37 repeats; mildly affected individuals or asymptomatic mutation 'carriers' 50–99 repeats; and the severely affected ('full mutation') individuals, 100 to ≥2000 repeats. Disease severity increases in successive generations (the phenomenon of genetic anticipation).
- Prenatal diagnosis is possible.

Congenital myopathies

These disorders are characterised by hypotonia and weakness at birth, with scoliosis, ptosis, and ophthalmoplegia often developing in late infancy/early childhood. In general, congenital myopathies have distinctive muscle biopsy findings, their names reflecting their myopathological features. In contrast, the muscle biopsy findings are dystrophic and nonspecific in congenital muscular dystrophies. The CPK is normal or slightly raised (moderately or markedly raised in congenital muscular dystrophies). The main disorders are as follows:

Nemaline myopathy
Muscle biopsy is diagnostic (characteristic nemaline bodies).

Central core disease (autosomal dominant)
Chromosome 19q13.1 is implicated, and muscle biopsy is diagnostic (central cores evident).

Centronuclear/myotubular myopathy
The most common type (the neonatal form) is X-linked. It has severe symptoms and a very high mortality, with muscle biopsy showing central nuclei and type 1 fibre predominance. The myotubularin gene (locus Xq28) is implicated.

Metabolic myopathies

Pompe's disease (infantile acid maltase deficiency or glycogen storage disease II)
Acid maltase releases glucose from glycogen, oligosaccharides, and maltose. Absence leads to glycogen storage. This autosomal recessive disorder presents in the first three months of life with rapidly progressive weakness, hypotonia, and enlargement of liver, heart, and tongue. CNS glycogen storage causes hyporeflexia and diminished alertness. Feeding and respiratory difficulties are common, and so is death before the age of two years. Diagnosis is by assaying acid maltase activity in muscle, lymphocytes, or urine. Muscle biopsy shows large vacuoles full of glycogen (PAS-positive) and strongly reactive to acid phosphatase. The gene defect maps to chromosome 17q23. There is no therapy.

Cytochrome c oxidase deficiency
At least two forms are recognisable, benign infantile myopathy and fatal infantile myopathy. Fatal infantile myopathy presents soon after birth with severe lactic acidosis, marked weakness, hypotonia, and respiratory and feeding difficulties. Most affected infants die before the age of one year. Muscle biopsy and histochemistry show ragged-red fibres with lipid and glycogen accumulation, and no cytochrome oxidase activity. The benign form is distinguished from the fatal form by immunological detection of the enzyme by enzyme-linked immunosorbent assay (ELISA) in muscle tissue (enzyme protein is absent in the fatal form).

Fatty acid oxidation defects
These disorders include the carnitine deficiency syndromes and fatty acid oxidation enzyme defects, which generally present in infancy with generalised weakness, hypotonia, lethargy, or coma. Muscle biopsy shows lipid accumulation and enzymatic deficiency in muscle tissue or cultured skin fibroblasts.

Mitochondrial myopathies

These are multisystem disorders with growth failure, muscle fatigue with exercise, myopathic facies, microcephaly, mental retardation, myoclonic seizures, ataxia, and stroke-like episodes. Fluctuating neurologic abnormalities are characteristic. The inheritance pattern is maternal (maternal transmission of mitochondrial DNA).

Nonlysosomal glycogenoses

Phosphofructokinase deficiency
Diagnosis is by muscle biopsy with immunohistochemistry (glycogen deposition, absence of phosphofructokinase), and enzyme assays (diminished muscle phosphofructokinase activity).

Phosphorylase deficiency
Muscle biopsy and immunohistochemistry are diagnostic (myopathic changes, glycogen deposition, and absent phosphorylase activity).

Prader–Willi syndrome

- This syndrome presents with profound hypotonia at birth, feeding difficulties necessitating tube feeding, but no respiratory difficulties.
- The cry is weak and high pitched.
- Facies are characteristic with a high forehead, dolichocephalic head, small almond-shaped eyes, open triangular mouth, fair hair, and blue eyes. Also characteristic are small hands and feet.
- Hypotonia gradually improves, and the infants achieve independent mobility after the age of two years.
- There is a tendency to gross generalised obesity after the child starts walking.
- Males have undescended testes and rudimentary scrotum, and are infertile.
- There is intellectual impairment with IQ in the low normal to mildly retarded range.

Diagnosis

Although the karyotype appears normal, specific DNA probes reveal in most cases a deletion of the proximal arm of the paternally inherited chromosome 15 (15q11–13). Most cases are sporadic. Patients without the deletion (15–20% of cases) have two copies of the maternal chromosome and no paternal contribution (an example of maternal disomy or genomic imprinting). These can be isodisomic, where the child receives two copies of the same autosome, or heterodisomic, where the child receives a pair of autosomes from a single parent. Infants with Angelman's syndrome have a similar deletion (15q11–13) but involving the maternal contribution, and those without the deletion may be disomic for the paternal chromosome.

Further reading

Darras BT. Neuromuscular disorders in the newborn. *Clinics in Perinatology* (1997) **24:**827–44.
Dubowitz V. *The Floppy Infant*, 2nd edn. Clinics in Developmental Medicine, No. 76. Cambridge: Cambridge University Press, 1980.
Dubowitz V. *Muscle Disorders in Childhood*, 2nd edn. London: WB Saunders, 1995.
Rosenberg RN, Pruiser SB, DiMauro S et al. *The Molecular and Genetic Basis of Neurological Disease*. Stoneham, MA: Butterworth-Heinemann, 1993.

Related topics of interest

- feeding difficulties
- hypotonia
- neurological evaluation
- neuromuscular disorders—neurological.

Neuromuscular disorders—neurological

Neuromuscular disease in the newborn period is uncommon and often presents a major diagnostic challenge. As weakness is one of the primary presentations of neuro-muscular disorders, it is useful to go through the exercise of determining whether the weakness is primarily due to a 'peripheral' neuromuscular disorder or a primary central neurological disorder. Primary neuromuscular disorders are often associated with a normal level of consciousness, decreased or normal tendon reflexes, poor limb recoil, and minor dysmorphic features or congenital anomalies, whereas central neu-rological disorders have associated decreased consciousness, seizures, cranial nerve signs, normal or brisk reflexes, strong limb recoil, a tendency for muscle tone to improve with time, and major congenital anomalies. Inquiry into the family history (including consanguinity, delayed milestones, and childhood deaths) is most import-ant. Polyhydramnios, decreased foetal movements, breech presentation, abnormal labour, and birth asphyxia also suggest neuromuscular disease. Inquire from the mother and examine for signs of myotonic dystrophy or myasthenia gravis.

Clinical features

- Reduced tone, power, and muscle bulk.
- Myotonia, fasciculations, facial diplegia, and ptosis.
- Examine parents (for example, for myotonia and easy muscle fatigue in mother) with myotonic dystrophy and myasthenia gravis.
- Common congenital anomalies include micrognathia, prominent forehead, high-arched palate, undescended testes, congenital dislocation of the hips, scoliosis, and contractures.

Investigations

Biochemical

- creatine phosphokinase (CPK)—elevated with skeletal and cardiac muscle damage; may need to assay CPK isoenzyme levels to distinguish between brain, cardiac, and muscle
- aspartate aminotransferase (AST)—persistently elevated in neuromuscular disor-ders with liver involvement, as in Pompe's disease
- CSF—raised CSF protein in peripheral nerve disease
- serum lactate—raised in mitochondrial cytopathies.

Genetic

An increasing number of recognised gene deletions may be detected by molecular genetic techniques which also enable prenatal diagnosis to be made. DNA may be extracted and stored for future genetic analysis.

Imaging

- radiographs—thin ribs; cardiomegaly, as in metabolic cardiomyopathy

- cranial CT/MRI/ultrasound—brain malformation as in cerebral dysgenesis and decreased white matter in congenital muscular dystrophy; dilated ventricles in congenital myotonic dystrophy
- muscle ultrasound—assessing muscle bulk; adipose or connective tissue infiltration increases muscle echogenicity.

Neurophysiology
- nerve conduction velocity—diminished in peripheral neuropathy
- electromyogram (EMG)—assesses intrinsic muscle electrical activity (for example, shows fibrillation in peripheral neuropathy and anterior horn cell disease, and fasciculations in anterior horn cell disease). Maternal electrophysiology studies may be more informative than the infant's (as in myotonic dystrophy and myasthenia gravis).

Histopathology
Needle and open muscle biopsy for immunohistochemistry and electron microscopy may give definitive diagnosis.

Management

Supportive care is required—supplemental oxygen, assisted ventilation, prevention of contractures by physiotherapy, and nasogastric tube feeding. Prolonged assisted ventilation, prematurity, and multiple congenital anomalies are associated with poor outcome.

Anterior horn cell disease

Spinal muscular atrophies (SMA)
The three clinical variants are based on rate of progression and age at onset of disease:

1. acute spinal muscular atrophy, SMA type I, or Werdnig–Hoffmann disease
2. intermediate SMA or SMA type II
3. chronic SMA, SMA type III, or Kugelberg–Welander disease.

After cystic fibrosis, SMA is the second commonest lethal autosomal recessive disorder, with an incidence of one in 6000 births.

In SMA type 1, there is progressive, severe degeneration of anterior horn cells in spinal cord and cranial nerve motor nuclei. The clinical features are diminished foetal movements, respiratory distress at birth, alertness, paradoxical respiratory movements, and frog-leg position, with contractures being uncommon. Cranial nerve involvement results in impaired sucking and swallowing with atrophy and fasciculations of the tongue. Examination shows hypotonia, areflexia, and weakness affecting the lower extremities, earlier and more severely than the upper extremities and proximal muscles more than distal ones. As the disease advances, there is paralysis of the bulbar muscles, loss of the cough reflex, and an inaudible cry. EMG shows spontaneous fasciculations and fibrillations. CPK is normal or mildly to moderately elevated (up to five times upper limit of normal). There is rapid deterioration and respiratory death in the first two years of life.

All three types of autosomal-recessive SMA have been mapped to a single locus on chromosome 5q11.2–13.3 with preferential deletion of two genes, the survival motor neuron and the neuronal apoptosis inhibitory protein gene. Prenatal and postnatal genetic diagnosis is therefore now possible. Current treatment of SMA type 1 is supportive only, given the poor prognosis. Most patients with SMA types II and III are normal at birth and usually sit unsupported (but never stand), death occurring after age two years (SMA type II) or adulthood (SMA type III).

Peripheral nerve disease

Examples include giant axonal neuropathy, inflammatory neuropathies, metabolic neuropathies (Leigh's disease), and sensory neuropathies (such as congenital sensory neuropathy) characterised by hypotonia and generalised weakness, more pronounced distally with absent tendon reflexes. Cranial nerve and respiratory muscle involvement, feeding difficulties, and joint contractures are common. CSF protein may be raised. CSF and plasma lactate are raised in Leigh's disease. Muscle biopsy shows denervation.

Neuromuscular junction disorders

Transient neonatal myasthenia gravis

This develops in 15% of infants of mothers with myasthenia gravis. Maternal anti-acetylcholine receptor antibodies or immunocytes cross the placenta, and symptomatic infants may also synthesise acetylcholine receptor antibodies. Clinical features are severe hypotonia (69%), weak suck, dysphagia, ptosis (50%), ophthalmoplegia, and respiratory failure (65%). Diagnosis is confirmed by demonstrating high serum concentration of acetylcholine receptor antibody in newborn infants and reversal of symptoms with edrophonium chloride (Tensilon test)—0.04–0.15 mg/kg i.m. or s.c. injection (preferred route) or 0.04 mg/kg IV. Clinical improvement is evident within minutes and lasts 10–15 min. Exchange transfusion may be helpful in severe cases. For treatment, use pyridostigmine (5–10 mg orally, four-hourly) or neostigmine (1–5 mg orally, four-hourly).

Congenital myasthenic syndromes

These can be classified according to the site of the defect, that is, presynaptic (familial infantile myasthenia, autosomal recessive), postsynaptic or synaptic (congenital end-plate acetylcholinesterase deficiency, autosomal recessive; classic slow-channel syndrome, autosomal dominant; congenital acetylcholine receptor deficiency, autosomal recessive), or mixed. Presenting symptoms in infancy include fluctuating weakness, weak cry and suck, generalised hypotonia, respiratory distress, and feeding difficulties. Tests for antiacetylcholine receptor antibodies are negative. The Tensilon test is positive except in the classic slow-channel syndrome and in congenital end-plate acetylcholinesterase deficiency. The diagnosis is based on history and examination, EMG studies, the Tensilon test, response to acetylcholinesterase inhibitors, and muscle biopsy. Long-term treatment with neostigmine or pyridostigmine may be used if the Tensilon test is positive.

Metabolic and toxic junction disorders

Hypermagnesaemia from therapy with magnesium sulphate for maternal eclampsia may produce severe weakness, apnoea, bulbar dysfunction, and autonomic dysfunction. Aminoglycosides may produce a very similar picture.

Infantile botulism

Infants are normal at birth but develop symptoms between the ages of ten days and six months. This results from intestinal absorption of ingested *Clostridium botulinum* toxin. Clinical features include marked weakness, hypotonia, absent reflexes, bulbar dysfunction, ophthalmoplegia, constipation, and respiratory insufficiency. Examination reveals diffuse hypotonia and weakness, ptosis, mydriasis, reduced gag reflex, and preservation of deep tendon reflexes. Diagnosis is by culturing *C. botulinum* from stools, and EMG shows increasing response to repetitive nerve stimulation. Respiratory support and antitoxin therapy may be required. Symptoms last 2–6 weeks.

Further reading

Darras BT. Neuromuscular disorders in the newborn. *Clinics in Perinatology* (1997) **24:**827–44.

Dubowitz V. *The Floppy Infant*, 2nd edn. Clinics in Developmental Medicine No. 76. Cambridge: Cambridge University Press, 1980.

Dubowitz V. *Muscle Disorders in Childhood*, 2nd edn. London: WB Saunders, 1995.

Rosenberg RN, Pruiser SB, DiMauro S et al. *The Molecular and Genetic Basis of Neurological Disease*. Stoneham, MA: Butterworth-Heinemann, 1993.

Related topics of interest

- feeding difficulties
- hypotonia
- neurological evaluation
- neuromuscular disorders—muscular.

Nitric oxide therapy

The discovery of nitric oxide (NO) as an endogenous biological mediator and the elucidation of its biological roles has been one of the most significant recent developments in medicine. NO is now recognised to be involved in the physiology of almost every life form and organ system, being involved in functions as diverse as central and autonomic neurotransmission, hormonal release, bacterial cell killing, platelet inhibition, and smooth muscle relaxation. Of particular interest to the care of newborns is the role of NO in smooth muscle relaxation.

NO and vascular biology

Vascular endothelial cells synthesise NO from the amino acid L-arginine and oxygen by the enzyme NO synthase (NOS). The released NO, a lipophilic molecule, travels freely through cell membranes and can act on the neighbouring vascular smooth muscle cells immediately beneath them. Within the vascular smooth muscle, NO binds to the enzyme, soluble guanylate cyclase (sGC), stimulating it to produce cyclic guanylate monophosphate (cGMP) from guanosine triphosphate. cGMP activates protein kinases and leads ultimately to the dephosphorylation of myosin light chains and muscle relaxation. Any NO released from the abluminal surface of the endothelial cell into the bloodstream is rapidly bound to haemoglobin and converted to nitrate, which is finally excreted in urine.

NO in the perinatal period

- NO mediates the normal pulmonary vascular adaptation at birth.
- Inhibition of endogenous NO synthesis results in the failure of the postnatal pulmonary vascular adaptation and the development of PPHN.
- Hypoxia and pulmonary hypertension, which characterise PPHN, inhibit release of endogenous NO.
- A lower synthetic rate of NO has been reported during the acute phase of PPHN, and, L-arginine, a substrate for NO synthesis, may be deficient in some infants with PPHN.
- Inhaled NO therapy therefore circumvents a deficiency in the two substrates for NO synthesis, oxygen and L-arginine, and supplies the vasodilator directly to the pulmonary vasculature.
- Inhaled NO is effective in reversing the hypoxaemia due to PPHN.
- Infants with congenital heart disease and pulmonary vascular disease have endothelial dysfunction and impaired endogenous NO production manifest as pulmonary hypertension. This is responsive to inhaled NO therapy.
- Inhaled NO therapy has become the therapy of choice in disorders characterised by PPHN.

Advantages of inhaled NO over intravenous vasodilators

- selective pulmonary vasodilation without systemic hypotensive effects
- improves ventilation-perfusion matching (may be made worse by IV vasodilators)
- vasodilatory effect rapidly instituted and terminated (onset of pulmonary vasodilation may be slow with IV agents, and any systemic hypotensive effects profound and slow to reverse, especially with tolazoline).

Disadvantages of inhaled NO therapy

- cost of administration equipment and, more recently, the gas itself, following the granting of a patent to the suppliers
- equipment may not be readily portable—problems with transferring infants receiving treatment (for example, to ECMO centre) if portable NO administration equipment is not available
- dependence on NO, even in the absence of obvious beneficial effect
- undefined NO toxicology profile in newborns, both in the short term and long term
- considerable expertise required to administer the therapy safely
- potential toxicity to attendant medical and nursing staff.

Administration of inhaled NO

The following requirements must be met:

- Reliable equipment is on hand to monitor continuously the concentration of administered NO and NO_2.
- The duration of contact and mixing between NO and the administered oxygen before inhalation by the patient is minimal (sufficient to allow adequate mixing of NO and O_2, but not the excessive oxidation of NO to NO_2).
- NO and NO_2 are scavenged from the exhaust gases to avoid environmental contamination.
- Full intensive care monitoring and support exist, including blood methaemoglobin measurement.
- Adequate environmental and safety checks are in place.
- Staff administering NO therapy must be familiar with the equipment, the safe administration and monitoring of NO therapy, and the potential adverse effects.

Clinical applications for inhaled NO

- PPHN of any cause, including CHD
- conditions characterised by ventilation-perfusion mismatch with or without PPHN:
  —pneumonia
  —paediatric acute respiratory distress syndrome (ARDS)
  —respiratory distress syndrome
  —aspiration syndromes (MAS, blood, and vomitus)
  —CLD (acute deteriorations, as with pneumonia).

Evidence for the efficacy of inhaled NO

To date, over 12 randomised trials involving over 1000 term or near-term infants have been completed. ECMO use was decreased in the NO-treated groups (one fewer ECMO patient for every six patients treated with NO). However, up to 40% of infants failed to respond to NO.

- Inhaled NO improves outcome in hypoxic term or near-term infants ($\geq$34 weeks' gestation) by reducing the incidence of the need for ECMO (mortality is not reduced).
- Inhaled NO has been demonstrated to improve survival and reduce the incidence of CLD in preterm infants. The incidence of intracranial and pulmonary haemorrhages is not altered by the use of inhaled NO.
- Inhaled NO was an effective therapy for the pulmonary hypertensive crises which complicate surgery for congenital heart disease. However, formal prospective, randomised controlled trials are awaited.
- Inhaled NO has not been demonstrated to improve the outcome (or reduce mortality) in neonatal and paediatric ARDS, congenital diaphragmatic hernia (CDH), or CLD.

Clinical notes

- As NO inhibits platelet aggregation, NO therapy may be inappropriate in haemorrhagic disorders (such as recent severe IVH or pulmonary haemorrhage). However, inhaled NO does not increase the incidence of pulmonary or intracranial haemorrhages.
- The efficacy of NO is independent of the baseline oxygenation index (OI) and the primary pulmonary diagnosis except for infants with CDH, whose outcome is not improved.
- The clinical response to NO is most dramatic in those with the most severe hypoxaemia, and whether the infants have clear evidence of PPHN or not does not affect the outcome.
- A starting dose of 10 ppm in infants of <34 weeks' gestation and 20 ppm in older infants is probably optimal. If there is no response to 40 ppm NO, further increments in the dose are unlikely to produce a response.
- Once a satisfactory response has been obtained, gradually wean the NO dose to the lowest effective dose (maintenance therapy may be possible with 1 ppm or less).
- Final weaning of inhaled NO is likely to succeed when the administered NO concentration is <5 ppm, the OI is $\leq$5, or the FiO_2 is $\leq$0.45. Weaning may be further facilitated by the coadministration of IV prostacyclin (10 ng/kg per min), dipyridamole (0.4 mg/kg per min over 10 min, three doses repeated 12-hourly), or sildenafil (0.3–1 mg/kg 6-hourly).
- On average, responders to NO require treatment for a total of under seven days.
- Monitor methaemoglobin levels at least daily (normal level under 2%). Reduce the NO dose if methaemoglobin levels exceed 2% and treat methaemoglobinaemia with IV methylthioninium chloride.

- Prescribing NO on a drug treatment chart encourages adherence to the treatment regimen.
- Providing a local policy and/or guidelines facilitates the safe administration of NO by all members of staff.
- NO therapy is more effective when administered by HFOV than with conventional ventilation.

Further reading

Barrington KJ, Finer NN. Inhaled nitric oxide for respiratory failure in preterm infants. *Cochrane Database Systematic Reviews* (2001) (4):CD000509.

Dobyns EL, Cornfield DN, Anas NG et al. Multicenter randomised controlled trial of the effects of inhaled nitric oxide therapy on gas exchange in children with acute hypoxemic respiratory failure. *Journal of Pediatrics* (1999) **134:**406–12.

Edwards AD. The pharmacology of inhaled nitric oxide. *Archives of Disease in Childhood* (1995) **72:**F127–30.

Finer NN, Barrington KJ. Nitric oxide for respiratory failure in infants born at or near term. *Cochrane Database Systematic Reviews* (2001) (4):CD000399.

Mupanemunda RH, Edwards AD. Treatment of newborn infants with inhaled nitric oxide. *Archives of Disease in Childhood* (1995) **72:**F131–4.

Schreiber MD, Gin-Mestan K, Marks JD, et al. Inhaled nitric oxide in premature infants with the respiratory distress syndrome. *New England Journal of Medicine* (2003) **349:**2099–107.

Sokol J, Jacobs SE, Bohn D. Inhaled nitric oxide for acute hypoxemic respiratory failure in children and adults. *Cochrane Database Systematic Reviews* (2003) (1):CD002787.

Zapol WM, Bloch KD (eds). *Nitric Oxide and the Lung.* New York: Marcel Dekker, 1996.

Related topics of interest

- congenital diaphragmatic hernia
- extracorporeal membrane oxygenation
- persistent pulmonary hypertension of the newborn
- mechanical ventilation
- meconium aspiration syndrome
- pulmonary hypoplasia

Nutrition

The provision of adequate oxygen, nutrition, and warmth to the vulnerable, small preterm infant forms the basis of modern neonatal medicine. A foetus in utero doubles its weight from 500 to 1000 g between 22 and 27 weeks, and in the following four weeks (27–31 weeks) acquires a further 500 g of weight, a rate of growth unmatched at any other time in the normal human life span. Achievement of similar growth rates for new VLBW infants presents a formidable nutritional challenge due to the relative inability of these infants to metabolise nutrients and excrete waste products. Furthermore, as the majority of energy and nutrient stores are laid down in the third trimester, preterm delivery puts the VLBW infant at considerable disadvantage. Nutritional goals for extremely preterm infants are therefore to supply energy nutrients not only to meet basic needs but also to promote growth. The optimal diet for preterm infants is one that supports growth at intrauterine rates but without imposing stress on the infants' immature metabolic and excretory functions.

Parental nutritional requirements

In the immediate postnatal period, the extremely preterm infant experiences marked tissue catabolism from stress, infection, and undernutrition, reflected by a 5–15% weight loss in the first week of life. Should the energy intake be increased beyond that required for maintenance, the infant starts gaining weight by the end of the first week of life, with birth weight being regained in 10–17 days.

- Energy intakes of 110–165 kcal/kg per day are required to meet maintenance energy needs and growth (100 ml/kg per day of 10% dextrose provides only 40 kcal/kg per day).
- Undernutrition affects pulmonary maturation, growth, immunity, long-term growth, and neurodevelopment.
- The plasma concentration of most amino acids falls precipitously within hours after birth if protein is not administered.
- Nutritional support should be commenced in the ELBW infant (or the sick, more mature infant) at the earliest opportunity.
- Delayed onset of IV nutrition (total parenteral nutrition [TPN]) is accompanied by a loss of endogenous protein of 0.5–1 g/kg per day.
- Early amino acid intake in ELBW infants reverses the nitrogen loss (as little as 1.15 g amino acid/kg per day with energy intake under 30 kcal/kg per day may improve nitrogen retention).
- As insulin secretion depends on the plasma concentration of certain amino acids (such as leucine and arginine), low plasma levels of amino acids not only limit protein metabolism but also predispose to hyperglycaemia (reduced glucose uptake secondary to reduced insulin secretion in response to low plasma concentration of the amino acids responsible for stimulating insulin).
- Commence TPN in ELBW as soon as is possible after birth if the infant is not receiving enteral feeds.

- The TPN content of proteins, lipids, carbohydrates, electrolytes, minerals, vitamins, and trace elements can be adjusted as the total amount of TPN administered and the duration of TPN administration increase. Maximum amounts of lipid and protein are 3 and 4 g/kg per day, respectively.
- Lipid emulsions should be given as a 20% solution, rather than 10%, as this results in lower plasma concentrations of phospholipid, cholesterol, and triglycerides.
- Certain nutritional deficiencies at this critical period in life may have a profound influence on the development of disease in later childhood and adulthood.

Administration and monitoring of parenteral nutrition

- Central venous catheters inserted percutaneously into a central position are preferable to peripheral vein infusions, which carry the risk of skin necrosis from extravasation of nutrient infused into subcutaneous tissue.
- Central venous catheters allow administration of hyperosmolar solutions (as when fluid volumes must be restricted with a symptomatic PDA) for prolonged periods.
- However, TPN administration via central venous catheters has several complications, including:
  —sepsis (*S. epidermidis*, *Candida*, and *Malassezia*)
  —cholestatic jaundice (10–14%)
  —cardiac arrhythmia
  —pleural effusion or chylothorax
  —intracardiac thrombi
  —pulmonary embolism
  —thrombosis of the major vessels in which catheter is placed
  —perforation of the inferior vena cava with abdominal ascites (TPN found when abdomen is drained).
  —cardiac tamponade (following perforation of the right atrial wall)
  —impaired immunity
  —cholelithiasis
- Regular biochemical monitoring is required (initially daily U and E and blood glucose with weekly liver-function tests, and then less frequently once the infant is in a steady metabolic state).

Initiation and advancement of enteral feeds

- Intraluminal nutrition is necessary for normal gastrointestinal structure and functional integrity.
- Enteral feeds have direct trophic effects and indirect effects secondary to release of intestinal hormones.
- The provision of minimal enteral feedings (trophic feedings) primes the gastrointestinal tract prior to more substantial enteral nutrition. This results in a reduction of feeding intolerance, earlier attainment of full enteral feeding, reduced levels of serum bilirubin, and a reduction in the incidence of cholestasis.
- Intermittent gavage feeds (nasogastric or orogastric) are a convenient way of safely providing enteral feedings to ELBW infants who are relatively stable.

- Gradually reduce TPN volumes as more feeds are tolerated enterally.
- Rapid advancement of enteral feeds (>20 ml/kg per day) is associated with increased risk of NEC.
- Infants may be fed with an indwelling umbilical artery catheter (UAC). This is *not* associated with an increased incidence of NEC.
- Mother's own milk is ideal food for the preterm or term infant. It is better tolerated and confers some immunological protection as well as neurodevelopmental advantages. If it is not available, donor breast milk may be used.

Breast versus formula feeds

- Whenever possible, breast milk should be used for feeding preterm infants, especially SGA and VLBW infants.
- The incidence of NEC may be up to six times greater in formula-fed infants.
- Observational studies suggest that breast-feeding may advantage the infant in cognitive and intellectual development compared to infants fed formula milk. This was evident at 18 months and 7.5–8 years even after adjusting for social and educational differences between groups. This advantage was related to being fed milk by tube in the neonatal period, and not with subsequent breast-feeding, and was dose-related to the proportion of breast milk consumed.
- Breast milk should be fortified when given to preterm infants, as this improves growth and bone mineral content.
- In the absence of breast milk, preterm formula should be used.
- Long-chain polyunsaturated fatty acids (LCP) may have important roles in brain and retinal development and are present in breast milk. Most infant formulas do not yet contain LCP, and addition of this should perhaps be recommended.
- Additional supplements of carbohydrate (such as Maxijul, SHS International, UK), or carbohydrate and fat (Duocal, SHS International) may be required in enterally fed infants when weight gain is poor.
- Breast-feeding is contraindicated if the mother has HIV infection or is taking certain medications (such as cytotoxics and illicit drugs).

Further reading

American Society for Parenteral and Enteral Nutrition: Guidelines for the Use of Parenteral and Enteral Nutrition in Adult and Pediatric Patients, Section VII: Nutrition support for Low-Birth-Weight Infants. *Journal of Parenteral and Enteral Nutrition* (1993) **17**:335A–495A.

Barker DJP. *Mothers, Babies and Health in Later Life*, 2nd edn. Edinburgh: Churchill Livingstone, 1998.

Cooke RJ (ed.). Neonatal nutrition. *Seminars in Neonatology* (2001) **6**(5).

Cowett R (ed.). Nutrition and metabolism in the micropremie. *Clinics in Perinatology* (2000) **2**(1).

Morgan JB, Dickerson JWT (eds). *Nutrition in Early Life*. Indianapolis, IN: Wiley, 2003.

Schanler RJ (ed.). Breastfeeding 2001. I. The evidence for breastfeeding. *Pediatric Clinics of North America* (2001) **48**(1).

Tsang RC, Lucas A, Uauy R et al (eds). *Nutritional Needs of the Preterm Infant: Scientific Basis and Practical Guidelines*. Baltimore, MD: Williams & Wilkins, 1993.

Ziegler EE, Thureen PJ, Carlson SJ. Aggressive nutrition of the very low birthweight infant. *Clinics in Perinatology* (2002) **29**:225–44.

Related topics of interest

- breast-feeding
- feeding difficulties
- fluid and electrolyte therapy
- gastrooesophageal reflux
- necrotising enterocolitis
- trace elements and vitamins.

Oesophageal anomalies

Oesophageal atresia and tracheooesophageal fistula

Oesophageal atresia (OA) and tracheooesophageal fistula (TOF) are due to a failure of early embryonic differentiation of the oesophagus and trachea. At least five types are recognised, the commonest being oesophageal atresia with distal tracheooesophageal fistula (87%). Oesophageal atresia without fistula is the second commonest type (8%), followed by the 'H' type TOF (4%).

OA presents with excessive dribbling of saliva and episodes of cyanosis and respiratory distress on the first day of life. The lack of foetal swallowing during the pregnancy usually causes polyhydramnios, and this in turn may cause preterm labour and delivery. The diagnosis is confirmed by failure to pass a nasogastric tube into the stomach. Radiographs of the chest and abdomen will show the tube lodged in the blind end of the upper oesophageal pouch. At least 85% of babies with OA have a TOF. Usually, this connects with the lower oesophagus, and so air enters the stomach and may cause distension. The incidence is approximately 1:3500. Familial occurrence is infrequent.

Clinical features

Respiratory distress results from airway obstruction by secretions, aspiration of secretions or milk into the lungs, or a distended abdomen. When OA occurs without a TOF, or with one that connects with the upper pouch, no air enters the abdomen, which is then scaphoid rather than distended. There may be associated abnormalities of the *v*ertebrae, an imperforate *a*nus, *t*racheo*o*esophageal fistula, and *r*enal abnormalities to constitute the acronymic VATER syndrome. Infants who have an 'H'-type TOF, but no oesophageal atresia, usually present after the neonatal period with frequent lower respiratory infections and/or respiratory difficulties during feeds. Cinefluoroscopy and bronchoscopy/oesophagoscopy reveal the fistula.

Management

Prior to surgery, the infant is best nursed head-up at 45°, and the oesophagus is aspirated either with a multiple end-hole suction catheter (Replogle), or by aspirating a wide-bore NG tube every 5 min. If possible, ventilation should be avoided, as it can cause excessive gastric distension.

The operation of choice is a primary end-to-end anastomosis as soon as the baby is stable. A nasogastric silastic feeding tube is passed through the anastomosis at the time of surgery. This NG tube must be very secure; another cannot be passed postoperatively for fear of damaging the anastomosis. Postoperative nutrition is initially parenteral, but as the bowel recovers, enteral feeding can be started slowly. Prior to commencing oral feeds, a barium swallow is performed to check the integrity of the anastomosis.

When primary anastomosis cannot be achieved, a gastrostomy is created for decompression and feeding, and to allow intermittent insertion of a bougie to stretch the lower oesophageal pouch. The upper pouch can also be stretched intermittently. An oesophagostomy is created in the neck to allow external drainage of the saliva and allow sham feeding. In time, end-to-end anastomosis can be achieved.

Complications

Postoperative complications include stenosis of the circumferential oesophageal scar: this is treated by dilation. A persistent, brassy 'TOF-cough' may persist for years and is due to the abnormalities of the trachea. These infants may be especially difficult to feed, particularly if a long period elapses without oral feeds. Gastrooesophageal reflux is common and requires medical and sometimes surgical therapy. The anastomosis may also break down with recurrence of the fistula.

Family support group and information

Tracheo-Oesophageal Fistula Support
St George's Centre
91 Victoria Road
Netherfield
Nottingham NG4 2NN, UK
Tel 0115 961 3092
www.tofs.org.uk

Further reading

Ein SH, Shandling B. Pure esophageal atresia: a 50 year review. *Journal of Pediatric Surgery* (1994) **29:**1208–11.
O'Neill JA Jr, Rowe MI, Grosfeld JL et al. *Pediatric Surgery*, 5th edn. St Louis, MO: Mosby, 1998.
Puri P (ed.). *Newborn Surgery*, 2nd edn. London: Arnold, 2003.
Stringer MD, Oldham KT, Mouriquand PDE et al. *Pediatric Surgery and Urology: Long-Term Outcomes*. Philadelphia: WB Saunders, 1998.

Related topics of interest

- congenital malformations and birth defects
- feeding difficulties
- gastrooesophageal reflux
- neonatal surgery.

Orthopaedic problems

Developmental dysplasia of the hip (DDH)

Although its strict definition is 'a partial or complete displacement of the femoral head from the acetabulum', the term 'developmental dysplasia of the hip (DDH)' is now used to embrace a spectrum of abnormalities embracing dislocation, subluxation, and even dysplasias. Congenital hip instability is found in 15–20 per 1000 babies. Most of these resolve spontaneously. Unscreened and untreated, about one in 1000 babies go on to develop a dislocated hip. Risk factors include:

- female sex
- a family history
- breech presentation
- neuromuscular disease.

There has been concern that some neonatal screening programmes failed to reduce the incidence of DDH needing surgery, but a consensus view has emerged that screening will minimise, but not prevent, the late diagnosis of DDH. Debate continues as to the most efficacious, cost-effective, and feasible way to screen all babies. At present, screening is by physical examination alone, ultrasound scan (which may be universal or for selected high-risk babies), or both.

Physical examination

- Is the hip dislocated at the start of the examination? If so, full abduction of the thigh with forward pressure on the greater femoral trochanter from the middle finger will reveal a positive Ortolani's sign (a clunk as the femoral head relocates into the acetabulum), or will prove impossible, indicating an irreducible hip.
- Can the hip be dislocated, that is, is it unstable? Barlow's manoeuvre attempts to lift the femoral head anteriorly from the acetabulum and then displace it lateroposteriorly. If the joint subluxates, movement may be felt with the impression of the femoral head sliding laterally. Ortolani's test will then be positive, even if it was negative when the hips were first abducted.

The management of each hip must be planned, and in centres where ultrasound scanning is only selectively available for those with a recognised risk factor or abnormal examination, a scheme similar to that below will be followed:

- clinically normal and low risk   no action—discharge
- clinically normal and high-risk history follow-up and early scan
- clinically abnormal or suspicious   follow-up and early scan
- dislocated or dislocatable   refer to physiotherapist and orthopaedic surgeon for splinting and investigation.

Ultrasound scanning detects not only dislocated hips but also shallow acetabula and dysplasia of the femoral head and acetabulum. While congenital dislocation of the hips can be treated and the outcome for that treatment (and missed cases) is clear, there is no treatment for dysplastic hips, but now that they can be detected early, their natural history will become clearer.

Treatment

The underlying principle is that the femoral head is held within the acetabulum so that the two can grow together and mould to each other. In unstable hips, this can be achieved by gently splinting the legs in abduction until the joint is stable. Splinting can be left for several weeks in an unstable hip, and then applied only to those with continuing clinical or sonographic abnormalities. If abduction can be achieved only with some force, there is a risk of avascular necrosis of the femoral head secondary to the pressure generated by the pull of the stretched adductor muscles. Therefore, some hips are splinted after an adductor tenotomy to relieve the pressure. In irreducible congenital dislocation of the hips, an open surgical reduction is necessary.

Talipes

This is the inability to place the foot plantigrade on a flat surface. Risk factors include a family history, neuromuscular disease, and oligohydramnios. The legs (and spine) must be carefully checked for signs of neuromuscular disease. Talipes is described by the position of the foot: plantar-flexed (equino-), dorsiflexed (calcaneo-), and hooked or twisted inwards (varus) or everted (valgus). Many feet with talipes need only massage and stretching exercises. Strapping can be used to bring an equinovarus foot into a better position. It is applied so as to pull on the foot when the knee is extended. More severe talipes may need serial plasters and surgery.

'Positional talipes' is an oxymoron. Whatever the posture of the foot at rest, talipes is 'positional' if the foot can be placed plantigrade on a flat surface in midposition without force. It does not need treating.

Fractures

Fractures tend to occur in three groups of babies:

- babies with congenital bone abnormalities
- preterm babies with osteopaenia of prematurity
- healthy, large term babies with difficult deliveries.

The third group is the commonest. Neonatal fractures heal rapidly with extensive callus formation. Very little treatment is needed apart from analgesia if necessary and gentle immobilisation of the fractured bone if possible.

Skull	Cephalhaematoma may rarely be associated with a fracture. If confirmed on radiograph, consider CT scanning.
Humerus	May be fractured during a difficult extraction. This is very painful and produces pseudopalsy and crepitus. Use a vest to splint arm to chest wall. Check vascular and nerve supply to forearm and hand. The bone should heal with no long-term problems.
Clavicle	May be fractured during delivery. Often not diagnosed until the callus is palpable, although the baby may be irritable initially. Difficult to diagnose on radiograph prior to callus formation because of curvature of the clavicle. No specific treatment is necessary.
Ribs	Fractures may occur spontaneously or during physiotherapy in babies

Femur
     with osteopaenia of prematurity. Diagnosis is usually retrospective when callus is seen on chest radiograph. Fractures may occur during breech extraction, or postnatally in infants with neuromuscular disorders. This is very painful with accompanying crepitus. Bleeding into the thigh may cause shock. Healing and remodelling will occur without Gallows traction. Support the limb gently during handling and nappy changes.

Note that fractures outside the immediate perinatal period may be a sign of nonaccidental injury. There should always be a high index of suspicion when young infants (even while in hospital) present with fractures. The history should tally with the injury and a skeletal survey, with or without a cranial CT scan (depending on the history and examination), may be necessary. Ophthalmoscopy for retinal haemorrhages should be remembered.

Further reading

American Academy of Pediatrics. Clinical practice guideline: early detection of developmental dysplasia of the hip. Committee on Quality Improvement, Subcommittee on Developmental Dysplasia of the Hip. *Pediatrics* (2000) **105:**896–905.
Broughton NS (ed.). *A Textbook of Pediatric Orthopedics*. Philadelphia: WB Saunders, 1997.
Jones DA. *Hip Screening in the Newborn*. London: Butterworth-Heinemann, 1998.
Lennox IAC, McLauchlan J, Murali R. Failures of screening and management of congenital dislocation of the hip. *Journal of Bone and Joint Surgery* (1993) **75:**72–5.

Related topics of interest

- birth injuries
- childbirth complications and foetal outcome
- congenital malfomations and birth defects
- postnatal examination.

Outcomes of neonatal intensive care

Although neonatal intensive care is a relatively new speciality, it has witnessed striking improvements in the survival of sick newborn infants, particularly at the lowest birth weights, where survival had been so poor. For instance, the numbers of survivors per 1000 live births, in white, singleton infants weighing less than 1000 g has increased 70-fold, between 1960 and 1983 (US data). There is continuing debate however, on whether we are improving survival at the cost of contributing more handicapped individuals to society. Outcome studies have often been institution based, tracking small numbers of subjects and with restricted variability in socioeconomic and environmental factors. Infants have been assessed at different ages, using different instruments; often without control groups and often too narrowly focused to elucidate accurately the specific factors that affect outcome.

Ideally, birth-weight and gestational-age-specific outcome data should be derived from geographically defined populations to allow for a more accurate prediction of the survival and morbidity of infants of any given gestational age by estimated or actual birth weight. Several recent population-based studies have now reported outcomes in very-low-birth-weight (VLBW) infants. To remain relevant, such outcome data sets require regular updating to allow for improvements in survival.

Improving survival—stable morbidity

The marked improvement in the survival of VLBW and ELBW infants has been achieved without a concomitant increase in morbidity in the survivors. The reported trends and prevalence of CP in industrialised nations have been inconsistent. A large meta-analysis of 111 outcome studies of VLBW infants born since 1960 found no significant change in the rate of CP between earlier cohorts (1960–77) and later-born cohorts (1978–86). Yet other studies have reported that mental retardation and severe visual impairment, rather than CP, now constitute the major neurodevelopmental impairment in VLBW infants. In general, major neonatal morbidity increases with decreasing gestational age and birth weight. Approximately 50–60% of VLBW infants will have normal outcomes, and 40–50% will have some degree of impairment, ranging from mild or moderate (20–30%) to severe (20%), with these children remaining at high risk of learning difficulties at school age.

Outcome—birth to hospital discharge

The neonatal morbidities that have a major influence on later development include CLD, severe brain injury, retinopathy of prematurity (ROP), NEC, and nosocomial infections. Morbidity increases with decreasing gestational age and birth weight, and it varies depending on the patient demographics and variation in clinical practice. The majority of survivors below 26 weeks' gestation have one or more of the above complications. CLD is associated with sudden unexpected death, poor nutrition and growth, poor feeding skills, prolonged hospital stays, and episodes of nosocomial infection, which all contribute to poorer long-term outcomes. In current world literature, CLD (defined as oxygen dependence at 36 weeks' postmenstrual age) occurs in 57–86% of infants at 23 weeks' gestation, 33–89% at 24 weeks' gestation, and 16–71% at 25 weeks' gestation. Ultrasonographic signs of brain injury, such as severe periventricular and intraventricular haemorrhage, periventricular infarction, PVL, and persistent ventriculomegaly, increase the risks of mental and motor impairments. Rates of severe ultrasound abnormality vary from 10–83% at 23 weeks' gestation and 9–64% at 24 weeks' gestation to 7–22% at 25 weeks' gestation. Severe ROP is associated with later visual impairment and functional disability. Severe ROP is reported in 25–50% of infants born at 23 weeks' gestation, 13–33% at 24 weeks' gestation, and 10–17% at 25 weeks' gestation. In ELBW infants who survive to a postmenstrual age of 36 weeks, a simple count of the three commonest neonatal morbidities, CLD, brain injury, and severe ROP, strongly predicts the risk of later death or neurosensory impairment. Sepsis also remains a major cause of neonatal morbidity, being associated with longer hospital stays, higher rates of CLD, and poor growth. Similarly, NEC is associated with sepsis, poor growth, and a significant mortality.

- The EPICure study evaluated the outcome for all infants born at 20–25 weeks in the UK and Ireland between 1 March 1995 and 31 December 1995. Of the 811 infants born before 26 weeks' gestation and admitted for neonatal intensive care, 61% died before discharge from hospital. Respiratory complications, intracranial haemorrhage, sepsis, and NEC accounted for 91% of all deaths. At 36 weeks' postmenstrual age, 74% of infants were receiving supplementary oxygen, and later 32% were discharged with home oxygen therapy. ROP requiring treatment was reported in 14%.
- The American NICHD Neonatal Research Network prospectively collected perinatal data on an inborn cohort of 4438 infants weighing 501–1500 g at birth and 195 infants weighing 401–500 g at birth during 1995–6 to determine neonatal morbidity and mortality. Survival to discharge was 54% for infants 501–750 g at birth, 86% for those 751–1000 g, 94% for those 1001–1250 g, and 97% for those 1251–1500 g. The overall incidence of CLD was 23%, proven NEC 7%, and severe (grade 3 or 4) intracranial haemorrhage 11%. In infants weighing 401–500 g mortality was 89%, almost all survivors developing CLD. Poor postnatal growth was a major concern, occurring in 97% of VLBW infants and 99% of ELBW infants.
- Birth-weight and gestational-age-specific survival data sets have yet to be produced for the UK national population. However, such data have been produced for a geographically defined population of the Trent region, which is considered representative of England and Wales. Table 1 shows survival data for the Trent region (European infants) admitted for neonatal care with comparative geographically based data from the EPICure study, the Australian state of Victoria, and the Australian and New Zealand Neonatal Network. For comparison, Table 2 provides recent survival and morbidity data for the national population of New Zealand, and Table 3 provides survival data for nine regions covering a third of all births in France during 1997. Obviously, data on outcome vary *between* and *within* individual countries. Australia, New Zealand, and the USA report better outcomes than the UK.

Table 1 Survival rates by gestational age—data are percentage survival (with 95% confidence intervals).

Source	Gestation (completed weeks)	22	23	24	25	26	27	28	29	30	31	32
Trent Health Region, UK (NNU admissions) 1994–1997	Female	8 (4–14)	16 (10–23)	29 (22–36)	46 (39–52)	63 (57–68)	77 (73–81)	87 (84–90)	93 (90–95)	96 (94–97)	98 (96–99)	99 (97–100)
	Male	6 (3–12)	13 (8–19)	24 (19–31)	40 (34–46)	58 (52–63)	73 (68–77)	84 (81–87)	91 (89–93)	95 (93–96)	97 (96–98)	98 (97–99)
Victoria, Australia (all live births) 1994–1997		3 (0–10)	25 (17–26)	46 (37–55)	72 (64–77)	85 (80–90)	82 (77–88)	91 (87–94)	92 (88–94)	96 (94–97)	97 (95–98)	97 (96–98)
Australian and New Zealand Neonatal Network (NNU admissions) 1994–1997		17 (6–36)	32 (25–40)	59 (54–64)	73 (70–77)	82 (79–85)	90 (88–92)	93 (92–95)	95 (94–96)	97 (96–98)	99 (98–99)	NA
EPICure (NNU admissions) 1995		9 (0–21)	20 (13–27)	34 (28–39)	52 (47–57)							

Table 2 Outcomes for all high-risk New Zealand newborn infants in 1998–9.

Gestational age (weeks)	<24	24–25	26–27	28–29	30–31	32–33	34–36	37–38	39–40	>40
Survived to hospital discharge (%)	42	72	87	95	97	99	99	99	91	95
Survival free of major morbidity (%)	11	28	28	81	90					

Table 3 The Epipage study, a population based cohort study of all births between 22 and 32 weeks during 1997 in nine regions covering a third of all births in France.

Gestational age (weeks)	22	23	24	25	26	27	28	29	30	31	32
All births (n)	102	137	115	204	239	289	338	324	480	599	846
Total stillbirths (%) Σ	84	78	63	42	34	20	16	16	13	8	8
Live births (%) Σ	16	22	37	58	66	80	84	84	87	92	92
Labour ward deaths (%) §	100	80	36	21	11	5	1	1	2	1	0
Admitted to NICU (%) §	0	20	64	79	89	95	99	99	98	99	100
Survival to discharge (%) §	0	0	31	50	56	71	78	89	92	95	97

Σ Percentage of all births
§ Percentage of all live births

Outcome at 1–5 years

Children are considered to be severely disabled if they have a major neurological abnormality, such as CP, blindness, deafness requiring aids, or cognitive function that is less than two standard deviations below the mean. The rates of disability generally increase with decreasing gestational weight and birth weight. Overall, the rates of severe disability for infants of 23–25 weeks' gestation for regional populations are very similar at approximately 30%. Many of the severely disabled children have multiple impairments. In most studies, rates of subnormal cognitive function are higher than those of neuromotor or neurosensory impairment. SGA children have higher rates of neonatal complications, including CLD and severe ROP, making them more susceptible to poorer growth and neurodevelopmental outcome. As a group, infants of birth weight under 500g have a high mortality and very poor neurodevelopmental outcomes. The small proportion of survivors largely consists of female SGA infants.

There are now several international reports on outcomes in VLBW infants (and ELBW infants in particular).

- The EPICure study evaluated the outcome of all infants born before 26 weeks' gestation in the UK and Republic of Ireland from March to December 1995, when they reached a median age of 30 months (corrected for gestational age). Some 92% of the 308 surviving children were formally assessed. Overall, 49% had no disability, 23% had severe disability, and 25% had 'other' disabilities. Deaths accounted for 2% and missing data, 1%. 'Severe disability' was defined as one that was likely to put the child in need of physical assistance to perform daily activities. Disabilities that did not fall into this category were designated 'other disabilities'. Overall, 2% were blind or perceived light only, and 3% had hearing loss that required hearing aids.
- The Victoria Infant Collaborative Study Group (a population-based study) followed up infants born at 23–27 weeks' gestation in 1991–2 in the Australian state of Victoria. Of the 401 live births, 56% survived to two years, and 55% of the survivors were free of disability. The survival rate and survival rate free of disability rose with increasing gestational age. The rates of mild, moderate, and severe disability were 24%, 15%, and 6% respectively. When the same cohort was followed up to five years, survival was unchanged at 56%, 80% being free of a major sensorineural disability, while 20% had at least one major sensorineural disability. Only 2% were blind, and 0.9% required hearing aids for sensorineural deafness.
- The NICHD Neonatal Research Network (USA) followed up 1480 ELBW infants born in 1993–4 to 18–22 months' corrected age (78% were evaluated). Some 51% of the cohort had normal neurodevelopmental and sensory assessments. The probability of being classified as abnormal neurologically increased steadily as birth weight decreased. CP was diagnosed in 17% of the infants, 3% were blind, and 3% had hearing impairment requiring aids.
- More recently, all 211 surviving ELBW infants (from a cohort of 529 infants) born in Finland in 1996–7 were followed for two years. Overall, 42% had no abnormality, and 18% were severely impaired. Speech delay was present in 42%, motor impairments were present in 24%, 11% had CP, and 23% had ophthalmic abnormalities. One child was blind (0.5%), and two (1%) had lost vision in one eye.

Outcome at school age

At school age, a greater percentage of VLBW youngsters than normal-birth-weight children have a specific learning problem (especially in the visuomotor area) requiring special education services (up to ≥50%) compared with 7% for a full-term cohort of similar socioeconomic status.

- In one report of a cohort of ELBW teenagers from a geographically defined region in Canada born between 1977 and 1982, ELBW children did less well on Wide Range Achievement Tests—Revised Reading, Spelling and Arithmetic, a higher proportion receiving special education assistance and/or having repeated a grade. Another report found a linear relationship between IQ and birth weight, even when controlling for maternal IQ and social class. VLBW youngsters were also at increased risk of attention-deficit disorder and hyperactivity, which in turn affect overall academic achievement.
- Another recent study reported a 15-year, single-centre follow-up of 213 children born at less than 29 weeks' gestation during 1985–7 in New York (USA). At primary school age (mean age seven years), approximately 31% had no physical or educational impairment, and 21% had at least one severe disability. At secondary school age (mean age 14 years), 41% had no physical or educational impairment, and 19% had at least one severe disability. Neonatal intraventricular haemorrhage and low socioeconomic status were the strongest predictors of adverse outcome.

Outcome at adolescence and in young adulthood

There is always a trade-off between increasing length of follow-up and diminished relevance to contemporary infants, because of the improvements in perinatal care and survival rates in the intervening years. Current adolescents were born before the advent of surfactant, which has had a major impact on the survival of VLBW and ELBW infants.

- One recent report from Victoria, Australia, which followed up 79 of 88 (90%) survivors of 351 ELBW live-born children to the age of 14 years, reported that 46% had no disability, 14% were severely disabled, 15% were moderately disabled, and 25% were mildly disabled. Six per cent had bilateral blindness and 5% were deaf.
- A regional study from Canada reported on the outcome of 154 of 169 ELBW survivors aged 12–16 years. Learning difficulties were noted in 34%, hyperactivity in 9%, and seizures in 7%. Survivors made greater use of specialist and community resources than control participants.
- A recent report from Ohio, USA (2002) showed that in young adulthood (age ≥20 years) VLBW men (but not women) were less likely than normal-birth-weight controls to be enrolled in postsecondary study. VLBW participants had lower mean IQ, lower academic scores, higher rates of neurosensory impairment, and suboptimal height. They also had lower rates of pregnancy, and alcohol and drug use than normal-birth-weight controls.

Useful website

www.emedicine.com/ped/neonatology.htm
Part of the largest and most current online clinical knowledge base available to health professionals.

Further reading

Bregman J. Developmental outcome in very low birthweight infants: current status and future trends. *Pediatric Clinics of North America* (1998) **45:**673–90.

Cust AE, Darlow BA, Donoghue DA, on behalf of ANZNN. Outcomes for high risk New Zealand newborn infants in 1998–1999: a population-based, national study. *Archives of Disease in Childhood, Foetal and Neonatal Edition* (2003) **88:**F15–22.

D'Angio CT, Sinkin RA, Stevens TP et al. Longitudinal, 15-year follow-up of children born at less than 29 weeks' gestation after introduction of surfactant therapy into a region: neurologic, cognitive, and educational outcomes. *Pediatrics* (2002) **110:**1094–102.

Doyle LW, Morley CJ, Halliday J. Prediction of survival for preterm births—data on the quality of survival are needed. *British Medical Journal* (2000) **320:**647.

Draper ES, Manktelow B, Field DJ et al. Prediction of survival for preterm births by weight and gestational age: retrospective population based study. *British Medical Journal* (1999) **319:**1093–7.

Hack M, Fanaroff AA. Outcomes of children of extremely low birthweight and gestational age in the 1990s. *Seminars in Neonatology* (2000) **5:**89–106.

Hack M, Flannery DJ, Schluchter M et al. Outcomes in young adulthood for very-low-birth-weight infants. *New England Journal of Medicine* (2002) **346:**149–57.

Larroque B, Bréart G, Kaminski M, et al, on behalf of the Epipage study group. Survival of very preterm infants: Epipage, a population based cohort study. *Archives of Disease in Childhood, Foetal and Neonatal Edition* (2004) **89:**F139–44

Lemons JA, Bauer CR, Oh W et al. Very low birth weight outcomes of the National Institute of Child Health and Human Development Research Network, January 1995 through December 1996. NICHD Neonatal Research Network. *Pediatrics* (2001) **107:**E1.

Tommiska V, Heinonen K, Kero P et al. A national two year follow up study of extremely low birthweight infants born in 1996–1997. *Archives of Disease in Childhood, Fetal and Neonatal Edition* (2003) **88:**F29–35.

The Victorian Infant Collaborative Study Group. Outcome at 2 years of children 23–27 weeks' gestation born in 1991–92. *Journal of Paediatrics and Child Health* (1997) **33:**161–5.

Vohr BR, Wright LL, Dusik AM et al. Neurodevelopmental and functional outcomes of extremely low birth weight infants in the National Institute of Child Health and Human Development Neonatal Research Network, 1993–1994. *Pediatrics* (2000) **105:**1216–26.

Wood NS, Marlow N, Costeloe K et al. Neurologic and developmental disability after extremely preterm birth. *New England Journal of Medicine* (2000) **343:**378–84.

Related topics of interest

- cerebral palsy
- chronic lung disease
- extreme prematurity
- necrotising enterocolitis
- respiratory distress syndrome
- retinopathy of prematurity
- surfactant replacement therapy.

Patent ductus arteriosus

The natural history of a patent ductus arteriosus (PDA) in healthy term and preterm infants (regardless of gestational age) is that of spontaneous closure by the fourth day of life. Infants with RDS have delayed closure of the duct, causing clinical problems with increasing frequency as birth weight and gestational age decrease. The incidence of clinically significant PDA in preterm infants with RDS has been reported to vary from 7% (birth weight $>1500\,g$, or ≥33 weeks' gestation) to 51% (birth weight $<1000\,g$ or <28 weeks' gestation). The incidence of PDA also varies with the severity of RDS and is influenced by acute perinatal stress, hypoxia, acidosis, fluid therapy, surfactant therapy, and prenatal medication.

Pathophysiology

Normal postductal closure is mediated by a complex mechanism involving oxygen and other mediators. Hypoxia relaxes the ductus, whereas hyperoxia constricts the ductus. There are developmental changes in the sensitivity of the ductus to oxygen, increasing sensitivity being seen with increasing gestational age. Prostaglandins (PG), particularly PGE_2, also relax the ductus, the ductus of the immature infant being more sensitive to PG than that of the more mature infant. Furthermore, the ductus remains reactive to PG even after initial constriction, accounting for the PDA recurrence in preterm infants. Steroids decrease the sensitivity of the ductus to PGE; hence, prenatal administration of steroids decreases the incidence of PDA. During the acute stage of RDS, PGE levels are elevated, and this may influence ductal patency. With resolution of RDS, there is a reduction in pulmonary vascular resistance, a rise in pulmonary blood flow, and a congestive circulatory state. This may increase ventilatory requirements and increase the risk of developing CLD, NEC, IVH, and pulmonary haemorrhage.

Clinical features

The PDA in preterm infants may be subclinical (no murmur) or clinical (murmur present), while clinical PDA may be nonsignificant (no cardiopulmonary dysfunction) or significant (with cardiopulmonary dysfunction). In the absence of a ductus murmur, a PDA can be diagnosed noninvasively only by Doppler echocardiography. A nonsignificant clinical PDA presents with only a heart murmur (at the left sternal border, second intercostal space), which is largely systolic, although it may continue into the diastolic phase.

Significant clinical PDA
- precordial murmur (commonly purely systolic) in the pulmonary area
- hyperactive precordium
- bounding pulses
- resting tachycardia
- frequent apnoea
- carbon dioxide retention

- cardiomegaly on chest radiograph
- failure to wean off the ventilator at the expected time or unexplained deterioration of respiratory status.

Diagnosis

- pulmonary plethora or congestion with cardiomegaly on chest radiograph
- direct visualisation of PDA on two-dimensional doppler colour-flow echocardiography
- left atrial enlargement with increase in LA/Ao ratio (>1.3) on echocardiogram (normal values 0.66–1.06)
- high left ventricular function index (shown by left ventricular shortening fraction) (normal value $34 \pm 3\%$).

Management

- Optimise oxygenation.
- Restrict fluids to 80–120 ml/kg per day.
- Correct anaemia (maintain haematocrit at >40%).
- Administer diuretics for fluid overload or congestive heart failure. Use furosemide 0.5–1 mg/kg per dose once or twice daily (1–3 mg/kg IV for congestive heart failure). For maintenance therapy, use chlorothiazide 20 mg/kg per dose once or twice daily with amiloride 0.2 mg/kg, as furosemide causes significant electrolyte imbalance. Monitor electrolytes. Note that furosemide also promotes ductal patency by stimulating renal PGE_2 production.
- Spontaneous closure may occur in 22–28% of patients with the above measures.

Pharmacological closure of ductus should be employed if the above measures are not sufficient. Indometacin, a PG synthetase (cyclooxygenase type 1) inhibitor, has been the primary agent used for many years. A dose of 0.2 mg/kg intravenously over 30 min 8–12-hourly for a total of three doses (or 0.3 mg/kg IV 12-hourly × 3 for infants over four weeks of age), or the prolonged low-dose regimen of 0.1 mg/kg per dose daily for six days, is generally used. However, indometacin decreases platelet aggregation (increasing the risk of haemorrhage), cerebral blood flow (but with no long-term neurological deficits), gastrointestinal perfusion (increasing the risk of NEC, gastrointestinal haemorrhage, or perforation), and renal blood flow (causing transient renal dysfunction with reduced glomerular filtration rate and urine output, and dilutional hyponatraemia, necessitating a 20% reduction in administered fluids during treatment). Prolonged low-dose administration causes less renal dysfunction, has a lower recurrence rate (~50% less), and is equally effective. The renal side effects of indometacin may also be prevented by the simultaneous administration of furosemide (1 mg/kg) without reducing its efficacy. The overall efficacy of indometacin in effecting ductal closure during the first 14 days of life (in infants of <1750 g) is approximately 70%. After 14–21 days, efficacy is reduced, and the drug is ineffective in infants aged over six weeks. Efficacy is also reduced, in both the very small preterm infant (<800 g birth weight) and infants of high postconceptional age.

In view of the above side effects of indometacin, ibuprofen, another nonsteroidal anti-inflammatory drug, is now also being used, at a dose 10 mg/kg IV followed by 5 mg/kg 24 and 48 h later. Ibuprofen appears to be as effective as indometacin but with fewer cerebral, gastrointestinal, and renal side effects. Second courses may be given to infants who do not respond to the first course or those with recurrent PDA, although the response is often poor. Nonresponse to a single course in infants under 1000 g birth weight is often an indication for surgery.

Relative contraindications for pharmacological therapy

- shock
- necrotising enterocolitis
- haemorrhagic disease
- thrombocytopenia (platelets <50 000/mm^3)
- recent (<48 h) intraventricular haemorrhage
- renal impairment (blood urea >14 mmol/l, creatinine >140 μmol/l, or persistent oliguria of <1 ml/kg per h).

Surgical closure of PDA

Prior to surgery, detailed echocardiography should be performed to exclude associated congenital heart disease with duct-dependent lesions. Indications for surgery are a strong contraindication or side effect to indometacin or ibuprofen therapy, failure to respond to indometacin or ibuprofen therapy (once in infants of birth weight <1000 g or twice in infants >1000 g), or the presence of a large, clinically significant PDA (detected echocardiographically) in an infant of birth weight under 1000 g. Ductal ligation may be performed on the neonatal unit in small preterm infants, obviating the need to transport such infants to operating theatres, on- or off-site, with the attendant complications of hypothermia, interruption of vascular access, and accidental extubation. Surgery has a more predictable outcome and may be preferable in very small preterm infants, but complications include pneumothorax, pleural effusion (serous or chylous), excessive intraoperative blood loss, and phrenic and recurrent laryngeal nerve injuries.

Prevention

- Antenatal corticosteroids reduces the severity of RDS *and* the incidence of clinically significant PDA.
- The early (<48 h of life) administration of dexamethasone therapy to preterm infants results in a decreased incidence of PDA. Corticosteroids decrease the sensitivity of ductal tissue to the relaxing effects of PG. However, in view of the current concerns about postnatal dexamethasone therapy and adverse neurodevelopmental outcome, alternative strategies would be preferable.
- Fluid restriction (<140 ml/kg per day) during the first week of life reduces the incidence of clinically significant PDA.
- Inappropriate use of plasma expanders for hypotension may predispose to the development of a clinically significant PDA.

- Prophylactic administration of indometacin decreases the incidence of clinically significant PDA without convincingly improving morbidity and mortality, and is therefore not generally recommended.
- Prophylactic ductal ligation in infants of birth weight under 1000 g does not reduce mortality or morbidity (apart from decreasing the incidence of NEC) and would result in surgery being performed in many infants who do not require it.

Further reading

Burch M, Archer N. *Pediatric Cardiology*. London: Chapman & Hall, 1998.

Cooke L, Steer P, Woodgate P. Indometacin for asymptomatic patent ductus arteriosus in preterm infants. The Cochrane Library, Issue 2. Chichester: John Wiley & Sons, 2004.

Gavilanes AWD, Heineman E, Herpers MJHM et al. Use of neonatal intensive care unit as a safe place for neonatal surgery. *Archives of Disease in Childhood, Fetal and Neonatal Edition* (1997) **76:**F51–3.

Knight DB. The treatment of patent ductus arteriosus in preterm infants. A review and overview of randomised trials. *Seminars in Neonatology* (2001) **6:**63–73.

Ohlsson A, Walia R, Shah S. Ibuprofen for the treatment of patent ductus arteriosus in preterm and/or low birth weight infants. The Cochrane Library, Issue 2. Chichester: John Wiley & Sons, 2004.

Rennie JM, Cooke RWI. Prolonged low dose indomethacin for the persistent ductus arteriosus of prematurity. *Archives of Disease in Childhood* (1991) **66:**55–8.

Shah SS, Ohlsson A. Ibuprofen for the prevention of patent ductus arteriosus in preterm and/or low birth weight infants. The Cochrane Library, Issue 2. Chichester: John Wiley & Sons, 2004.

Skinner J. Diagnosis of patent ductus arteriosus. *Seminars in Neonatology* (2001) **6:**49–61.

Skinner J, Alverson D, Hunter S (eds). *Echocardiography for the Neonatologist*. Edinburgh: Churchill Livingstone, 2000.

Van Overmeire B, Smets K, Lecoutere D et al. A comparison of ibuprofen and indomethacin for closure of patent ductus arteriosus. *New England Journal of Medicine* (2000) **343:**674–81.

Related topics of interest

- chronic lung disease
- congenital heart disease—congestive cardiac failure
- congenital heart disease—cyanotic defects
- fluid and electrolyte therapy
- necrotising enterocolitis
- neonatal surgery
- respiratory distress syndrome.

Periventricular leucomalacia

Periventricular leucomalacia (PVL) refers to necrosis of white matter dorsal and lateral to the external angles of the lateral ventricles, involving particularly the centrum semiovale (frontal horn and body), and the optic (trigone and occipital horn) and acoustic (temporal horn) radiations. The incidence of PVL at autopsy shows great variation with autopsies showing PVL in up to 75% of preterm infants. During life, one recent report gave a peak incidence of 15.7% at 28 weeks' gestation, falling to 4.3% at 32 weeks' gestation (overall 9.2%), when PVL was determined by cranial ultrasonography. PVL is most often seen in preterm infants, infants with cardiorespiratory disturbance, and infants with a postnatal survival of more than a few days (commonly 1–3 weeks). Recently, an association has also been recognised between ventilation-induced hypocapnia and PVL, particularly in the preterm infant.

Neuropathology

PVL has distinctive pathological features, comprising both focal periventricular necrosis and more diffuse cerebral white-matter injury. The focal necrotic lesions occur primarily in the distribution of the end zones of the long penetrating arteries. The two commonest sites for PVL focal necrosis are in the white matter near the trigone of the lateral ventricles and around the foramen of Monro. These sites are the arterial end and border zones (that is, watershed areas) between the terminal branches of the long penetrating branches of the middle cerebral artery and the posterior cerebral artery (peritrigonal white matter) or the anterior cerebral artery (frontal white matter), respectively.

The more diffuse regions of cerebral white-matter injury are characterised by a diffuse loss of oligodendrocytes and a corresponding increase in hypertrophic astrocytes. These diffuse lesions are less likely to undergo major cystic changes, and therefore more commonly go undetected by cranial ultrasonography during life. Diminished cerebral white-matter volume and an increase in ventricular size are more readily noted.

Pathogenesis

Three major interacting factors have important roles in the pathogenesis of PVL, namely:

1. the intrinsic vulnerability of the cerebral white matter in the preterm newborn
2. a pressure-passive cerebral circulation
3. the unique periventricular vascular anatomy in preterm newborns.

Infection and inflammatory cytokines may also have minor roles. The periventricular vascular supply in preterm infants is derived from deep-penetrating basal cerebral arteries, which have few side branches and anastomoses, making these areas most susceptible to falls in perfusion pressure and cerebral blood flow. With increasing gestational age, there is an increase in anastomoses of the periventricular vasculature, making these deep periventricular regions less susceptible to ischaemia. An additional factor in the pathogenesis of PVL is the presence of a pressure-passive cerebral circulation where cerebral blood flow falls with a decrease in blood pressure. This cerebrovascular autoregulatory defect predisposes the periventricular arterial border zones and end zones in cerebral white matter to ischaemia. A third important parameter is the inherent vulnerability of cerebral white matter to injury, due to the marked sensitivity of the early differentiating oligodendrocytes to free-radical attack. Large numbers of free radicals are generated under conditions of ischaemia-reperfusion, which is central to the pathogenesis of PVL.

More recently, French and American studies have provided support for the concept that both prenatal (chorioamnionitis) and postnatal infections may cause neurochemical mediated injury to the white matter (by inflammatory markers such as cytokines), and provide an additional pathway to PVL.

Diagnosis

The principal diagnostic tool is cranial ultrasonography. The acute lesions appear as bilateral echodensities, or 'flares', distributed diffusely in the periventricular white matter or localised to the main sites of predilection for PVL, namely, around the foramen of Monro or near the trigone of the lateral ventricles. The localised echodensities may resolve over the next 1–3 weeks or be replaced by multiple small echolucent cysts, giving rise to a 'Swiss cheese appearance'. After 1–3 months, well-delineated cysts disappear with gliosis and collapse of cyst walls, leaving enlarged ventricles and decreased cerebral myelin. Ultrasonography, however, is relatively insensitive and may miss up to 70% of PVL detected by histopathology, especially small focal areas of necrosis and more diffuse white-matter injury (MRI has greater diagnostic precision). However, once detected, periventricular cysts are the most sensitive and specific neurosonographic predictors of cerebral palsy in preterm infants. The parasagittal measurements of the anteroposterior dimensions of cystic PVL best predict which infants will have quadriplegia (more common with cystic PVL of ≥20mm) and the more severe cognitive and sensory impairments.

Prognosis

Developmental sequelae, including the type of cerebral palsy, degree of functional motor deficits, and associated disabilities, are closely linked with the location and extent of the cystic PVL. Cysts that are limited to the frontal or anterior periventricular region have not usually been associated with cerebral palsy. Bilateral multiple cysts involving the middle (centrum semiovale) or posterior periventricular regions have been associated with cerebral palsy and other disabilities. The periventricular locus of PVL is such that it affects the descending fibres from the motor cortex, primarily those subserving the function of the lower limbs (giving rise to spastic diplegia), with more severe lesions progressively involving the motor fibres of the upper limbs and finally intellectual functions as well, leading to corresponding marked intellectual deficits. PVL may also impair subsequent cortical neuronal organisation and cognitive function. In surviving infants with cystic PVL, the prevalence of all types of cerebral palsy has ranged from 38% to 93%, spastic cerebral palsy being present in all (but 21–69% being diplegia, 27–71% quadriplegia, and 0–33% hemiplegia). In general, once cystic PVL and ventricular dilation (indicative of white-matter atrophy) have developed, 60–90% of such infants will develop spastic diplegia and other neurological deficits.

Prevention

As postnatally acquired PVL is primarily due to cerebral ischaemia, avoidance of systemic hypotension and hypocarbia is important. Infants with a pressure-passive cerebral circulation are especially susceptible to PVL. Near-infrared spectroscopy (still largely a research tool) is currently the main technique for detecting this circulatory abnormality.

Further reading

Fazzi E, Orcesi S, Caffi L et al. Neurodevelopmental outcome at 5–7 years in preterm infants with periventricular leukomalacia. *Neuropediatrics* (1994) **25:**134.

Gannon CM, Wiswell TE, Spitzer AR. Volutrauma, $PaCO_2$ levels and neurodevelopmental sequelae following assisted ventilation. *Clinics in Perinatology* (1998) **25:**159–75.

Perlman J (ed.). Perinatal brain injury. *Clinics in Perinatology* (2002) **29**(4).

Perlman JM, Risser R, Broyles RS. Bilateral cystic periventricular leukomalacia in the premature infant: associated risk factors. *Pediatrics* (1996) **97:**822–7.

Rogers B, Msall M, Owens T et al. Cystic periventricular leukomalacia and type of cerebral palsy in preterm infants. *Journal of Pediatrics* (1994) **125:**S1–8.

Saliba E (ed.). Perinatal brain injury. *Seminars in Neonatology* (2001) **6**(2).

Volpe JJ. Brain injury in the premature infants—neuropathology, clinical aspects, pathogenesis and prevention. *Clinics in Perinatology* (1997) **24:**567–87.

Zupan V, Gonzalez P, Tacaze-Masmonteil T et al. Periventricular leukomalacia: risk factors revisited. *Developmental Medicine and Child Neurology* (1996) **38:**1061–7.

Related topics of interest

- cerebral palsy
- complications of mechanical ventilation
- extreme prematurity
- germinal matrix-intraventricular haemorrhage
- outcome of neonatal intensive care
- respiratory distress syndrome
- seizures.

Persistent pulmonary hypertension of the newborn

Since the original description by Gersony and colleagues of the 'PFC' syndrome in the late 1960s, there have been considerable advances in our understanding of the developmental biology and pathophysiology of persistent foetal circulation, now known as persistent pulmonary hypertension of the newborn (PPHN). However, the clinical management of this disorder is often frustrating, not least because the diagnostic criteria are inadequately standardised and the optimal therapy is often disputed. Adding to the confusion is that PPHN is not a single disease entity but a complex of diverse causes, all with a similar clinical picture. Therefore, it is unlikely that a single therapeutic intervention will cure all infants with PPHN.

In PPHN, the high foetal pulmonary vascular resistance and pulmonary arterial pressure do not fall after birth or they subsequently rise. As pulmonary arterial pressure exceeds the systemic arterial pressure, right-to-left shunting occurs across the patent foramen ovale (PFO) (right atrium to left atrium) or through the PDA (pulmonary artery to aorta), leading to systemic hypoxaemia.

The disorder occurs in term and preterm infants. The incidence varies worldwide from approximately one in 1500 to as often as two to six in 1000 live births. It is more common in the USA, where it may account for 3.4% of all neonatal admissions (~10 000 newborns annually), and it is the most common cause of death in infants of birth weight over 1000 g.

Pathophysiology

There are physiological (or functional) factors and anatomical (or structural) factors which contribute to the development of PPHN.

Physiological factors

These produce pulmonary vasoconstriction via local vasoactive mediators, such as prostaglandins, thromboxanes, leucotrienes, bradykinin, endothelin-1, and platelet activating factor. There are a normal number of arteries and normal muscularisation.

- MAS
- RDS
- hypothermia
- hypoglycaemia
- perinatal asphyxia
- bacterial pneumonia
- severe hypoxia or acidosis
- polycythaemia-hyperviscosity syndrome.

Anatomical factors

Decreased number of arteries with decreased cross-sectional area of pulmonary vascular bed
- CDH
- primary pulmonary hypoplasia

- peripheral pulmonary artery stenosis
- congenital alveolar capillary dysplasia.

Normal number of arteries but with increased muscularisation of arteries
- post-maturity
- placental insufficiency
- chronic foetal hypoxia.

Clinical features

- lability of oxygenation
- prominent right ventricular impulse with narrowly split and loud second heart sound
- tricuspid, mitral, or pulmonary incompetence murmur
- hepatomegaly and signs of heart failure
- lung fields commonly clear or oligaemic
- blood gas: severe hypoxaemia with mild acidosis slightly elevated or normal carbon dioxide
- ECG—right ventricular dominance, right axis deviation, and right atrial enlargement.

Diagnosis of PPHN

There is no specific ideal test for PPHN. When hypoxaemia is out of proportion to the degree of parenchymal lung disease and there is no evidence of cyanotic CHD, consider PPHN as a diagnosis. The following signs are helpful:

- Lability of oxygenation, unprovoked wide swings in PaO_2.
- Preductal and postductal PaO_2 differences. Simultaneous preductal and postductal monitoring of oxygen saturation or PaO_2 shows a difference of 5–10% or >2.5 kPa, respectively.
- Hyperoxia-hyperventilation test. A brief (~10 min) period of hyperventilation induces alkalosis and pulmonary vasodilation with a consequent rise in PaO_2. This manoeuvre is associated with increased risk of pneumothorax and further lung damage, particularly as hyperventilation tends to be continued should oxygenation improve.
- Two-dimensional Doppler echocardiography is the most useful and accurate diagnostic technique. Right-to-left shunting of blood through the PDA and PFO can be visualised and the magnitude of pulmonary hypertension estimated from the flow velocity of the regurgitant jet at the pulmonary or tricuspid valve. CHD (especially anomalous venous drainage) can also be excluded at the same time.

Management—general

Stabilise the patient to prevent swings in oxygenation and other vital parameters
- Identify and correct any physiological abnormalities likely to increase pulmonary vascular resistance (such as hypoglycaemia and acidosis).
- Avoid excessive handling.
- Maintain systemic arterial pressure.

- Sedate (opiates and benzodiazepines)—where necessary paralyse to facilitate ventilation.

Maintain systemic arterial pressure
Correct hypotension with volume expanders (normal saline, albumin, FFP, and blood) and/or commence inotropes (dopamine and dobutamine).

Reduce pulmonary arterial pressure
There is a choice of IV and inhaled agents (see below).

Assess severity of the impairment of gas exchange
This helps predict the outcome and gauge response to therapy. Two parameters may be used to predict the outcome in infants failing conventional ventilator support: the oxygenation index (OI) or the alveolar-arterial oxygen (AaDO$_2$) gradient.

$$OI = \frac{\text{mean airway pressure (cmH}_2\text{O)} \times \text{FiO}_2 \times 100\%}{\text{postductal } PaO_2 \text{ (mmHg)}}$$

or

$$OI = \frac{\text{mean airway pressure (cmH}_2\text{O)} \times \text{FiO}_2 \times 100\% \times 0.13}{\text{postductal } PaO_2 \text{ (kPa)}}$$

The alveolar-arterial oxygen (AaDO$_2$) gradient is represented by the equation:

$$AaDO_2 = FiO_2(P - 47) - PaO_2 - PaCO_2[FiO_2 + (1 - FiO_2)/R]$$

where P is the barometric pressure (mmHg), 47 is the partial pressure of water vapour (mmHg), R is the respiratory quotient (0.8), FiO$_2$ is the fractional inspired oxygen concentration, PaO$_2$ is the arterial PO$_2$ (mmHg), and PaCO$_2$ is the arterial PCO$_2$ (mmHg). When FiO$_2$ is 100%, and assuming P$_A$CO$_2$ (alveolar PCO$_2$) is equivalent to PaCO$_2$, the equation reduces to

$$AaDO_2 = 713 - (PaO_2 + PaCO_2)\text{ mmHg, where } P = 760\text{ mmHg (sea level)}.$$

An OI of greater than 40, or an AaDO$_2$ gradient of greater than 620 mmHg, for 8 h correlates with 80% predicted mortality. The OI and AaDO$_2$ are equally effective as predictors of outcome.

Management of ventilation

- Administer surfactant (whether patient has pneumonia, MAS, or idiopathic PPHN). MAS, requires several doses of surfactant.
- Hyperventilation is now obsolete, as it is associated with increased pulmonary morbidity from chronic lung disease and adverse neurodevelopmental outcome (especially sensorineural hearing impairment) and impaired psychomotor development). Hypocapnia decreases CBF.
- Induced metabolic alkalosis may be preferable to hyperventilation-induced alkalosis. However, no studies have evaluated the efficacy of this therapy. Hypernatraemia may ensue from repeated sodium bicarbonate administration.

- 'Conservative' ventilation may be equally effective or superior to hyperventilation. This is deliberate hypoventilation allowing high $PaCO_2$ in order to diminish lung injury. The target pH is ≥ 7.25 as compared to ≥ 7.5 with hyperventilation.
- High-frequency ventilation, particularly high-frequency oscillatory ventilation (HFOV), may be superior to conventional ventilation in improving outcome, as HFOV improves lung recruitment. High-frequency jet ventilation (HFJV) may be as effective as HFOV.
- Vasodilator therapy has a definite role in improving oxygenation in PPHN.

Intravenous vasodilators

Intravenous vasodilators may be less effective than inhaled vasodilators, as the former produce concomitant hypotension. The most commonly used intravenous vasodilators are as follows:

- sodium nitroprusside 0.2–6 µg/kg per min
- prostacyclin (epoprostenol) 1–40 ng/kg per min
- PGD$_2$ 1–25 µg/kg per min
- nitroglycerine 0.5–12 µg/kg per min
- tolazoline 1–2 mg/kg bolus, followed by 1–2 mg/kg per h
- magnesium sulphate 200 mg/kg over 20–30 min followed by 20–150 mg/kg per h to maintain serum magnesium concentration of 3.5–5.5 mmol/l.

Inhaled vasodilators

Inhaled vasodilator therapy is dominated by nitric oxide (NO), the recently discovered potent endogenous vasodilator. To date, over 12 randomised trials involving over 1000 term or near-term infants have been completed. ECMO use was decreased in the NO-treated groups (one fewer ECMO patient for every six patients treated with NO). However, up to 40% of infants failed to respond to NO.

- Inhaled NO improves outcome in hypoxic term or near-term infants (≥ 34 weeks' gestation) by reducing the incidence of the need for ECMO (mortality is not reduced).
- Inhaled NO has been demonstrated to improve survival and reduce the incidence of CLD in preterm infants. The incidence of intracranial and pulmonary haemorrhage is not altered by the use of inhaled NO.
- Inhaled NO is an effective therapy for the pulmonary hypertensive crises which complicate surgery for congenital heart disease. However, formal prospective, randomised, controlled trials are awaited.
- Inhaled NO has not been demonstrated to improve the outcome (or reduce mortality) in neonatal and paediatric acute respiratory distress (ARDS), congenital diaphragmatic hernia (CDH), or CLD.

Nebulised prostacyclin has also been used as a selective pulmonary vasodilator with good effect. It has not, however, been subjected to as much detailed study as inhaled NO.

Extracorporeal membrane oxygenation

ECMO is indicated when medical therapy has failed. However, this should be done well before the infant is moribund, as the infant would then be too unstable to transport and would face increased risk of sudden cardiorespiratory decompensation and death during transport. An OI of 30 (or perhaps lower) or an AaDO$_2$ of $\geq$600 mmHg is a useful baseline criterion for ECMO eligibility. The eligibility criteria for ECMO are summarised as follows:

- gestational age of $\geq$34 weeks and weight >2000 g
- absence of intracranial haemorrhage
- absence of congenital heart disease
- reversible lung disease
- fewer than 10–14 days of mechanical ventilation
- failure of maximal medical treatment (that is, supporting cardiac output with volume expansion or pressor support and respiratory support, which includes surfactant therapy, inhaled NO, and, where relevant, HFOV).

The best outcome is for neonates with MAS (overall survival 95%), while other neonatal respiratory conditions have an overall survival rate of 80%. The lowest survival rate, of about 50%, is among patients with sepsis, CDH, or cardiac disorders. Paediatric conditions tend to be more variable, and overall survival is approximately 50%. ECMO treated infants do not have increased morbidity (86% of survivors being neurodevelopmentally normal), compared with infants treated with conventional ventilator therapy.

Prognosis

Deaths from PPHN have decreased in recent years, perhaps due to earlier diagnosis and treatment, with an overall survival rate of approximately 80%.

Further reading

Abman SH. New developments in the pathogenesis and treatment of neonatal pulmonary hypertension. *Pediatric Pulmonology Suppl* (1999) **18**:201–4.

Clark RH, Kueser TJ, Walker MW et al. Low-dose nitric oxide therapy for persistent pulmonary hypertension of the newborn. Clinical Inhaled Nitric Oxide Research Group. *New England Journal of Medicine* (2000) **342**:469–74.

Finer NN, Barrington KJ. Nitric oxide for respiratory failure in infants born at or near term (Cochrane Review). Cochrane Database Systematic Reviews 2001; **2**: CD000399.

Kinsella JP, Abman SH. Inhaled nitric oxide: current and future uses in neonates. *Seminars in Perinatology* (2000) **24**:387–95.

Lotze A, Mitchell BR, Bulas DI et al. Multicenter study of surfactant (beractant) use in the treatment of term infants with severe respiratory failure. Survanta in Term Infants Study Group. *Journal of Pediatrics* (1998) **132**:40–7.

Related topics of interest

- congenital diaphragmatic hernia
- extracorporeal membrane oxygenation
- mechanical ventilation
- meconium aspiration syndrome
- nitric oxide therapy.

Polycythaemia

Marked polycythaemia gives rise to the hyperviscosity syndrome, which is associated with significant morbidity. Blood viscosity is determined by haematocrit, red cell deformability, and plasma viscosity, the haematocrit being most important. Polycythaemia is present when the central venous haematocrit is ≥65%. Peripheral venous haematocrits are significantly higher than central ones. The haematocrit rises in the first 24h as plasma volume decreases. Prevalence rates of 2–4% have been reported. It is more common in babies born at high altitude. It is the hyperviscosity secondary to polycythaemia that causes most of the clinical problems.

Aetiology

The causation may be passive (foetus receives a transfusion of red cells) or active (foetus produces excessive red cells in response to intrauterine stimuli).

Passive
- twin-to-twin transfusion
- maternal–foetal transfusion
- delayed clamping of cord.

Active
- maternal diabetes
- neonatal thyrotoxicosis
- severe maternal heart disease
- congenital adrenal hyperplasia
- Beckwith–Wiedemann syndrome
- chromosomal abnormalities, especially trisomies 13, 18, and 21
- intrauterine hypoxia (hence elevated levels of erythropoietin), especially placental insufficiency or pre-eclampsia, small-for-gestation infants, post-term infants, and maternal smoking.

Pathophysiology

It is unclear whether these symptoms are due primarily to the sluggish circulation and poor oxygen delivery or the accompanying hypoglycaemia. Hypoglycaemia is due in part to the high red cell mass and low plasma volume, as well as low intraerythrocytic glucose level which reduces the overall glucose content of blood. In severe polycythaemia, sludging of the red cells and platelets in a sluggish peripheral circulation may occur, resulting in tissue hypoxia and thrombosis. This is most serious in the brain, where it may cause convulsions and infarcts.

Clinical features

- irritability
- vomiting

- poor feeding
- easily startles
- tremulousness
- difficulty in arousal
- hypotonia and lethargy
- signs commonly appear when the normal physiological reduction in plasma volume occurs (first 24 h).

Complications

Early
- hypoglycaemia and hypocalcaemia.
- hyperbilirubinaemia (kernicterus)
- thrombocytopenia
- respiratory distress
- renal vein thrombosis
- cardiac and renal failure
- seizures
- NEC
- distal bowel obstruction
- priapism and testicular infarction

Late
- low IQ
- spastic diplegia
- neurodevelopmental delay
- speech and fine motor abnormalities.

Investigations

- FBC
- blood glucose
- serum calcium
- serum bilirubin
- U and E (in presence of poor renal function)
- head ultrasound scan (in presence of seizures)
- abdominal radiograph (suspected NEC or obstruction)
- coagulation screen (in the presence of thrombocytopenia)
- determine haematocrit by centrifugation (calculated values from automatic electronic counters are inaccurate and lower than values obtained by centrifugation).

Management

A partial exchange transfusion replaces infants' whole blood with fresh-frozen plasma (FFP) or 4.5% human albumin (when FFP is not readily available), aiming for a haematocrit of 55%. However, crystalloids (as in normal saline solution) may also be used effectively, especially if there is hypervolaemia secondary to twin–twin transfusion. The blood volume to be exchanged approximates 20 ml/kg. Alternatively, use the following formula: exchange volume = total infant's blood volume (85 ml × birth weight) × (observed haematocrit minus desired haematocrit) ÷ observed haematocrit. Perform the partial exchange in small volumes (5–10-ml aliquots), using peripheral veins (using umbilical vessels increases the risk of NEC).

For significant symptoms, perform a partial exchange transfusion promptly. For mild or minor symptoms, keep the infant well hydrated and warm. Screen high-risk infants by performing capillary haematocrit, and if this is ≥65–70%, perform venous haematocrit. Screen for and treat hypoglycaemia. If symptoms do not develop within 48 h and the baby is feeding well, complications are unlikely.

Further reading

Black VD. Neonatal hyperviscosity syndromes. *Current Problems in Paediatrics* (1987) **17:**73–130.

Christensen RD. *Hematologic Problems of the Neonate*. Philadelphia: WB Saunders, 2000.

Delaney-Black V, Camp BW, Lubchenco LO et al. Neonatal hyperviscosity association with lower achievement and IQ scores at school age. *Pediatrics* (1989) **83:**662–7.

Oski FA, Naiman JL (eds). *Hematologic Problems in the Newborn*, 5th edn. Philadelphia: WB Saunders, 1998.

Ramamurthy RS. Postnatal alteration in haematocrit and viscosity in normal infants and in those with polycythemia. *Journal of Pediatrics* (1989) **114:**169–70.

Werner EJ. Neonatal polycythemia and hyperviscosity. *Clinics in Perinatology* (1995) **22:**693–710.

Related topics of interest

- anaemia
- intrauterine growth restriction
- jaundice
- transfusion of blood and blood products.

Postnatal examination

All infants, including those allowed home within a few hours of birth, should have a full examination within the first day of life. Ideally, the mother should be present to enable her to ask any questions she may have. In addition, any problems noted can then be discussed immediately.

History

As always, the examination must be complemented by a history. Quickly note the maternal obstetric and medical histories (such as hepatitis B infection). Note also significant social problems (such as drug abuse and other child protection issues) and the family history (including tuberculosis). Finally, run through the pregnancy details and note any complications (such as polyhydramnios and abnormal foetal scans), labour (such as intrapartum pyrexia), and delivery, including details of the resuscitation, Apgar scores, and birth weight. Progress since birth (feeding, passage of stools or urine, and any other problems noted) should also be quickly reviewed.

Initial examination

Note age at time of examination. Check weight, length, and head circumference and plot on percentile chart if necessary. Undress the infant completely and check whether the appearance of the infant and posture are normal. Note the colour (such as pale, cyanosed, jaundiced, or plethoric), skin condition (such as dry or peeling), and any blemishes. Examine each region in turn, starting with the head.

Head and neck
Note shape of skull and check sutures, fontanelle, and the rest of the scalp (cephalhaematoma?), facies (any asymmetry or other anomalies), eyes (shape, size, and epicanthic folds), iris (colobomata), cornea (diameter over 11 mm and hazy in congenital glaucoma), cataracts (absent red retinal reflex), ears (shape and size; are they low-set?), nasal airway (check patency), mouth (check hard and soft palate intact), and neck (any soft tissue swellings; are clavicles intact?).

Chest
Check shape, and breathing pattern and effort. Check heart sounds (murmurs?).

Abdomen and genitalia
Note liver, spleen, and kidney size, and number of cord vessels. Feel femoral pulses. Check that anus is patent and genitalia are normal with descended testes. If genitalia are ambiguous, say so and do not assign a sex!

Spine and limbs
Check that the spine is straight with no dimples and hairy patches. Check that the upper and lower limbs are of normal shape, have full range of movements, and are

symmetrical with normal palmar creases. Check that the hips have full range of movements and do not dislocate.

Activity and behaviour
Note muscle tone and activity (symmetrical movements) with appropriate reflexes (grasp, suck, Moro, and step) and normal cry. Asymmetrical movements may suggest birth-injury-related palsies (such as Erb's palsy) or a fracture.

Special notes
Infants should pass meconium within 48h. Failure to do so suggests bowel obstruction (vomiting and abdominal distension) or anorectal anomalies (such as imperforate anus). Passing a small finger per rectum may encourage passage of a meconium plug followed by meconium. Consider the possibility of Hirschsprung's disease or CF in infants with a meconium plug and delayed passage of meconium (>48h). Serum immunoreactive trypsin level, stool tryptic activity, or a sweat test may be required in the follow-up period. Urine should also be passed within 48h of birth; otherwise, look for evidence of urinary obstructions (enlarged bladder and urethral valves) or reduced urine production (such as renal agenesis, renal vein thrombosis, or acute tubular necrosis).

Ascertain that the infant has received vitamin K prophylaxis. BCG vaccination should be given where appropriate (as in family history of tuberculosis) and infants born to hepatitis B-positive mothers should receive hepatitis B vaccine (0.5 ml i.m. at birth and repeated at age one and two months. Infants whose mothers are e-antigen positive and e-antibody negative should also receive human anti-hepatitis B immunoglobulin (200 IU by deep i.m. injection) within 24h of birth to confer immediate protection until the vaccine is effective. This should be followed by a full course of vaccinations, with review at one year for a booster dose and to check for evidence of adequate immunity.

Discharge examination

This is similar to the initial examination with some additional points being noted.

- Feeding (breast or bottle) should be established.
- Any parental concerns should be addressed and any questions answered.
- Pending investigations should be discussed fully and details of follow-up arrangements finalised.
- Marked jaundice should be investigated and discharge allowed only if the serum bilirubin is falling or stable.
- Complete and sign (legibly) the discharge record, copies being forwarded to all appropriate personnel in the community.

Further reading

Clark DA. *Atlas of Neonatology*. Philadelphia: WB Saunders, 2000.
Fletcher MA. *Physical Diagnosis in Neonatology*. Philadelphia: Lippincott Williams & Wilkins, 1997.

Friedman MA, Spitzer AR. Discharge criteria for the term newborn. *Pediatric Clinics of North America* (2004) **51:**599–618.

Jones DA. *Hip Screening in the Newborn*. London: Butterworth-Heinemann, 1998.

Phillips AGS. *Neonatology: A Practical Guide*. Philadelphia: WB Saunders, 1996.

Rudolph A (ed.). *Atlas of the Newborn*, vols 1–5, 3rd edn. Oxford: Blackwell Science, 1997.

Thomas R, Harvey D. *Neonatology: Colour Guide*, 2nd edn. Edinburgh: Churchill Livingstone, 1997.

Related topics of interest

- assessment of gestational age
- birth injuries
- congenital anomalies and birth defects
- hepatitis B and C
- immunisation
- jaundice.

Pregnancy complications and foetal health

As maternal health is intricately linked with that of the foetus, serious complications of pregnancy invariably also affect the foetus. A selection of some of the common complications of pregnancy and their attendant effects on the foetus is presented.

Antepartum haemorrhage (APH)

This constitutes bleeding from the genital tract from 28 weeks' gestation up to delivery of the foetus. APH can have serious consequences for both the mother and foetus. It is associated with a marked increase in perinatal mortality and is also a significant cause of maternal mortality. The two main causes are placenta praevia and placental abruption. The latter is more serious and is associated with a twofold increase in mortality.

Placental abruption
This is due to placental separation with attendant maternal and foetal blood loss (often concealed) and foetal compromise.

Maternal clinical features
- painful bleeding from the genital tract
- foetal parts and heart rate difficult to ascertain
- uterus tense, tender, irritable, and at times hard
- blood loss out of proportion to mother's condition, progressing to shock.

Foetal risks
- intrauterine death
- preterm delivery (RDS)
- foetal blood loss and asphyxia.

Management
- immediate maternal resuscitation with fresh blood transfusion
- coagulation defects rectified
- foetal viability ascertained ultrasonically
- if foetus dead, labour induced (after resuscitating mother), aiming for vaginal delivery.

Placenta praevia
The placenta encroaches upon the lower uterine segment and may partially or completely cover the cervix.

Maternal clinical features
- recurrent painless bleeding from the genital tract
- maternal condition is proportional to blood lost.

Foetal risks
- The risk is that of preterm delivery (RDS).

Management
- position of placenta ascertained ultrasonically
- emergency delivery by caesarean section for severe bleeding
- expectant management aiming to prolong pregnancy to 37–38 weeks for minor haemorrhages
- elective caesarean section at 37–38 weeks for all but minor degrees of placenta praevia.

Pre-eclampsia

Also called 'pregnancy-induced hypertension', pre-eclampsia (PE) is characterised by hypertension and proteinuria during pregnancy (mostly third trimester) and immediate puerperium. Severe PE consists of hypertension and proteinuria ($>0.25\,g/l$); mild PE is hypertension without proteinuria. With an incidence of up to one in ten pregnancies, PE and related hypertensive disorders are still a significant cause of maternal morbidity and death. PE may rapidly progress through the PE state to eclampsia, which is characterised by seizures. PE may also develop into a serious hypertensive disorder with elevated liver enzymes, epigastric pain, and low platelets (HELLP syndrome).

Maternal clinical features
- hypertension (blood pressure [BP] $\geq 140/90$)—mild PE
- hypertension with proteinuria—severe PE
- agitation, confusion, visual disturbance, epigastric pain, nausea, and vomiting with brisk reflexes—PE state
- seizures (with above)—eclampsia state.

Foetal risks
- preterm delivery
- acute or chronic placental insufficiency with IUGR
- placental abruption, foetal asphyxia, and intrauterine death.

Management
- bed rest in hospital
- prevention of disease progression to the most severe spectrum
- antihypertensive therapy (methyldopa, hydralazine, and beta-blockers)
- anticonvulsant therapy (diazepam, chlormethiazole, and magnesium sulphate)
- for severe disease, prompt delivery by caesarean section is often necessary.

Preterm rupture of membranes (PROM)

Before 34 weeks, management of PROM is conservative. Tocolytics (beta-mimetics) may be used temporarily, affording the opportunity to induce pulmonary maturity by corticosteroids.

Foetal risks
- preterm delivery
- limb contractures
- amnionitis and foetal infection
- respiratory distress syndrome
- periventricular leucomalacia and cerebral palsy
- pulmonary hypoplasia with prolonged and early PROM.

Management
Maternal antibiotics are administered, following high vaginal and cervical swabs.

Preterm labour and birth

This constitutes labour and birth before 37 weeks' gestation. Prematurity is the single largest contributor to the early neonatal mortality rate.

Aetiology and risk factors
- polyhydramnios
- incompetent cervix
- multiple pregnancy
- antepartum haemorrhage
- maternal infection (such as UTI)
- preterm rupture of membranes
- poor socioeconomic background
- PE and related disorders.

Management
- Perform a maternal ultrasound scan to assess foetal maturity, growth, and presentation and exclude obvious anomalies.
- Commence tocolysis if labour is not advanced (cervix under 4 cm) and gestation is under 34 weeks.
- The fetal fibronectin test is a useful test for preterm delivery. A negative test between 22 and 34 weeks gestation suggests that delivery is unlikely to occur within the next two weeks.
- Administer corticosteroids to reduce the incidence of RDS (neonatal death, IVH, and NEC). Two doses of 12 mg betamethasone should be given i.m. 24 h apart, to all women threatening to deliver between 24 and 34 weeks' gestation. The optimal treatment–delivery interval for administration of antenatal corticosteroids is after 24 h but less than seven days after the start of treatment. However, the use of repeat courses of antenatal corticosteroids has not been shown to be beneficial.

Prolonged pregnancy

Prolonged pregnancy (beyond 42 weeks' gestation) carries risks for both mother and foetus.

Foetal risks
- birth asphyxia
- chronic foetal malnutrition
- difficult and prolonged labour
- unexpected intrauterine death
- foetal distress and meconium aspiration
- perinatal mortality after 42 weeks' gestation is twice that at 38–42 weeks' gestation.

Management
- regular and careful assessment of foetal well-being
- induction of labour.

Polyhydramnios

In polyhydramnios, the amniotic fluid volume exceeds 2000 ml. Mild polyhydramnios usually has no obvious cause, whereas most severe polyhydramnios (amniotic fluid index over 24 cm or deepest pool ≥15 cm) has an identifiable cause. Polyhydramnios may be secondary to maternal factors (especially diabetes) or foetal factors (such as oesophageal atresia, multiple pregnancy, anencephaly, high intestinal obstruction, hydrops fetalis, Down's syndrome, diaphragmatic hernia, neuromuscular disorders, or Beckwith–Weidemann syndrome). Major malformations may be found in up to 40% of the infants, with 5% having chromosomal anomalies.

Maternal clinical features
- maternal discomfort
- uterine size appearing large for dates.

Foetal risks
- preterm labour
- preterm rupture of membranes
- abruption (following amnioreduction)
- twin–twin transfusion (in twin pregnancy).

Management
- Mothers should have a glucose tolerance test and detailed foetal scan.
- In severe polyhydramnios, foetal karyotyping may be required.
- Amnioreduction may relieve maternal discomfort (large volume taps may precipitate an abruption).
- Maternal indometacin (75–200 mg/day), which reduces foetal urine production, may be beneficial.
- Look for possible anomalies in the infant after birth.

Oligohydramnios

Midtrimester oligohydramnios is associated with increased mortality from premature rupture of membranes (pulmonary hypoplasia), urinary tract malformations (such as renal agenesis), and IUGR. Amnioinfusion of a warmed physiological solution permits better imaging of the foetus and confirms premature rupture of membranes. Abnormal karyotypes are present in 5–10%.

Foetal risks
- foetal death
- limb contractures
- pulmonary hypoplasia.

Management
- obtain detailed foetal scans
- obtain foetal karyotype where indicated
- perform an ultrasound examination of newborn infant's renal tract.

Gestational diabetes

This is defined as impaired glucose tolerance during pregnancy which reverts to normal after the puerperium. It is associated with an increased incidence of foetal malformations and perinatal complications.

Maternal clinical features
- polyhydramnios
- delivery complications
- hyperglycaemia and glycosuria.

Foetal risks
- polycythaemia
- sudden foetal demise
- hypertrophic cardiomyopathy
- diabetic embryopathy (such as caudal regression, anencephaly, meningocele, vertebral dysplasia, congenital heart disease, and small left colon).

Perinatal risks
- jaundice
- hypoglycaemia
- hypocalcaemia
- renal vein thrombosis
- RDS (relative surfactant deficiency)
- birth injury and asphyxia (large size)
- feeding difficulties (immature sucking and swallowing).

Management of the foetus/infant
- induction of labour at 38 weeks' gestation
- operative delivery if foetus is large
- early feeding (orally or intravenously with 10–15% dextrose)
- blood-glucose monitoring after birth for 24–48 h until blood sugars consistently ≥3 mmol/l

- respiratory distress, jaundice, and polycythaemia to be managed expectantly
- commence antibiotics (following cultures) if respiratory distress persists
- where appropriate, exclude other malformations (such as vertebral or cardiac) by appropriate radiographs and echocardiography.

Useful websites

www.marchofdimes.com
The March of Dimes Birth Defects Foundation – a US based charity concerned with pregnancy and the newborn.

www.safehands.org
A charity to help health professionals prevent deaths and suffering in pregnancy and childbirth.

Further reading

American College of Obstetricians and Gynecologists. Management of Preterm Labour, ACOG Practice Bulletin, Number 43, 2003.

Andersen HF. Use of fetal fibronectin in women at risk for proterm delivery. *Clinical Obstetrics and Gynecology* (2000) **43:**746–58.

Beischer NA, Mackay EV, Colditz PB. *Obstetrics and the Newborn*, 3rd edn. Philadelphia: WB Saunders, 1997.

Burrow GN, Ferris TF. *Medical Complications During Pregnancy*, 4th edn. Philadelphia: WB Saunders, 1995.

Chamberlain G, Steer P. *Turnbull's Obstetrics*, 3rd edn. Edinburgh: Churchill Livingstone, 2001.

Creasy R, Resnik R (eds). *Maternal–Fetal Medicine*, 4th edn. Philadelphia: WB Saunders, 1998.

Foley MR, Strong TH. *Obstetric Intensive Care: A Practical Manual*. Philadelphia: WB Saunders, 1997.

Lyell DJ. Hypertensive disorders of pregnancy: relevance for the neonatologist. *Neoreviews* (2004) **5:**240–6.

Reece EA. Maternal fuels, diabetic embryopathy: pathomechanisms and prevention. *Seminars in Reproductive Medicine* (1999) **17:**183–94.

Related topics of interest

- congenital malformations and birth defects
- childbirth complications and foetal outcome
- intrauterine growth restriction
- multiple pregnancy.

Prenatal diagnosis

The last decade has witnessed many significant advances in prenatal diagnosis. Improvements in ultrasound imaging techniques, the application of biochemical and DNA analysis and karyotyping to samples of foetal tissue obtained by chorionic villus sampling (CVS), amniocentesis, and foetal blood sampling have all greatly extended the scope of prenatal diagnosis to a host of structural malformations, chromosomal abnormalities, specific gene defects, and several metabolic disorders.

Structural malformations

In the UK, routine scans are performed at 18–19 weeks' gestation to screen for congenital malformations. Screening detects 55% of the major and 35% of minor malformations. The most commonly detected malformations are listed below on a systems basis:

CNS
- anencephaly
- encephalocele
- haemorrhage
- hydrocephalus
- open spina bifida
- hydranencephaly
- holoprosencephaly
- intracranial cysts
- Dandy–Walker malformation
- agenesis of the corpus callosum.

Cardiovascular system
- complex congenital heart disease
- hypoplastic left heart syndrome
- coarctation of the aorta
- transposition of the great vessels.

Respiratory system
- lung sequestration
- mediastinal tumours
- congenital diaphragmatic hernia
- congenital cystic adenomatoid malformation of the lung.

Gastrointestinal system
- gastroschisis
- bowel perforations with ascites and gut hyperechogenicity
- duodenal atresia (with 'double bubble', suggests trisomy 21)
- omphalocele (high incidence of cardiac and chromosomal abnormalities).

Genitourinary system

The commonest congenital anomalies are detected by ultrasound (20–30% of all). Lesions include renal agenesis, dilated renal pelvis, multicystic kidneys, and other features of an obstructive uropathy (such as thick-walled bladder and dilated upper urethra in posterior urethral valves).

Musculoskeletal system

Over 100 skeletal dysplasias are now diagnosable prenatally from the detection of abnormal skeletal shape (as in camptomelic and thanatophoric dysplasia) or bone mineralisation (as in hypophosphatasia and achondrogenesis), while fractures and callus formation may be seen in osteogenesis imperfecta (types II—IV). Akinesia and severe contractures may be seen in neuromuscular disorders such as arthrogryposis multiplex congenita.

Miscellaneous anomalies

Cleft lip (and palate) may be readily detected along with other soft-tissue anomalies, such as hydrops and cystic hygromas. The nuchal translucency test (carried out between 11 and 13 weeks gestation) detects foetuses at high risk of chromosomal abnormality (such as Down's syndrome) and structural heart disease.

Invasive diagnostic techniques

Amniocentesis

This is usually performed in the second trimester (at 15–16 weeks) under ultrasound guidance. The procedure has a 1% risk of spontaneous abortion. Up to 20 ml of amniotic fluid is aspirated, and cells from this are cultured (2–4 weeks) and then subjected to cytogenetic, DNA, or enzymatic analysis. The main disadvantage is the slow turnaround time, necessitating terminations at 20 weeks. Amniocentesis may also be used for amnioinfusion (oligohydramnios) and amniotic fluid drainage (polyhydramnios). This procedure is associated with pulmonary hypoplasia.

Chorionic villus sampling (CVS)

CVS has been in use over the last 15 years with great success. It is performed earlier than amniocentesis (8–12 weeks' gestation) and involves passing a catheter transcervically into the chorion frondosum and obtaining chorionic tissue by suction. More recently, CVS has been performed with a 2-mm diameter transcervical CVS forceps. The forceps is guided through the cervical canal under ultrasound guidance. Sampling is achieved by opening the forceps and closing while advancing the forceps further into the placenta and then withdrawing it. CVS can also be performed transabdominally with a double-needle technique. However, the reports of foetal limb reduction defects following CVS before ten weeks' gestation have resulted in the restriction of this procedure before ten weeks' gestation. The procedure-related loss is 2–3% in the younger women but ~6% in the older women. Rapid cytogenetic analysis can be made directly on the obtained tissue preparations or following 12–24-h cell cultures. Enzyme assays for inborn errors of metabolism can be performed directly on sampled chorionic tissues. Results are available sooner than after amniocentesis, allowing an easier first-trimester termination where indicated. Occasionally, however, a discrepancy may exist between chorionic and foetal karyotype, making later amniocentesis necessary.

Foetal blood sampling (FBS)
FBS of the umbilical vein close to its placental insertion under direct ultrasonic guidance is the commonest approach. Alternatively, blood may be sampled from the intrahepatic portion of the foetal umbilical vein. The procedure is performed after 17 weeks' gestation with a procedure-related loss of approximately 1%. This procedure can be used both for diagnostic purposes (as in haemoglobinopathies, coagulopathies, immunodeficiency syndromes, cytogenetic and DNA studies, and inborn errors of metabolism) and for monitoring foetal well-being or foetal therapy (as in monitoring acid–base status, intrauterine infection, red cell alloimmunisation, immune thrombocytopenia, and blood or platelet transfusion).

In vitro fertilisation and preimplantation diagnosis
It is now also possible to perform cytogenetic and DNA analyses from single cells obtained from human embryos as early as the eight-cell stage. The embryos can be sexed and several genetic disorders excluded before implantation.

Further reading

Allan L. Antenatal diagnosis of heart disease. *Heart* (2000) **83**:367–70.
Harrison MR, Evans M, Adzick NS et al. *The Unborn Patient: Prenatal Diagnosis and Treatment*, 3rd edn. Philadelphia: WB Saunders, 2000.
Kumar S, O'Brien A. Recent developments in fetal medicine. *British Medical Journal* (2004) **328**:1002–6.
Rodeck CH, Whittle M. *Fetal Medicine: Basic Science and Clinical Practice*. Edinburgh: Churchill Livingstone, 1998.
Whittle MJ, Connor JM (eds). *Prenatal Diagnosis in Obstetric Practice*, 2nd edn. Oxford: Blackwell Science, 1995.

Related topics of interest

- chromosomal abnormalities
- congenital malformations and birth defects
- haemolytic disease
- inherited metabolic disease—investigation and management
- intrauterine growth restriction.

Pulmonary air leaks

Pulmonary air leaks occur when there is high transpulmonary pressure, alveolar overdistension, and finally alveolar rupture. Following alveolar rupture, gas may track along the perivascular spaces into the pleura (pneumothorax), the interstitium (pulmonary interstitial emphysema [PIE]), the mediastinum (pneumomediastinum), and the pericardium (pneumopericardium), or through the diaphragmatic foramina into the peritoneum (pneumoperitoneum).

Pneumothorax

This is the commonest form of air leak, occurring in up to 1% of all newborns, though only 0.1% may be symptomatic. Pneumothoraces can occur spontaneously at birth or during resuscitation, but thereafter prevalence is increased in the presence of pulmonary disease (such as MAS or RDS) and assisted ventilation. Pneumothoraces are correlated with high mean and peak inspiratory pressures, long inspiratory times, and breathing out of phase with the ventilator.

Clinical features
Large tension pneumothoraces produce sudden deterioration in the infant's condition, causing pallor, hypotension, bradycardia, and hypoxaemia. Air entry is reduced on the affected side and the mediastinum shifted away from the affected side. Pneumothoraces are bilateral in 15–20% of cases, and if unilateral, are more commonly on the right. Pneumothoraces predispose infants to IVHs.

Management
Transillumination of the chest with a fibre-optic light shows increased transillumination on the affected side (but PIE may give similar appearance). Confirm by chest radiograph. In an emergency, needling both sides of the chest may produce immediate improvement. Pneumothoraces should be drained in symptomatic infants or infants receiving assisted ventilation. A chest drain (size 10–14FG) should be inserted under local anaesthesia, and the adequacy of drainage and position of the drain checked by radiography. Better drainage is often achieved if the drain is aimed anteriorly with the drain lying retrosternally. The risk of developing a pneumothorax may be reduced by using the lowest effective pressures, employing relatively fast ventilator rates with short inspiratory times, and sedating active babies.

Pulmonary interstitial emphysema (PIE)

PIE is primarily a disorder of preterm infants with RDS requiring high-pressure ventilation. Small airways rupture, with air dissecting into the interstitium and being trapped within the perivascular sheaths of the lung. This reduces pulmonary perfusion, producing a ventilation–perfusion mismatch, hypoxaemia, and hypercapnia. It becomes progressively more prevalent with decreasing birth weight.

Clinical features

PIE commonly presents with worsening gas exchange in a ventilated infant. The radiograph is diagnostic with unilateral or bilateral cystic radiolucencies and hyperinflation. The appearances on transillumination may resemble a large pneumothorax.

Management

Minimise ventilation pressures and reduce PEEP to maintain satisfactory gases (allow higher $PaCO_2$ if $pH \geq 7.25$). Use heavy sedation or paralysis, employ fast ventilator rates (short inspiratory times). High-frequency oscillatory ventilation may be beneficial. With unilateral PIE, place the infant on its side with the hyperinflated lung dependent. Selective bronchial intubation of the nonaffected lung may also be useful, especially if the left lung is affected. Alternatively, for localised disease, large cysts may be artificially punctured and a chest drain left in situ to drain the pneumothorax.

Pneumomediastinum

With an incidence of approximately one in 400, this is often seen in the presence of other air leaks in preterm ventilated infants, though, if isolated, it is usually asymptomatic. Diagnosis is made on the chest radiograph, which shows air around the cardiac silhouette and, on lateral views, a hyperlucent area behind the sternum. No therapy is required, as drainage is usually ineffective.

Pneumopericardium

This may arise from gas tracking from the mediastinum into the pericardial sac in a sick ventilated preterm infant, producing cardiac tamponade. There is rapid clinical deterioration with bradycardia, hypotension, cyanosis, and muffled heart sounds. Mortality is high. This may mimic a pneumothorax, but the chest radiograph is diagnostic, with gas completely surrounding the heart. Presence of gas beneath the heart differentiates this from a pneumomediastinum, where gas cannot track beneath the heart due to the attachment of the mediastinal pleura to the diaphragm. Small asymptomatic pneumopericardia may be observed only, but, if symptomatic, urgent pericardial taps should be performed (subxiphoid approach) with continuous monitoring of the cardiovascular status.

Pneumoperitoneum

This most commonly arises from perforation of the gut (mainly NEC), but it may also arise from within the chest (of ventilated infants), with the gas from air leaks tracking down diaphragmatic foramina into the peritoneum. A history of gastrointestinal disease or an abnormal gas pattern on abdominal radiograph suggests a surgical pneumoperitoneum rather than a transdiaphragmatic air leak. Marked abdominal distension may be drained by a needle tap or a drain left in situ.

Further reading

Fanaroff AA, Martin RJ. *Neonatal-Perinatal Medicine: Diseases of the Fetus and Infant*, 7th edn. St Louis, MO: Mosby, 2001.

Goldsmith JP, Karotkin EH (eds). *Assisted Ventilation of the Neonate*, 4th edn. Philadelphia: WB Saunders, 2003.

Greenough A, Milner AD (eds). *Neonatal Respiratory Disorders*, 2nd edn. London: Arnold, 2003.

Greenough A, Roberton NRC. Acute respiratory disease. In: JM Rennie, NRC Roberton (eds). *Textbook of Neonatology*, 3rd edn. Edinburgh: Churchill Livingstone, 1999: 481–607.

Halahakoon CN, Halliday HL. Other acute lung disorders. In: VYH Yu (ed.). *Baillière's Clinical Paediatrics*, Vol. 3/No. 1, *Pulmonary Problems in the Perinatal Period and their Sequelae*. London: Baillière Tindall, 1995: 87–114.

Kirkpatrick BV, Mueller DG. Respiratory disorders in the newborn. In: V Chernick, T Boat (eds). *Kendig's Disorders of the Respiratory Tract in Children*, 6th edn. Philadelphia: WB Saunders, 1998: 328–64.

Related topics of interest

- chronic lung disease
- complications of mechanical ventilation
- congenital diaphragmatic hernia
- mechanical ventilation
- meconium aspiration syndrome
- pulmonary hypoplasia
- respiratory distress syndrome.

Pulmonary haemorrhage

Massive pulmonary haemorrhage represents one end of a continuum of disorders characterised by pulmonary oedema. In the initial stages, rising capillary pressure leads to a rise in interstitial fluid, resulting in fluid loss into the alveoli and finally capillary haemorrhage. A sudden onset and a high mortality are characteristic. This is now largely a disorder of preterm infants ventilated for severe RDS and often a large PDA causing heart failure, with reported incidences of 1–12 per 1000 live births. Some 2–5% of babies with RDS develop some form of pulmonary haemorrhage. It is also seen in term infants, particularly in association with severe birth asphyxia, hypothermia, severe rhesus haemolytic disease, hydrops, left heart failure, fluid overload, sepsis, coagulation disorder, maternal diabetes, hypoglycaemia, and small-for-gestational-age infants. As the haemorrhagic fluid is protein rich, it inactivates surfactant, worsening gas exchange. This haemorrhagic fluid has a haematocrit of 10%. Although synthetic surfactant therapy for RDS may increase the incidence of *clinical* pulmonary haemorrhage, *pathologically* diagnosed (at autopsy) pulmonary haemorrhage is not increased. Risk factors for pulmonary haemorrhage in surfactant-treated infants include birth weight under 700 g, male sex, presence of a PDA, and prophylactic use of synthetic rather than natural surfactant.

Clinical features

Commonly, there is a sudden deterioration accompanied by the appearance of large amounts of pink/red frothy fluid or frank blood from the infant's oropharynx, or endotracheal tube if already intubated. There may be bleeding from other sites. The infant may be pale, hypotensive, bradycardic, cyanosed, apnoeic or with gasping respiration, and shocked. If in heart failure, the infant is tachycardic with an accompanying murmur (particularly with a PDA) and hepatosplenomegaly. There are widespread crepitations with reduced air entry. In surfactant-treated infants, blood-stained secretions may be the only sign.

Investigations

- *FBC*. Haemoglobin commonly below 10 gm/dl.
- *Clotting screen*. May be normal but commonly becomes deranged following a massive pulmonary haemorrhage.
- *Radiology*. Chest radiograph shows a 'white-out', or may be less striking, resembling RDS, and there may be cardiomegaly.
- *Blood gases*. Hypoxia and hypercapnia with a combined respiratory and metabolic acidosis are characteristic.
- *Bacteriology*. Perform an infection screen (without an LP).

Management

- Urgent resuscitation is required to prevent sudden death. Endotracheal intubation for mechanical ventilation and simultaneous volume expansion with blood or

plasma is a prerequisite. Also correct any underlying disorder(s). A high PEEP ($\geq 6\,cmH_2O$) and long inspiratory time ($\geq 0.5\,s$) may be beneficial.
- Transfuse FFP (10–15 ml/kg) and/or cryoprecipitate as indicated, with additional vitamin K to improve coagulation.
- Restrict fluids to 60–90 ml/kg per day when in congestive heart failure, adding diuretics (furosemide 1.5 mg/kg b.d.) when bleeding has stopped.
- Commence broad-spectrum antibiotics following cultures.
- Correct acidosis with bicarbonate.
- Frequent suctioning (up to several times in the hour) may be required in the initial stages to prevent the ET tube from blocking. The suction catheter should be measured so as to protrude only ~0.5 cm past the ET tube tip to avoid provoking fresh bleeding during suctioning.
- Maintain the blood pressure with infusions of colloid, blood, or inotropes.
- Additional surfactant therapy when pulmonary haemorrhage has occurred after the first dose may be beneficial (though controversial!).

Prevention

- Avoid acidosis.
- Avoid asphyxia.
- Avoid hypothermia.
- Avoid hypoglycaemia.
- Correct coagulation defects.
- Suction intubated infants with care.
- Avoid overtreating with surfactant.
- Wean ventilation pressure (PEEP) slowly in ELBW infants.
- Be careful to apply the above measures to growth-restricted infants, as they may be particularly at risk.

Further reading

Fanaroff AA, Martin RJ. *Neonatal-Perinatal Medicine: Diseases of the Fetus and Infant*, 7th edn, St Louis, MO: Mosby, 2001.

Greenough A, Milner AD (eds). *Neonatal Respiratory Disorders*, 2nd edn. London: Arnold, 2003.

Greenough A, Roberton NRC. Acute respiratory disease in the newborn. In: JM Rennie, NRC Roberton (eds). *Textbook of Neonatology*, 3rd edn, Edinburgh: Churchill Livingstone, 1999: 481–607.

Halahakoon CN, Halliday HL. Other acute lung disorders. In: VYH Yu (ed.). *Baillière's Clinical Paediatrics*, Vol. 3/No. 1, *Pulmonary Problems in the Perinatal Period and their Sequelae*. London: Baillière Tindall, 1995: 87–114.

Kirkpatrick BV, Mueller DG. Respiratory disorders in the newborn. In: V Chernick, T Boat (eds). *Kendig's Disorders of the Respiratory Tract in Children*, 6th edn. Philadelphia: WB Saunders, 1998: 328–64.

Kluckow M, Evans N. Ductal shunting, high pulmonary blood flow, and pulmonary haemorrhage. *Journal of Pediatrics* (2000) **137**:68–72.

Raju TNK, Langenberg P. Pulmonary haemorrhage and exogenous surfactant therapy: a meta-analysis. *Journal of Pediatrics* (1993) **123**:603–10.

Related topics of interest

- acute collapse
- persistent ductus arteriosus
- respiratory distress
- shock
- surfactant replacement therapy.

Pulmonary hypoplasia

This may be defined as an incomplete development of the lung, resulting in reduced lung weight and distending volume. There is an associated reduction in the number of airway divisions, alveoli, arteries, and veins. The true incidence of pulmonary hypoplasia is not known, as it is commonly underreported and the diagnosis frequently masked by other pulmonary disorders.

Primary pulmonary hypoplasia

This occurs in the absence of any other diseases or conditions that would impair lung development, such as oligohydramnios or absent renal function. The reported incidence is low, less than 1% of admissions to a neonatal unit being affected.

Secondary pulmonary hypoplasia

This may be ten times more common than primary pulmonary hypoplasia and may be present in 10–15% of early neonatal deaths.

Aetiology
Several mechanisms have been postulated from clinical observations and animal experiments. A reduction in amniotic fluid volume (such as chronic amniotic fluid leak before 26 weeks' gestation, Potter's syndrome, or even midtrimester amniocentesis) commonly leads to pulmonary hypoplasia. It has been postulated that prolonged thoracic compression, reduced foetal breathing movements, and reduced intrathoracic lung fluid pressure may all be mechanistically related to pulmonary hypoplasia. Reduced intrathoracic space has been shown experimentally to reduce lung development, in accord with clinical observations (as in congenital diaphragmatic hernia, pleural effusions, thoracic tumours, and asphyxiating thoracic dystrophy). Drug administration to pregnant mothers, especially angiotensin-converting enzyme (ACE) inhibitors has also been associated with pulmonary hypoplasia.

Clinical features

Unilateral pulmonary hypoplasia
This is usually asymptomatic and may be a chance finding in chest radiography. At times, however, there may be a mediastinal shift to the hypoplastic side, as may be evident clinically. Associated congenital malformations (cardiac, renal, skeletal, or gastrointestinal) may be the presenting complaint and may greatly increase the morbidity.

Bilateral pulmonary hypoplasia
Presentation is determined by the severity of the disorder. The mildly affected may have persistent tachypnoea and a chest radiograph showing a bell-shaped chest with well-inflated but small lungs. With severe pulmonary hypoplasia, resuscitation may be difficult or impossible with high inflation pressures ($>30\,cmH_2O$), 100% O_2, and persisting CO_2 retention.

Diagnosis

- high pressure ventilation with persisting CO_2 retention (as above)
- lung-function tests showing reduced functional residual capacity (FRC)—less than 60% of expected value, that is, 16 ml/kg body weight.

Management

Prenatal

Premature rupture of membranes before 25 weeks is associated with poor outcome. Elective delivery at 34 weeks may be recommended. Intrathoracic space-occupying lesions, such as cysts or effusions, should be drained in utero to prevent prolonged lung compression.

Postnatal

Severe pulmonary hypoplasia is incompatible with life. Less severe pulmonary hypoplasia may best be ventilated on high rates and low mean airway pressures. Persistent pulmonary hypertension of the newborn (PPHN) may be a complicating factor especially when there is associated lung disease (such as RDS, sepsis—especially group B streptococcus—or meconium aspiration). High-frequency oscillation and inhaled NO therapy may be beneficial, but infants with severe pulmonary hypoplasia respond poorly to inhaled NO. Associated congenital anomalies (such as congenital diaphragmatic hernia) may adversely affect the outcome. ECMO is contraindicated in severe pulmonary hypoplasia. Associated postural and limb deformities respond to physiotherapy and orthopaedic interventions.

Differential diagnosis

The following conditions may coexist and should be considered as alternative diagnoses:

- severe RDS
- primary PPHN
- group B streptococcus pneumonia
- neuromuscular disorders (such as myotonic dystrophy).

Prognosis

- Mortality is high, especially in primary pulmonary hypoplasia (over 50%).
- Associated anomalies (such as renal agenesis or congenital diaphragmatic hernia) increase mortality.
- Pneumothorax, PIE followed by CLD, and prolonged oxygen dependency are likely to develop in affected preterm infants.
- Long-term lung function may recover completely during the first few years of life or remain abnormal, depending on the original diagnosis.

Useful website

www.emedicine.com/pedtopic2627.htm
Part of the largest and most current online clinical knowledge base available to health professionals.

Further reading

Greenough A, Milner AD (eds). *Neonatal Respiratory Disorders*, 2nd edn. London: Arnold, 2003.

Kilbride HW, Thibeault DW. Neonatal complications of preterm premature rupture of membranes: pathophysiology and management. *Clinics in Perinatology* (2001) **28:**761–85.

Krumel TM. Congenital malformations of the lower respiratory tract. In: V Chernik, T Boat (eds). *Kendig's Disorders of the Respiratory Tract in Children*, 6th edn. Philadelphia: WB Saunders, 1998: 287–328.

Lauria MR, Gonik B, Romero R. Pulmonary hypoplasia: pathogenesis, diagnosis, and antenatal prediction. Obstetrics and Gynecology (1995) 86: 466–75.

Milner AD, Fox G. Congenital abnormalities of the respiratory system. In: VYH Yu (ed.). *Baillière's Clinical Paediatrics*, Vol. 3/No. 1. *Pulmonary Problems in the Perinatal Period and Their Sequelae*. London: Baillière Tindall, 1995: 171–202.

Winn HN, Chen M, Amon E. Neonatal pulmonary hypoplasia and perinatal mortality in patients with midtrimester rupture of amniotic membranes—a critical analysis. *American Journal of Obstetrics and Gynecology* (2000) **182:**1638–44.

Related topics of interest

- complications of mechanical ventilation
- congenital diaphragmatic hernia
- persistent pulmonary hypertension of the newborn
- respiratory distress
- resuscitation.

Renal and urinary tract disorders— nephrology

Nephrons develop from the fifth week of intrauterine life, and they are fully formed, though not fully functional, by 36 weeks' gestation. The infant glomerulus is a third of the size of the adult glomerulus, and although the tubules are functioning by 9 weeks, they are short and immature even at term. Consequently the newborn kidney is functionally immature. The glomerular filtration rate (GFR) and renal blood flow are low in the newborn period. After birth, the GFR increases as a function of post-conceptional age rather than postnatal age. As tubular function is immature, urine-concentrating ability is limited, as is the ability to excrete a water load. Unlike term infants, preterm infants are less able to conserve sodium and excrete hydrogen ions.

Presentation of renal and urinary tract disorders

Family history
- history of an inherited renal disorder, such as polycystic kidney disease—autosomal recessive and dominant—and Alport's syndrome (X-linked)
- history of metabolic disorder (autosomal recessive) with renal manifestation (such as cystinosis and tyrosinosis)
- history of vesicoureteric reflux (4% risk of reflux in first-degree relatives of index patient, but 50% risk of scarring present in index case).

Antenatal history
- abnormal kidneys on foetal anomaly scan at 17–20 weeks or later (as in dilated collecting system, multicystic kidney, and renal agenesis)
- oligohydramnios (renal agenesis, dysplasia, obstructed urinary tract, and Potter's syndrome)
- elevated alpha-fetoprotein in amniotic fluid.

Perinatal history
- placental weight over 25% of birth weight (congenital nephrotic syndrome, Finnish type, autosomal recessive, and associated with prematurity)
- single umbilical artery (urinary tract anomalies in ≤3%).
- delayed micturition (99% of healthy infants urinate by 48h), suggesting renal underperfusion (asphyxia, hypotension, congenital nephritis, urinary tract obstruction, renal agenesis, and tubular or cortical necrosis)
- oliguria (urinary output <20ml/kg per day or <1ml/kg per h) suggesting dehydration or any of the above factors
- haematuria (one in ten newborns have transient haematuria)—distinguish from haemoglobinuria or myoglobinuria; causes include cortical and medullary necrosis, acute renal failure, asphyxia, infection, and acute renal failure
- proteinuria (transient proteinuria up to 45mg/day is common); causes include renal vein thrombosis, infection, and idiopathic familial congenital nephrotic syndrome)

- leucocyturia (>3 white blood cells (WBCs) per high-power field is abnormal in a centrifuged urine sample)—suggests urinary tract infection or nephritis
- oedema (excessive water and salt intake, congenital nephrotic syndrome, obstructive uropathy, and acute renal failure)
- acidosis (metabolic acidosis with normal anion gap suggests renal tubular acidosis
- urinary tract infection (>10^5 organisms from two clean catch samples or any growth from a suprapubic aspiration sample)
- hypertension—mainly renovascular causes, especially renal artery thrombosis.

Specific disorders

Acute renal failure

Acute renal failure (ARF) is a sudden and severe reduction in GFR with loss of the renal ability to conserve electrolytes, concentrate urine and excrete wastes. Assume an infant is in ARF if urine output is <1 ml/kg per h for 24 h and/or creatinine is rising and above the normal range for gestation and postnatal age.

Prerenal failure (60% of ARF)
This is a functional response of normal kidneys to underperfusion. This is commonly due to renal underperfusion.

Renal underperfusion from hypovolaemia
- foetal/neonatal haemorrhage
- maternal antepartum haemorrhage
- inadequate fluid intake or increased losses (polyuria, insensible loss, gastrointestinal loss, or NEC).
- operative fluid loss

Renal underperfusion with normovolaemia
- asphyxia
- septic shock
- congestive cardiac failure.

Intrinsic renal failure (~40% of ARF)
This follows structural damage to renal tissue or vasculature. The main causes are shock and asphyxia.
- arterial or venous thrombosis
- acute tubular, medullary or cortical necrosis
- congenital renal anomalies (as in agenesis and dysplastic kidneys)
- congenital infection (such as toxoplasmosis or syphilis) and DIC.

Postrenal failure (<5% of ARF)
This follows mechanical or functional obstruction to urine flow.
- ureterocele
- pelviureteric or vesicoureteric junction obstruction
- urethral obstruction—(posterior urethral valves, urethral stricture, urethral diverticulum, tumours, and neurogenic bladder).

Clinical and biochemical features of renal failure
- oliguria and oedema
- hyperkalaemia (major cause of death from cardiac toxicity)
- hyponatraemia (dilutional)
- hypertension (from volume overload)
- metabolic acidosis (inability to excrete acids)
- hyperphosphataemia and hypocalcaemia.

Investigations
Blood
- U and E and creatinine
- albumin
- glucose
- calcium and magnesium
- acid–base status
- coagulation studies
- FBC and film
- blood culture (full septic screen if sepsis suspected).

Urine
- dipstick
- microscopy (casts)
- culture
- urea and creatinine
- electrolytes
- osmolarity.

Others
- weighing infant
- checking blood pressure
- renal ultrasound scan.

Management
Establish the diagnosis of renal failure and distinguish between the three main causes of renal failure, as their management differs. Confirm obstructive uropathy (postrenal failure) on ultrasound examination and refer to a urologist. Distinguishing prerenal from intrinsic renal failure may be difficult, but the following indices may be helpful. In prerenal failure, urine/plasma osmolarity is >2 (<1 intrinsic renal failure), urine sodium is <10 mmol/l (>40 mmol/l in intrinsic renal failure), urine/plasma urea is >10 (<10 in intrinsic renal failure), fractional sodium excretion (Fe_{Na}%) is <2% (>3% in intrinsic renal failure), and urinalysis commonly shows benign sediment (whereas red and white cells and casts are seen in intrinsic renal failure). Fe_{Na}% is calculated from the sodium and creatinine concentration of serum (S) and a spot urine (U) sample as follows: Fe_{Na}% $= (U/S)$ sodium $\times (S/U)$ creatinine $\times 100$. Once furosemide has been used, Fe_{Na}% becomes inaccurate. Prerenal failure requires prompt correction of renal underperfusion (associated with low BP, capillary refill time of >3s and core–peripheral temperature gap of >2°C), whereas established (intrinsic) renal failure requires a swift restriction of fluid intake. If the state of hydration is uncertain, give a

fluid challenge with colloid or normal saline (10–20 ml/kg IV over 30–60 min) followed by frusemide (2 mg/kg). If urine output improves (especially over 10 ml/kg over 3 h), there is renal underperfusion—continue with careful rehydration. If fluid volume is replete but there is hypotension, try an inotrope (such as dopamine 5–20 µg/kg per min). If fluid challenge fails, severely cut back fluids, replacing only insensible water loss plus measured fluid and electrolyte losses (weigh infant). Correct severe acidosis (pH < 7.2) and hyperkalaemia (serum potassium > 6 mmol/l ± ECG changes) with resonium enemas, 10% calcium gluconate (slow IV) insulin/dextrose infusion (one unit of insulin per 3 g of dextrose) at 0.15 units insulin/kg per hour or bicarbonate (IV). Monitor serum electrolytes and ECG regularly. Administer calcium supplements and phosphate-binding agents as required. If plasma sodium is < 120 mmol/l, potassium is > 8 mmol/l, bicarbonate is < 12 mmol/l, and creatinine > 630 µmol/l with severe fluid overload not responding to above measures, consider peritoneal dialysis. Treat suspected infection (after all cultures obtained) with non-nephrotoxic drugs. Hypertension (commonly due to fluid overload) responds to fluid restriction. As renal function improves, ease fluid and dietary restrictions; finally, remove them as renal function returns to normal.

Renal artery thrombosis

This is associated with a high umbilical artery catheter, sepsis, and hypercoaguable states. Physical signs include hypertension, haematuria, proteinuria, oliguria, congestive heart failure, and, if bilateral, minimal or absent renal function. Renal ultrasound scan is normal but radionucleotide ([131I] Hippuran) uptake is absent. Treat hypertension aggressively, as prospects for full recovery are good.

Renal venous thrombosis

This is associated with dehydration, asphyxia, hyperosmolality, polycythaemia and cyanotic CHD, and incidence is increased in IDMs. Common signs include flank or abdominal mass, haematuria, and thrombocytopenia. Ultrasonography shows enlarged kidney with thrombus in renal vein or extending into inferior vena cava. Management is supportive, with correction of predisposing factors and renal failure (if it develops). Prognosis is generally good.

Nephrotic syndrome

Nephrotic syndrome is rare in the newborn. Causes of neonatal nephrotic syndrome include nephrotic syndrome of Finnish type, epimembranous nephropathy due to renal vein thrombosis, congenital syphilis or hepatitis B, and diffuse mesangial sclerosis (DMS). In Finland, the prevalence is 1.2 per 10 000 births. The placenta is large (25% of birth weight—normal 18%), and clinical signs include oedema, heavy proteinuria, hypoalbuminaemia, and elevated cholesterol. The proteinuria is unresponsive to immunosuppressive drugs and corticosteroids. Renal histology shows diffuse proximal tubule dilation. There is severe failure to thrive and frequent bacterial infections. Management is symptomatic—salt restriction, diuretics, antibiotics for sepsis, and optimising calorie intake. Penicillin therapy is curative for the nephrotic syndrome due to congenital syphilis. If diagnosis is uncertain, renal biopsy is essential for an accurate diagnosis, prognosis, guiding therapy, and parental counselling.

Renal tubular acidosis (RTA)

This is a group of disorders caused by an impaired ability to acidify urine. Three types are recognised.

Distal RTA (type 1)

This is due to impaired distal acidification (an inability to lower urine pH below 5.5 in the face of systemic acidosis). Presenting clinical features include polyuria, hypercalciuria, potassium depletion, and failure to thrive.

Proximal RTA (type 2)

This is due to impaired HCO_3^- reabsorption in the proximal tubule with a decreased renal HCO_3^- threshold.

Hyperkalaemic RTA (type 4)

There is impaired acidification due to impaired renal ammoniagenesis. There is a normal ability to acidify urine after an acid load, but net acid excretion is subnormal due to decreased $NH4^+$ excretion. It is seen in infants with hypo- or pseudohypo-aldosteronism.

Suspect RTA when metabolic acidosis is accompanied by hyperchloraemia and a normal plasma anion gap, that is, $[Na^+ + K^+] - [Cl^- + HCO_3^-] = 8-16\,mmol/l$. A normal anion gap reflects HCO_3^- loss from kidneys or gastrointestinal tract. Distinguish proximal from distal RTA from the urine anion gap: a urine sample from a patient with hyperchloraemic metabolic acidosis and a negative urine anion gap suggest proximal RTA, while a positive anion gap suggests distal RTA. Oral alkali (sodium citrate or sodium bicarbonate) is the therapy of choice for RTA with oral diuretics (thiazide or frusemide) to reduce serum K^+ in type 4 RTA.

Bartter's syndrome

Bartter's syndrome consists of a number of related disorders with a similar pathophysiology but which differ with regard to age of onset, presenting symptoms, and the magnitude of urinary potassium, calcium, and prostaglandin excretion. Three types are recognised: the classic Bartter's syndrome, the hypocalciuric-hypomagnesemic Gitelman variant, and the antenatal hypercalciuric variant (hyperprostaglandin E syndrome). The antenatal variant is due to mutations in the genes encoding the sodium–potassium–chloride (Na–K–2Cl) cotransporter or the luminal K channel, the Gitelman variant is due to mutations in the gene encoding the sodium–chloride (Na–Cl) cotransporter, and the classic Bartter's syndrome is due to mutations in the Na–K–2Cl cotransporter gene NKCC2. The classic Bartter's syndrome is juxtaglomerular complex (JGC) hyperplasia, characterised by hypokalaemic alkalosis, hyperaldosteronism, hyperreninaemia (due to increased synthesis of renal prostaglandins, particularly E2), and low or low-normal BP. It may be inherited as an autosomal recessive trait or occur sporadically. Sodium (and water) and potassium loss is characteristic. Hypokalaemia stimulates renin secretion and aldosterone production. Volume depletion activates the renin–angiotensin–aldosterone feedback system, leading to JGC hyperplasia. Typical symptoms in infancy include polyuria, polydipsia, salt craving, dehydration, vomiting, failure to thrive, and marked muscle weakness, spasms, or tetany. Treatment includes sodium and potassium supplements, spironolactone (aldosterone antagonist), angiotensin-converting enzyme inhibitors (to counteract angiotensin II and aldosterone), indometacin, and calcium and magnesium (for muscle spasms and tetany).

Hypertension

Hypertension in infants and children is defined as a systolic and/or diastolic pressure ≥95th centile for age and sex on three separate occasions, but in newborns only systolic values are used. There is no evidence for a single precise starting point for treatment but therapy may be considered in a neonate with a systolic pressure constantly above 110–115mmHg. Over 75% of neonatal hypertension is secondary to renal artery thrombosis while approximately one in five may be due to renal artery stenosis. The correct cuff should be used (width ≥2/3 of upper arm length) with infant at rest. Symptoms and signs include those of underlying disorder and hypertension itself (hypertensive encephalopathy, seizures, and congestive cardiac failure). Treatment depends on the cause. Hypertension secondary to volume overload responds to fluid restriction, diuretics (such as furosemide 0.5–2mg/kg per dose 12-hourly or chlorothiazide 5–10mg/kg per dose 12-hourly), vasodilators (such as hydralazine 1–5mg/kg per day given 6-hourly, captopril 0.1–1.0mg/kg per day given 6-hourly) or β-blockers (such as propranolol 2–5mg/kg per day given 8-hourly). Monitor electrolytes when diuretics are used. For urgent control of hypertension, IV nitroprusside (0.5–5μg/kg per min) or diazoxide (3–5mg/kg) is useful. Investigate persistent hypertension to exclude renovascular disease, coarctation of the aorta, other intrinsic renal or postrenal disease, and adrenal disorders.

Useful websites

www.kidney.org
The National Kidney Foundation (US).

http://kidney.niddk.nih.gov
The National Kidney and Urologic Diseases Information Clearinghouse, a service of the National Institute of Diabetes and Digestive and Kidney Diseases, part of the US National Institutes of Health.

Further reading

Awuzu M, Hunley TE, Kon V. Pathophysiology of acute renal failure in the neonatal period. In: RA Polin, WW Fox (eds). *Fetal and Neonatal Physiology*, 2nd edn. Philadelphia: WB Saunders, 1998: 1691–6.

Broin LP, Satlin LM. Clinical significance of developmental renal physiology. In: RA Polin, WW Fox (eds). *Fetal and Neonatal Physiology*, 2nd edn. Philadelphia: WB Saunders, 1998: 1677–91.

Fanaroff AA, Martin RJ. *Neonatal-Perinatal Medicine: Diseases of the Foetus and Infant*, 7th edn, St Louis, MO: Mosby, 2001.

Postlethwaite RJ (ed.). *Clinical Paediatric Nephrology*, 2nd edn. Oxford: Butterworth-Heinemann, 1994.

Proesmans W (ed.). Therapeutic strategies in children with renal disease. *Baillière's Clinical Paediatrics*, Vol. 5, No. 4, London: Baillière Tindall, 1997.

Watkinson M. Hypertension in the newborn baby. *Archives of Disease in Childhood Fetal and Neonatal Edition* (2002) **86:**F78–81.

Related topics of interest

- acid–base balance
- blood pressure
- fluid and electrolyte therapy
- renal and urinary tract disorders—urology.

Renal and urinary tract disorders—urology

Polycystic kidney disease (PCKD)

This can occur in an autosomal dominant form (adult polycystic disease [ADPCKD]) or an autosomal recessive form (infantile polycystic disease [ARPCKD]). In ARPCKD, the main site of dilation is the collecting tubules. The severe form is rapidly fatal at or soon after birth. An IV pyelogram is characteristic (mottled nephrogram and retention of contrast with delayed excretion). The kidneys are massive, and patients surviving the first month experience increasing renal failure and hypertension. Liver biopsy shows hepatic fibrosis with biliary dysgenesis. The ARPCKD gene on chromosome 6 (called PKHD1) has recently been identified, but a diagnostic kit is not yet available.

ADPCKD is more common (90% of all PCKD) and presents similarly with renal failure and reduced renal function with progressive renal insufficiency. Although symptoms may present in childhood, they more commonly present in adulthood. Nephrosonography shows bilateral large and small renal cysts. Imaging studies cannot accurately distinguish ARPCDK from ADPCKD. In ADPCKD, there is usually a family history of PCKD, and parents often show hepatic or renal cysts when imaged (CT or ultrasound scans). ADPCKD has a better prognosis than ARPCKD. Two genes associated with ADPCKD have recently been identified, PKD1 on chromosome 16 (which produces the protein polycystin-1) and PKD2 on chromosome 4 (which produces the protein polycystin-2). A mutation in PKD1 or PKD2 can lead to cyst formation.

Renal cystic dysplasia

When the disorder is unilateral, the term 'multicystic kidney' is used. There are large cysts with little renal tissue. It is commonly detected prenatally. Always examine the contralateral kidney carefully, as anomalies (such as pelviureteric junction [PUJ] obstruction) are common. The nonfunctional kidney may require surgical removal (risk of neoplasia). Renal cystic dysplasia is associated with other anomalies such as the Zellweger cerebrohepatorenal syndrome and the Meckel–Gruber syndrome. A technetium-99m-labelled dimercaptosuccinic acid (^{99m}Tc-DMSA) scan is required to determine whether the kidney is functional.

Renal agenesis

The complete absence of both kidneys is rare (one in 10000 births). There is oligohydramnios and associated pulmonary hypoplasia with Potter's facies, bowed legs, clubbed feet, and no kidneys evident on prenatal scans; affected infants die perinatally or are stillborn.

Posterior urethral valves

This occurs only in males. The bladder is distended and urine stream is poor. Diagnosis is confirmed by renal ultrasound and micturating cystourethrogram (MCUG), though most patients still present acutely unwell with a UTI. The immediate management consists of draining the urinary tract via an indwelling catheter, commencing broad-spectrum antibiotics and IV fluid and electrolyte therapy. A paediatric urologist will be required to resect the valves. Some infants, however, eventually develop renal failure and require renal transplantation.

Hydronephrosis

This is readily diagnosed antenatally (renal pelvis AP diameter over 8–10mm after 34 weeks) and should be confirmed postnatally (24–48h) only if bilateral – otherwise at six weeks when GFR would have increased. Antibiotic prophylaxis should be commenced (trimethoprim 2mg/kg once daily) until MCUG has been performed to rule out vesicoureteric reflux. To determine whether a dilated kidney is obstructed, [^{99m}Tc] mercapto-acetyl-triglycerine-3 (MAG-3) with a diuretic may be helpful. If obstruction is suspected, seek a paediatric urological opinion. Otherwise, regular follow-up with repeat renal ultrasound scans is required with a high index of suspicion for intercurrent UTIs. In time, the hydronephrosis resolves along with the need for antibiotic prophylaxis. If the AP diameter remains <10mm it is seldom of significance.

Hypospadias

In hypospadias, the urethral meatus may be positioned just below the glans or far back at the root of the penis. In severe cases, the penis is short and curved (due to chordee), resembling a large clitoris, and causing problems in assigning a sex to the infant. It is vital, then, that the infant's karyotype, endocrine status, and pelvic anatomy be ascertained (ultrasound or laparotomy). Infants should not be circumcised prior to surgical repair.

Vesicoureteric reflux

Vesicoureteric reflux (VUR) is the consequence of an incompetent vesicoureteric valve mechanism and may resolve spontaneously or, infrequently, lead to chronic renal insufficiency. There is an important genetic component to nonobstructive or 'idiopathic' VUR. One-third of the siblings of affected children will also have VUR, while 60% of the offspring of parents with VUR will also be affected. VUR also occurs in apparently healthy infants and children (asymptomatic VUR), the incidence falling from birth to the age 4 years, and is more common in boys (4:1). VUR associated with UTI (symptomatic VUR) is, however, predominantly found in girls, with a 4:1 preponderance. VUR is more common in infants presenting with UTI (30–50%) and in infants with prenatal hydronephrosis. VUR can cause morphological (renal scars) and functional renal damage. Renal damage is more likely with gross VUR and bladder dysfunction (such as neurogenic bladder). Renal scars are caused by intrarenal reflux, bacterial infection (UTI), and/or obstruction acting in concert. The rapidly growing kidney (as in infants and toddlers) is most susceptible to morphological damage. VUR predisposes to arterial hypertension.

Diagnosis of VUR

MCUG is the reference standard. It visualises the urethra, bladder, and renal pelvis, permitting grading of severity of reflux. Indirect radionuclide voiding cystography (such as MAG-3 renogram) is less reliable and can be used only in the older, continent child. MCUGs should be considered in all infants presenting with prenatal dilation of the renal pelvis, family history of VUR, UTI, and acute pyelonephritis.

Management of VUR

The goal of medical therapy is to avoid UTIs by using antibiotic prophylaxis and regulation of bladder and bowel emptying. Optimum duration of prophylaxis is not known, but it is influenced by severity of VUR, intercurrent UTIs, and associated anatomic abnormalities (see below). Surgery is indicated in patients with dilating VUR (grade of ≥III), recurrent breakthrough infections, failure of medical therapy, or are noncompliant with medical treatment. However, medical and surgical treatments are almost equally effective in protecting kidneys from new damage or the progression of pre-existing damage. In 4.2% of patients, surgery is complicated by obstruction. Follow up until VUR resolves or risk of complications is minimal.

Urinary tract infection

This is confirmed by the finding of a pure growth of a single pathogen at a count of at least 10^5 colony-forming units/ml urine in at least two clean specimens of urine, or any growth from a suprapubic aspirated urine specimen. Pus cells may be present or absent. Absence of growth from an appropriately handled bag specimen can rule out UTI. The commonest predisposing factor is urinary stasis (VUR, bladder dysfunction, infrequent or incomplete voiding, or outflow obstruction as in urethral valves). In the first 2–3 months of life, UTI occurs predominantly in boys, at 3–12 months of age boys and girls are equally affected, and above one year girls are predominantly affected.

Clinical features

In infants, symptoms are nonspecific including:

- fever
- jaundice
- failure to thrive
- feeding difficulties
- vomiting and diarrhoea
- occasionally, severe illness with cyanosis, hypotension, and shock.

Immediate investigations

- dipstix urinalysis (UTI more likely when leucocyte and nitrite tests both positive)
- blood and urine cultures
- FBC
- U and E and creatinine

- lumbar puncture (if particularly unwell)
- renal ultrasound scan.

Urine microscopy of a fresh, uncentrifuged, clean sample identifies infection (eight organisms per high-power field, or 10^7 organisms/ml) and allows treatment to be started while awaiting culture results. Dipslides can also give reliable results within 24 h.

Management

Aim to establish a prompt diagnosis, rapid treatment, and detection of any underlying cause that might predispose to further infection or lead to long-term renal damage. If there is a strong suspicion of a UTI, start treatment once a clean sample has been obtained.

- Administer antibiotics covering common causative organisms (*Escherichia coli*, *Enterococcus* spp., *Klebsiella* spp., *Streptococcus faecalis*, *Proteus* spp., and *Pseudomonas* spp.).
- Commence initial antibiotic combination (such as ampicillin and gentamicin) until sensitivities are available and then switch to the most appropriate antibiotic(s), for 5–7 days (uncomplicated UTI) or ten days (systemically unwell).
- If infant is systemically unwell, use IV antibiotics until the infant is improved and has been apyrexial for 24–36 h before reverting to oral antibiotics.
- Maintain on prophylactic antibiotics (such as trimethoprim 2 mg/kg once daily) until vesicoureteric reflux is excluded.
- Monitor fluid and electrolytes in infants presenting with dehydration or systemic illness.
- Monitor BP.
- Check post-treatment urine sample without stopping prophylaxis. Persistence of infection, mixed infection, or early recurrence with resistant strain suggests bladder dysfunction or outflow obstruction.

Follow-up investigations (several weeks later)

- Perform MCUG (to detect VUR).
- Perform DMSA scan after ≥3 months (to identify renal scarring).
- Do urinalysis and urine microscopy at follow-up.
- Check BP at follow-up (hypertension and proteinuria are markers of progressive renal disease).
- Continue long-term prophylaxis if reflux or scarring present until child is 2–3 years.
- Advise parents to have infant reassessed if fever or symptoms recur despite prophylaxis.
- Reinfection with an organism sensitive to prophylactic therapy suggests noncompliance; infection with resistant organism requires full-dose treatment and adjustment of prophylaxis.
- In the absence of renal anomalies, follow-up is required for at least one year and ideally until the child has been infection-free for two years.

Imaging in renal disorders

Ultrasound scan is a mandatory first-line investigation in any renal disorder. *Intravenous urography (IVU)* is the investigation of choice in elucidating suspected anatomic abnormality. *[^{99m}Tc]-DMSA* is the investigation of choice in elucidating suspected renal parenchymal damage (scars). *MCUG* is the investigation of choice in determining the presence and severity of VUR. *MAG-3 renogram* is the investigation of choice when determining the quantitative excretory function of individual kidneys and possible outflow obstruction (when a diuretic is also administered).

Useful websites

www.pkdcure.org
The Polycystic Kidney Disease Foundation (USA).

www.kidney.org
The National Kidney Foundation (USA).

http://kidney.niddk.nih.gov
The National Kidney and Urologic Diseases Information Clearinghouse is a service of the National Institute of Diabetes and Digestive and Kidney Diseases, part of the US National Institutes of Health.

Further reading

Belman AB, King LR, Kramer SA. *Clinical Pediatric Urology*, 4th edn. London: Martin Dunitz, 2001.

Dick PT, Feldman W. Routine diagnostic imaging for childhood urinary tract infections: A systematic overview. *Journal of Pediatrics* (1996) **128:**15–22.

Obling H. Vesico-ureteral reflux (VUR). In: W Proesmans (ed.). *Therapeutic Strategies in Children with Renal Disease. Baillière's Clinical Paediatrics*, Vol. 5, No. 4, London: Baillière Tindall, 1997: 521–38.

Smellie JM. Management and investigation of children with urinary tract infection. In: RJ Postlethwaite (ed). *Clinical Paediatric Nephrology*, 2nd edn. Oxford: Butterworth-Heinemann, 1994.

Thomas DFM (ed). *Urological Disease in the Foetus and Infant: Diagnosis and Management*. Oxford: Butterworth-Heinemann, 1997.

Verrier Jones K. Vesico-ureteric reflux: a medical perspective on management. *Pediatric Nephrology* (1996) **10:**795–7.

Related topics of interest

- fluid and electrolyte therapy
- infection—neonatal
- renal and urinary tract disorders—nephrology.

Respiratory distress

Respiratory problems, manifest as respiratory distress, are the commonest cause of admission of newborns to the neonatal unit in the perinatal period. Respiratory distress arises from inadequate in utero maturation of the lung and of mechanisms controlling respiration, or from disease processes present before or after birth which compromise pulmonary function. The causes and management of respiratory distress vary depending on the gestational and chronological age of the infant.

Aetiology

Preterm infants

Respiratory
- pneumothorax
- surfactant deficiency
- pulmonary haemorrhage
- airway abnormalities (such as choanal atresia)
- congenital lung malformations (such as cystic adenomatoid malformation [CAM]).

Infection
- pneumonia
- septicaemia
- meningitis.

Miscellaneous
- cold stress
- hypoglycaemia
- inherited metabolic disease (such as congenital lactic acidosis).

Term infants

Respiratory
- pneumothorax
- pleural effusion
- primary ciliary dyskinesia
- transient tachypnoea of the newborn
- congenital surfactant protein B deficiency
- meconium and other aspiration syndromes
- airway abnormalities (such as choanal atresia, TOF)
- congenital malformations (such as CAM, pulmonary lymphangectasia, pulmonary hypoplasia, congenital diaphragmatic hernia, and congenital nasolacrimal duct obstruction [congenital dacryocystocele]).

Cardiovascular
Congenital heart defects which lead to heart failure (as in hypolastic left heart syndrome, obstructed total anomalous pulmonary venous drainage, and severe coarctation).

Infection
- pneumonia
- septicaemia
- meningitis.

Miscellaneous
- cold stress
- polycythaemia
- maternal drugs (such as opiates)
- birth trauma and birth asphyxia
- inherited metabolic disease (such as organic acidaemias)
- neuromuscular disorders (such as spinal muscular atrophy type I and myotonic dystrophy).

Clinical features

The characteristic features are tachypnoea, grunting, nasal flaring, and cyanosis, which may be superseded by apnoea or acute collapse. In addition, cardiac murmurs, abnormal peripheral pulses, or signs of cardiac failure may also be present if there is an underlying congenital heart defect.

Investigations

Pulse oximetry
It is useful to determine the arterial oxygen saturations as a guide to the severity of hypoxaemia and the urgency of intervention.

Temperature
Exclude hypothermia or pyrexia.

Biochemistry
Blood glucose (exclude hypoglycaemia) and CRP (raised in infection).

Arterial blood gases
This is essential to determine the degree of respiratory failure and decisions on the next most appropriate interventions to be made. Capillary or venous blood gases may be misleading in an infant with poor peripheral perfusion. Inordinate persistent metabolic acidosis may point to a metabolic disorder.

Chest radiograph
Rule out pneumothorax, effusions, pulmonary oedema, abnormal cardiac silhouette, congenital diaphragmatic hernia, bell-shaped chest as seen in neuromuscular disorders, ground-glass appearance with RDS, CAM, congenital pneumonia, or aspiration.

Blood culture and CRP
Always perform blood cultures with serial CRPs when sepsis is suspected.

FBC and film
Sepsis is suggested by low or high white blood cell count and thrombocytopenia.

Full septic screen
This should be performed when there is a high suspicion of sepsis.

ECG and echocardiogram
These are conducted for suspected congenital heart disease.

Management

Management is determined by the underlying diagnosis. Aim to correct acid–base disturbance and alleviate hypoxaemia and respiratory failure. Warm cold infants and correct hypoglycaemia. Preterm infants with the RDS and significant hypoxaemia should be intubated for surfactant administration and mechanical ventilation. However, some infants with milder RDS may be immediately extubated after surfactant administered and maintained on CPAP. More mature infants (>28 weeks' gestation) with mild RDS may be managed on CPAP or headbox oxygen with recourse to mechanical ventilation when the FiO_2 exceeds 0.6, if blood gases are unsatisfactory or there is apnoea. Transient tachypnoea of the newborn usually resolves with minimal support (supplemental oxygen). Unless the supplemental oxygen requirements are modest, an arterial line should be sited for blood-gas monitoring in oxygen-dependent infants. Suspected sepsis should be promptly treated with an appropriate combination of broad-spectrum antibiotics until blood cultures are available. Pneumothoraces and symptomatic effusions should be drained appropriately with repeat radiographs to determine the adequacy of the procedure.

Infants with suspected congenital heart disease or malformations requiring corrective surgery are best managed in specialist centres and may require ventilation for safe transportation. PGE_1 or PGE_2 should be commenced in infants with suspected duct-dependent congenital heart lesions (starting at 5 ng/kg per min and increasing to 10–20 ng/kg per min in 5-ng/kg per min increments), and a paediatric cardiology opinion sought.

Further reading

Avery GB, Fletcher MA, MacDonald M. *Neonatology: Pathophysiology and Management of the Newborn*, 5th edn. Philadelphia: Lippincott Williams & Wilkins, 1999.
Fanaroff AA, Martin RJ. *Neonatal-Perinatal Medicine: Diseases of the Foetus and Infant*, 7th edn. St Louis, MO: Mosby, 2001.
Gluckman PD, Heyman MA (eds). *Pediatrics and Perinatology. The Scientific Basis*, 2nd edn. London: Arnold, 1996.
Greenough A, Milner AD (eds). *Neonatal Respiratory Disorders*, 2nd edn. London: Arnold, 2003.
Hamvas A, Cole S, deMello DE et al. Surfactant protein B deficiency: antenatal diagnosis and prospective treatment with surfactant replacement. *Journal of Pediatrics* (1994) **125:**356–61.
Kirkpatrick BV, Mueller DG. Respiratory disorders in the newborn. In: V Chernick, T Boat (eds). *Kendig's Disorders of the Respiratory Tract in Children*, 6th edn. Philadelphia: WB Saunders, 1998: 328–64.

Royal College of Paediatrics and Child Health. Guidelines for Good Practice. *Management of Neonatal Respiratory Distress Syndrome*. December 2000.

Taeusch HW, Ballard RA, Gleason CA (eds). *Avery's Diseases of the Newborn*, 8th edn. Philadelphia: WB Saunders, 2005.

Yost CC, Soll RF. Early versus delayed selective surfactant treatment for neonatal respiratory distress syndrome. The Cochrane Library, Issue 2. Chichester: John Wiley & Sons, 2004.

Related topics of interest

- acid–base balance
- congenital diaphragmatic hernia
- congenital heart disease—congestive heart failure
- infection—general
- intubation
- maternal drug abuse
- mechanical ventilation
- meconium aspiration syndrome
- respiratory distress syndrome
- resuscitation.

Respiratory distress syndrome

Respiratory distress syndrome (RDS), previously called hyaline membrane disease, is the single most important medical disorder in preterm infants, affecting 40–50% of all infants born before 32 weeks' gestation. Avery and Mead first demonstrated in 1959 that the lungs of infants with RDS were uncompliant due to surfactant deficiency. Attempts to prevent RDS have therefore concentrated on ways of enhancing the action or accelerating production of surfactant. Accelerating lung morphologic maturity is also essential.

The incidence and severity of RDS is inversely proportional to gestational age (or birth weight). In infants under 27 weeks' gestation, RDS is almost universal and after 27 weeks, but before 32 weeks, RDS may affect two in three infants. After 32 weeks, RDS is less frequent and tends to be moderate regardless of other risk factors. Mortality during the acute phase is now largely confined to ELBW infants (<1000 g).

Factors influencing risk and severity of RDS

- *Gender*—girls have a lower risk, less severe disease, and a lower mortality than boys.
- *Race*—black infants have a lower incidence and severity than white infants matched for age and birth weight.
- *In utero stress*—risk is lower in disorders associated with placental insufficiency (such as IUGR, but not pre-eclampsia).
- *Multiple pregnancy*—multiple pregnancy increases the risk of RDS (especially in second twins).
- *Maternal habits*—smoking, alcohol ingestion, and maternal narcotic addiction reduce the incidence of RDS in preterm infants.
- *Antenatal factors*—premature rupture of membranes (sepsis and pulmonary hypoplasia).
- *Perinatal factors*—delivery by caesarean section prior to onset of labour, asphyxia, acidosis, and hypothermia all increase the risk of developing RDS.
- *Diabetes mellitus*—poor control increases risk of RDS.
- *Genetic factors*—a familial predisposition exists as well as the recently recognised surfactant protein B deficiency in congenital alveolar proteinosis.

Prevention of RDS

Prevention of prematurity is the ideal preventive strategy.

- If premature birth is inevitable, prenatal corticosteroid therapy is the most effective currently available intervention to reduce the incidence, severity, and mortality of RDS. Meta-analysis of randomised, controlled trials to date shows a reduction in risk of RDS of 40–60% and a reduction in mortality of 50%. Antenatal corticosteroids reduce the risk of developing periventricular haemorrhage and necrotising enterocolitis, and may protect against neurologic abnormality. Steroids should be given to all mothers at risk of premature delivery at 24–34 weeks' gestation with any of the following:

　　　—threatened preterm labour
　　　—antepartum haemorrhage
　　　—preterm rupture of membranes
　　　—any condition requiring elective preterm delivery.
- Treatment consists of preferably two doses of betamethasone 12 mg given i.m. 24 h apart. Optimal benefit begins 24 h after initiation of therapy and lasts at least seven days. Steroid therapy for less than 24 h still reduces the incidence of RDS and IVH and mortality. However, the use of repeated courses of antenatal corticosteroids has not been shown to have any significant advantages.
- The use of antenatal corticosteroids in multiple pregnancies is recommended, although it has not been shown to reduce significantly the incidence of RDS.
- The use of antenatal corticosteroids in pregnancies complicated by insulin-dependent maternal diabetes mellitus or gestational diabetes is uncertain.
- Corticosteroid administration does not appear to increase the risk of foetal or maternal infection, irrespective of whether the membranes were intact or ruptured at the time of treatment. Follow-up studies between six and 12 years of age have shown no adverse neurological or cognitive effects in children who received prenatal corticosteroids.
- Despite earlier promising studies, large randomised trials of thyrotrophin-releasing hormone (TRH)–corticosteroid combination therapy have not shown additional benefit, and this therapy is not recommended for clinical practice. Indeed, the most recent *Cochrane Review* demonstrated that coadministration of TRH with corticosteroids increased the incidence of adverse outcomes for both mothers and babies.
- Corticosteroid therapy is contraindicated in the following disorders:
　　　—porphyria
　　　—tuberculosis
　　　—systemic infection (with caution advised in suspected chorioamnionitis).

Pathology of RDS

Lung histopathology of infants dying from RDS shows:

- hyaline membranes (sloughed cell debris in a protein matrix formed at the junction of respiratory bronchioles and alveolar ducts)
- atelectasis in association with overdistended airspaces (gives the radiographic 'ground-glass' appearance)
- pulmonary capillary engorgement
- interstitial and alveolar oedema
- haemorrhages.

Pathophysiology and lung mechanics in RDS

The following features characterise RDS:

- delayed clearance of foetal lung fluid
- deficiency and inactivation of surfactant
- increased permeability of epithelial and endothelial barriers
- areas of atelectasis and ventilation–perfusion mismatch from intra- and extrapulmonary shunting of pulmonary blood flow.

Features of RDS

- expiratory grunt
- tachypnoea and nasal flaring
- intercostal and sternal recession
- apnoeas and cyanosis
- reduced lung compliance with increased work of breathing
- abnormal gas exchange (hypoxaemia and hypercapnia) commonly requiring supplemental oxygen or assisted ventilation
- abnormal chest radiograph—lung reticulogranular pattern (ground-glass appearance) and air bronchograms with small lung volumes.

Management of RDS

The main principles of management include:

- provision of adequate oxygenation and blood-gas exchange by administering supplemental oxygen with or without assisted ventilation, while minimising barotrauma and volutrauma, and preventing air leaks
- administration of surfactant either as prophylactic therapy at birth for infants at high risk of RDS, (as at ≤28 weeks' gestation or ≤1250 g birth weight) or as early rescue therapy
- supporting the cardiovascular system to maintain adequate cardiac output and tissue perfusion
- provision of adequate fluid therapy to maintain normal electrolyte and blood-glucose homeostasis
- maintaining adequate temperature control
- treating sepsis with appropriate antibiotics
- preventing intracranial haemorrhage
- avoiding unnecessary handling of the infant and providing sedation and/or analgesia.

Maintaining adequate blood gas exchange

This may be achieved by instituting continuous positive airway pressure (CPAP) or mechanical ventilation (see 'Mechanical ventilation'). Excessive CPAP (> 6 cm H_2O) may be detrimental (produces excessive FRC, reducing compliance and reducing pulmonary blood flow). Mechanical ventilation may be provided as positive pressure ventilation or high-frequency oscillatory ventilation. The aim of assisted ventilation should be to maintain adequate oxygenation (PaO_2 7.5–10 kPa), correct acidosis and avoid hypo- and hypercapnia. Note, however, that there is increasing evidence that gentler ventilation which tolerates higher levels of $PaCO_2$ (permissive hypercapnia) is associated with a lower incidence of CLD. Indeed, the avoidance of mechanical ventilation by using CPAP combined with prophylactic surfactant reduces the risk of CLD.

Synopsis of surfactant therapy

Surfactant became widely available for clinical use in Europe and North America in 1989–90, and this was marked by a striking reduction in neonatal mortality. The main benefits of surfactant therapy are as follows:

- major reduction in neonatal mortality (overall 40% reduction).
- that natural surfactants produce more rapid improvements in gas exchange and are superior to synthetic surfactants in reducing mortality
- reduction in the incidence of pneumothoraces
- variable reduction in the incidence of CLD
- reduction in the incidence of IVH (rescue therapy with synthetic surfactants)

Potential complications of surfactant therapy

- Hyperoxia—wean ventilation and oxygen accordingly.
- Maldistribution of surfactant to one lung must be avoided.
- Incidence of PDA and pulmonary haemorrhage may be increased in the extremely preterm infants. The risk of pulmonary haemorrhage may be greater with synthetic surfactants (such as Exosurf).
- Avoid destabilising the infant (that is, avoid desaturations, blood pressure perturbations, and blocking the endotracheal tube) during therapy (more likely when large volumes are administered at once).
- There is transmission of infectious agents (such as bovine spongiform encephalitis [BSE], or 'mad cow disease', in bovine-derived surfactants, which could cause the nvCJD in humans). Bovine surfactants are made from BSE-free herds.
- Immunological injury from the immunogenicity of surfactant proteins has not been reported. Surfactant therapy may reduce this risk by reducing the alveolar–capillary leaks associated with RDS and its treatment.

Surfactant is, however, ineffective in a third of all infants treated, partly due to maldistribution and surfactant inactivation. See 'Surfactant replacement therapy'.

Useful websites

www.emedicine.com/ped/neonatology.htm
Part of the largest and most current online clinical knowledge base available to health professionals.

www.neonatology.com
Neonatology on the web—an extensive resource on neonatology.

Further reading

Crowley P. Antenatal corticosteroid therapy: a meta-analysis of the randomized trials, 1972 to 1994. *American Journal of Obstetrics and Gynecology* (1995) **173**:322–5.

Donn SM, Wiswell TE (eds). Advances in mechanical ventilation and surfactant therapy. *Clinics in Perinatology* (2001) **28**(3).

Greenough A, Milner AD (eds). *Neonatal Respiratory Disorders*, 2nd edn. London: Arnold, 2003.

Jobe AH. Pathophysiology of respiratory distress syndrome and surfactant metabolism. In: RA Polin, WW Fox (eds). *Foetal and Neonatal Physiology*, 2nd edn. Philadelphia: WB Saunders, 1998: 1299–313.

Kattwinkel J, Bloom BT, Delmore P et al. Prophylactic administration of calf lung surfactant extract is more effective than early treatment of respiratory distress syndrome in neonates of 29 through 32 weeks' gestation. *Pediatrics* (1993) **92:**90–8.

Penney GC, on behalf of the Royal College of Obstetricians and Gynaecologists. Antenatal corticosteroids to prevent respiratory distress syndrome: guidelines. www.rcog.org.uk/clingov1.

Robertson JB, Taeusch HW (eds). *Surfactant Therapy*. New York: Dekker, 1995.

Royal College of Paediatrics and Child Health. Guidelines for Good Practice. *Management of Neonatal Distress Syndrome*. December 2000.

Thome UH, Carlo WA. Permissive hypercapnia. *Seminars in Neonatology* (2002) **7:**409–19.

Soll RF, Morley CJ. Prophylactic versus selective use of surfactant in preventing morbidity and mortality in perterm infants. The Cochrane Library, Issue 2. Chichester: John Wiley & Sons, 2004.

Yost CC, Soll RF. Early versus delayed selective surfactant treatment for neonatal respiratory distress syndrome. The Cochrane Library, Issue 2. Chichester: John Wiley & Sons, 2004.

Related topics of interest

- chronic lung disease
- complications of mechanical ventilation
- mechanical ventilation
- patent ductus arteriosus
- pulmonary air leaks
- surfactant replacement therapy.

Resuscitation

Everyone remembers the ABCD of any resuscitation:

- *A*irway
- *B*reathing
- *C*irculation
- *D*rugs.

But the first 'A' of neonatal resuscitation is for *a*nticipation. Every maternity unit must have in place equipment, guidelines, and trained staff to anticipate the need to resuscitate newborn babies. At its most basic, equipment is needed to keep the baby warm, to suck out the airways, and to ventilate the baby's lungs with air or oxygen. The time to prepare equipment is immediately *after* use, but check it again on arrival. The unit's guidelines must anticipate a wide variety of circumstances relating to the complications of pregnancy and delivery and different gestations at birth. Take precautions to reduce the risk of HIV transmission at all deliveries. Staff trained in advanced resuscitation must be resident to resuscitate the unexpectedly flat baby at birth and the unbooked preterm delivery, as well as attending the deliveries of babies recognised in advance as being at some risk. These usually include:

- all babies with a suspected congenital abnormality, which may cause immediate clinical problems
- all preterm deliveries under 36 completed weeks' gestation
- all caesarean sections under general anaesthetic
- babies born to HIV-positive mothers
- all breech presentations
- all multiple deliveries
- all deliveries with foetal distress:
  —thick meconium
  —type II dips
  —scalp pH under 7.2.

Particularly skilled resuscitators should attend deliveries of under 29 weeks' gestation, anticipated severe asphyxia, and known severe abnormalities or hydrops.

The aims of neonatal resuscitation can be summarised as: WOMB.

- Keep the baby *W*arm.
- Ensure *O*xygenation.
- Return the baby to the *M*other.
- Encourage early *B*reast-feeding.

At birth, assess the heart rate, respiratory effort, tone, and colour. This will help you decide what help, if any, is needed. Do not expose the baby unnecessarily. Remember the order of resuscitation:

1. *A*irway
2. *B*reathing
3. *C*irculation
4. *D*rugs.

Airway

The head should be in a neutral position—neither flexed nor overextended—and the jaw gently pulled forward to stop the tongue from obstructing the back of the pharynx.

Breathing

- If the breathing is shallow or irregular, but the heart rate is over 100, ensure the head is in a neutral position to open the airway, stimulate gently, reassess.
- If respiratory effort is absent, and the heart rate is falling or under 100 and airway manoeuvres have not helped, then start ventilation with a correctly fitting face mask and T-piece. Give five inflation breaths, each lasting three seconds. Use pressures of 20 to 30 cmH$_2$O. Check that the chest wall moves with the inflation breaths. If it does, reassess the heart rate, tone, colour and respiratory effort of the baby. If these are improving maintain the airway and allow a spontaneous improvement to occur. If there is not adequate response but the five inflation breaths have been achieved then give 30 seconds of regular ventilatory breaths, each lasting 0.5 to one second.
- If there is no movement of the chest wall during the inflation breaths do not proceed to ventilation breaths but recheck the airway, consider a jaw thrust (one or two persons), or insert a Geudel airway and/or inspect the airway to ensure that no foreign body is present. Give five inflation breaths again.
- If the baby responds to the ventilation breaths, particularly with a rise in the heart rate, then oxygenated blood is reaching the myocardium and the baby will soon pick up. Continue to give gentle ventilation breaths until you are satisfied that the baby is taking over the breathing.
- Recent evidence shows no differences in outcome between newborn infants resuscitated with 21% or 100% oxygen.

Circulation

- If the baby does not respond to ventilation breaths (but the chest wall is seen to rise and fall) then chest compressions (or external cardiac massage, ECM) may be necessary to move oxygenated blood from the lungs to the heart. To do this, encircle the chest with both hands so that the thumbs overlap over the sternum 1 cm below the imaginary line drawn between the nipples. Adequate compression of the chest is achieved by halving the distance between the rib cage and the spine with each compression. Give three compressions to every breath and aim to achieve approximately 90 compressions per minute. Reassess after 30 seconds.
- If the baby does not respond to chest compressions and it is clear that there is an airway and air is moving in and out of the lungs then drugs may be necessary.
- At this point experienced resuscitators often choose to intubate. However using the T-piece and mask technique, probably as few as 0.5 per 1000 babies will need intubation for resuscitation. Rather more than this are intubated because a number of doctors feel that this achieves a more secure airway and they can be more confident of inflating and ventilating the lungs.

- If intubation is used, then again the resuscitator must be confident that five effective inflation breaths have been given, each of three seconds, followed by regular 0.5 to one second ventilatory breaths. Resuscitation would then proceed as before using chest compression and drugs if necessary should the baby not respond.

Drugs

- Only use drugs after adequate ventilation and ECM fail to improve the baby's condition.
- Only four drugs are needed: adrenaline, sodium bicarbonate, glucose and naloxone. Table 1 gives the doses for these.
- Adrenaline, sodium bicarbonate and glucose are best given intravenously.
- Venous access can be quickly achieved by cannulation of the umbilical vein using a clean though—in this extreme emergency situation—not necessarily sterile procedure. It takes less than 20 seconds to insert an umbilical venous catheter and this can be done while others continue ventilation and chest compressions. All drugs given into the umbilical catheter must be flushed through with normal saline to ensure that they reach the baby's circulation.
- If venous access cannot be achieved then adrenaline can be given down an endotracheal tube in a dose ten times greater than the intravenous dose.
- Drugs given through the umbilical venous catheter will go straight to the right atrium, and as persistent foetal circulation will still be present, thence to the left atrium, the left ventricle and the coronary arteries. There is some concern that large boluses of bicarbonate given in this way may go up the aortic arch to the carotid arteries and cause cerebral damage. Sodium bicarbonate therefore should be given as a slow infusion, not a bolus.

Table 1 Drug doses for resuscitation.

Drug	Dose	Route	Comments
Epinephrine 1 in 10000	0.1 ml/kg then 0.3 ml/kg (10 μg/kg then 30 μg/kg)	IV	Repeat dose or give via UVC if inserted
	1 ml/kg	Endotracheal	
Sodium bicarbonate	2 mmol/kg (2 ml/kg of 8.4%)	IV	Slowly over 5–10 min, diluted to 4.2% in 5% dextrose
Glucose	0.2 g/kg (1 ml/kg of 20%)	IV	
Naloxone	100 μg/kg	i.m.	Not for babies of opiate-dependent mothers.

Special groups of babies

Preterm and low birth weight
- Keep the baby warm!
- Ask for theatre/delivery room temperature to be increased. Work under overhead heater in draught-free area.
- Dry rapidly while assessing baby's state. Change wet sheets for warm dry ones.
- Keep exposure to a minimum. Use prewarmed transport incubator to transfer the baby to NICU.
- Preterm babies of <30 weeks gestation may be best wrapped in polythene bags even before the baby is dried. This prevents evaporative heat loss, the major source of cooling during resuscitation. Keep the baby wrapped until a normal temperature is achieved under a radiant heater on the neonatal unit.

Caesarean-section babies
- Foetal lungs secrete fluid. This is reversed in term babies by catecholamine surges during labour—then the lungs are compressed in the birth canal, and only small amounts of fluid are left in the lungs prior to the first breath.
- Caesarean-section babies have excess lung fluid at birth and may 'drown' if it is not aspirated. If intubation is needed, suck out the trachea before ventilating.

Meconium-stained liquor
Approximately 8–10% of babies are born through meconium-stained liquor. Aspiration of this can lead to MAS, with potentially fatal consequences. Light meconium staining seldom causes problems, and intubation and suction are then unnecessary, but for babies delivered through heavily stained liquor with or without particulate matter, a combined midwifery-paediatric approach can be used:

1. The oropharynx is sucked out when the head is delivered either on the perineum or through a caesarean incision. However, if the baby is vigorous and crying nothing will be gained by inspecting the vocal cords and step 2 should be undertaken only if the baby is quiet and apnoeic.
2. The resuscitator visualises the cords and if there is evidence of meconium around the cords, then the trachea may be sucked out, either by inserting a FG10 suction catheter through the cords or by passing a catheter down through the endotracheal tube. Suction pressures of up to 100 mmHg are used through as large a catheter as possible.
3. If necessary, standard resuscitation can now start with a reduced chance of forcing meconium into the lungs with the first few positive pressure breaths.

There is no evidence that either compression of the chest after birth or saline lavage during resuscitation is beneficial.

Hydrops fetalis—see 'Hydrops fetalis'
Infants of HIV-positive mothers
- The safest way to deliver infants of HIV-positive mothers is by caesarean section.
- Resuscitation should be as atraumatic as possible with minimal damage to the baby's mucosa, thus reducing the risk of infection by infected maternal blood.

- Resuscitators should wear gloves, plastic aprons, gowns, and appropriate footwear and eye protection.
- No mouth-operated suction should be used.
- Once the baby is stable, wash off maternal blood and *only then* give i.m. vitamin K. This is to reduce the risk of infecting the infant.

Extremely preterm babies at the threshold of viability

Resuscitation of the very preterm infant is both technically and ethically difficult. The legal age of viability in the UK is 24 weeks' gestation, but some infants of less than 24 weeks survive, and for some gestation is uncertain. Units should have specific guidelines for the care of women in established labour at (say) 20–23 weeks when delivery is inevitable. A possible set of guidelines is offered below:

- On admission, the obstetric registrar is informed. When established labour is diagnosed and gestation confirmed as 'X' or above, the paediatric registrar is informed and management of the case is agreed by both teams. (In the author's unit, 'X' is 23 weeks, a figure chosen after audit of our outcomes and the EPICure study.)
- If unbooked and/or gestation is uncertain, the paediatric registrar will be present at birth. Active resuscitation will occur unless the baby is *very* small and immature.
- The plan of management is discussed with the parents by the obstetrician and recorded in the mother's notes.
- The management will fall into one of the following categories:

No active resuscitation
- There is no monitoring.
- Appropriate analgesia is chosen.
- Appropriate and sensitive support is given to the parents. It is important that they understand that the baby may breathe for some time after delivery.
- The paediatrician will not be present at delivery.
- The baby is dried, wrapped in a blanket, and given to the parents to hold. He/she will stay with the parents either on the delivery suite or on the postnatal ward (bereavement room) until there are no signs of life—unless otherwise requested.
- Follow unit guidelines for bereaved parents, including requesting a postmortem.

Active resuscitation
- No continuous electronic monitoring—because no emergency section will be performed.
- Intermittent auscultatory monitoring—some babies die during labour, and they will not be resuscitated if this is confirmed and there is no heart beat at birth.
- Mother nursed in delivery room with resuscitation equipment.
- The most senior paediatricians attend to assist resuscitation and support parents.
- The fact that intensive care has been started does not mean it has to be continued.

Termination of pregnancy for foetal abnormalities

Stopping resuscitation in asphyxiated babies

- On available evidence, it is reasonable to stop if a baby has no spontaneous respiratory effort after 30 min of appropriate resuscitation.
- In the absence of a heart beat, it is reasonable to stop after 10 min of appropriate resuscitation.

Useful websites

www.aap.org/nrp/nrpmain.html
American Academy of Pediatrics—Neonatal Resuscitation Program.

www.neonatology.com
Neonatology on the web—an extensive resource on neonatology.

Further reading

Ginsberg HG, Goldsmith JP. Controversies in neonatal resuscitation. *Clinics in Perinatology* (1998) **25:**1–15.

International Guidelines 2000 for Emergency Cardiovascular Care: Neonatal Resuscitation. *Circulation* (2000) **102** [suppl1]: 343–57.

International Guidelines for Neonatal Resuscitation: An excerpt from the Guidelines 2000 for Cardiopulmonary Resuscitation and Emergency Cardiovascular Care: International Consensus on Science. *Pediatrics* (2000) **106:**e29.

Kattwinkel I, Denson S, Zaichkin J et al. *Textbook of Neonatal Resuscitation*, 4th edn. Dallas, TX: American Academy of Pediatrics, 2000.

Perlman J, Niermeyer S (eds). Neonatal Resuscitation. *Seminars in Neonatology* (2001) **6:**(3).

Richmond S (ed). *Resuscitation at Birth—Newborn Life Support Provider Course Manual.* London: Resuscitation Council (UK), 2001.

Royal College of Paediatrics and Child Health, Royal College of Obstetricians and Gynaecologists. *Resuscitation of Babies at Birth.* London: BMJ Publishing, 1997.

Saugstad OD, Ramji S, Irani SF et al. Resuscitation of newborn infants with 21% or 100% oxygen: follow-up at 18 to 24 months. *Pediatrics* (2003) **112:**296–300.

Ushay HM, Notterman DA. Pharmacology of pediatric resuscitation. *Pediatric Clinics of North America* (1997) **44:**207–33.

Yeo CL, Tudehope DI. Outcome of resuscitated apparently stillborn infants: a ten year review. *Journal of Paediatrics and Child Health* (1994) **30:**129–33.

Related topics of interest

- acute collapse
- death of an infant
- extreme prematurity
- HIV/AIDS.

Retinopathy of prematurity

Retinopathy of prematurity (ROP) is a disorder of the developing retinal vasculature in which the normal progression of the newly forming vessels (vasculogenesis) is interrupted, resulting in the development of new abnormal blood vessels (neovascularisation), which may heal by completely involuting with normal vascularisation of the retina (regression) or progress to a chronic phase (cicatricial ROP), with scarring, retinal detachment, and visual loss. In 95% of cases, ROP regresses spontaneously, but progressive disease is the leading cause of blindness in preterm infants.

Epidemiology and natural history

Over the past two decades, the incidence of ROP has increased due to the increasing survival of ELBW infants (birth weight under 1000 g). The NIH-sponsored multicentre trial of cryotherapy for ROP (CRYO-ROP Study), carried out on an estimated 15% of all births in the USA in which the infants weighed less than 1251 g, has provided insight into the epidemiology and natural history of ROP.

- Some degree of ROP developed in <10% of those weighing >1500 g at birth, 47% weighing 1000–1250 g at birth, 78% weighing 750–999 g at birth, and 90% of those <750 g birth weight.
- In >90%, the condition regressed and healed before the onset of blinding disease, only 6% of all infants developing severe disease ('threshold ROP') requiring treatment.
- When left untreated, ~50% developed visual loss, but cryotherapy reduced the incidence of unfavourable outcome by ~50% among infants at threshold.
- The most preterm infants were more susceptible to ROP.
- The timing of the development of threshold ROP was related to postconceptional age (median 37 weeks) rather than chronological (postnatal) age.
- Cryotherapy reduced the incidence of blinding disease.

Aetiology and risk factors

- The aetiology of ROP is multifactorial.
- The degree of immaturity of the eye is the most important risk factor.
- The second strongest factor is oxygen therapy. A correlation exists between ROP and the concentration and duration of oxygen therapy, but wide variations in arterial oxygen tension may be a greater risk factor than the absolute level of hyperoxia. ROP has occurred in infants who never received supplemental oxygen, term infants with cyanotic CHD, and, rarely, even in stillborn infants.
- Severe ROP develops in the sickest infants (that is, it correlates with asphyxia, acidosis, shock, sepsis, blood transfusions, IVH, PVL, and CLD).
- Once the retina is fully vascularised, ROP can no longer develop.

Classification

In 1984, the International Classification of ROP (ICROP) was introduced, allowing the location, severity, and extent of disease to be described accurately. It was updated in 1987 to include the sequelae of ROP.

- *Disease location* is described by the use of three distinct zones of the retina centered on the optic disc. Zone 1 is the area closest to the optic disc; zone 3 is the most peripheral region and denotes complete vascularisation to the edge of the retina; zone 2 is intermediate.
- *Extent of disease* is recorded in clock hours of retina involved.
- *Disease severity* is divided into five stages. In stage 1, a visible demarcation line is seen separating vascular from avascular retina. In stage 2, a ridge develops from the line in stage 1 (the mesenchymal arteriovenous shunt). In stage 3 disease, there is extraretinal fibrovascular proliferation, with new vessels projecting from the ridge or retina (neovascularisation) into the vitreous. Stage 4 is partial retinal detachment, and stage 5 is total retinal detachment.
- 'Plus' (+) disease denotes disease progression with increasing dilation and tortuosity of the arterioles and a vitreous haze, and can occur at any stage of disease.

Screening

- Screening aims to identify infants at risk of severe disease and those who would benefit from the available therapies.
- ROP rarely develops before 4–6 weeks after birth.
- Current UK guidelines for ROP screening include the following criteria: any baby ≤1500 g birth weight or ≤31 weeks' gestational age, although it has been suggested that these be altered to <1250 g birth weight or ≤29 weeks' gestation.
- Two-weekly (or more frequent) follow-up examinations are performed until complete retinal vascularisation occurs.
- Once retinal vessels reach zone 3 (the most peripheral zone), severe ROP and visual sequelae are unlikely, whereas when severe disease (stage 3+) occurs in zone 1, prospects for vision are poor even with treatment.
- Stages 1 and 2 disease spontaneously regresses in 95% of cases. At stage 3+, 50% regress spontaneously, the other half progressing to retinal detachment without treatment.
- Stage 3+ is the *threshold* for treatment.

Treatment

- The treatment of choice is retinal ablative therapy of the peripheral avascular retina with cryotherapy or laser therapy (the currently preferred treatment).
- Cryotherapy reduces the incidence of adverse sequelae in severe disease by 50%.
- Retinal ablation eliminates the angiogenic stimulus for the abnormal neovascularisation produced in the avascular region. The peripheral retina is sacrificed in order to preserve the already vascularised retina and the macula in particular.
- Cryotherapy involves freezing the avascular portion of the retina (plus the sclera and choroid) under local or general anaesthetic.

- Adverse effects include conjunctival and eyelid oedema, subconjunctival haemorrhage, retinal and preretinal bleeding, apnoea, bradycardias (oculocardic reflex with eyelid pressure), desaturations, and respiratory and cardiorespiratory arrest.
- Diode indirect laser photocoagulation is equally effective, safer, and easier to apply, especially for zone 1 disease, which is difficult to reach with a cryoprobe. Laser therapy is better tolerated with fewer systemic complications, less ocular destruction, more discrete retinal scars, and less discomfort for the infants.
- Partial (stage 4) or total retinal detachment (stage 5 disease) has a poor prognosis for vision, as therapy (scleral buckling and vitrectomy) is ineffective.

Prevention

- Supplemental antioxidants (such as vitamin E) are ineffective.
- There is no safe range for arterial oxygen tensions though it is recommended that arterial PO_2 be maintained $<10\,$kPa.
- Maintaining oxygen saturations of 70–90% in infants of <28 weeks gestation during the first eight weeks of life may significantly reduce the incidence of threshold (treatable) ROP.
- Surfactant therapy has indirectly increased the incidence of ROP through increased survival of ELBW infants.

Long-term outcome

Sequelae of progressive ROP
- Progressive ROP leads to severe visual impairment or total visual loss.
- Late retinal detachments may still occur after initial successful treatment.

Sequelae of regressed ROP
- Generally, the higher the stage at the time of regression, the worse the sequelae, which include myopia (near-sightedness), visual field defects, strabismus, amblyopia, glaucoma, and late retinal detachments.
- ROP severity is also strongly associated with the development of strabismus (squint), crossed eyes (esotropia) being the most common.
- Should the eyes be unequally affected, the infant may suppress the use of the worse eye and develop a lazy eye (amblyopia), which should be aggressively treated to preserve binocular vision.

Useful websites

www.emedicine.com/ped/neonatology.htm
Part of the largest and most current online clinical knowledge base available to health professionals.

www.neonatology.com
Neonatology on the web – an extensive resource on neonatology.

Further reading

Fielder AR, Reynolds JD. Retinopathy of prematurity: clinical aspects. *Seminars in Neonatology* (2001) **6:**461–75.

Hunter BG, Mukai S. Retinopathy of prematurity: pathogenesis, diagnosis and treatment. *International Ophthalmology Clinics* (1992) **32:**163–84.

McColm JR, Fleck BW. Retinopathy of prematurity: causation. *Seminars in Neonatology* (2001) **6:**453–60.

Palmer EA. Results of U.S. randomised clinical trial of cryotherapy for ROP (CRYO-ROP). *Documenta Ophthalmologica* (1990) **74:**245–51.

Report of a Joint Working Party of the Royal College of Ophthalmologists and the British Association of Perinatal Medicine. Retinopathy of prematurity: guidelines for screening and treatment. *Early Human Development* (1996) **46:**239–58.

Smith LE. Pathogenesis of retinopathy of prematurity. *Seminars in Neonatology* (2003) **8:** 469–73.

Stout AU, Stout TJ. Retinopathy of prematurity. *Pediatric Clinics of North America* (2003) **50:**77–87.

Tin W. Optimal oxygen saturation for reterm babies. Do we really know? *Biology of the Neonate* (2004) **85:**319–25.

Tin W, Milligan DWA, Pennefather P, et al. Pulse oximetry, severe retinopathy, and outcome at one year in babies of less than 28 weeks gestation. *Archives of Disease in Childhood Fetal and Neonatal Edition* (2001) **84:**F106–10.

Ziavras E, Javitt JJ. Retinopathy of prematurity. In: TJ David (ed.). *Recent Advances in Paediatrics*, No. 13, Edinburgh: Churchill Livingstone, 1995: 177–91.

Related topics of interest

- chronic lung disease
- extreme prematurity
- outcomes of neonatal intensive care
- respiratory distress syndrome.

Sedation and analgesia on the neonatal intensive care unit

Although neonatal intensive care relies heavily on the use of sophisticated and expensive instrumentation for the constant remote monitoring of sick infants, several other necessary procedures require the infants to be directly handled. Many of these procedures (such as tracheal intubation, insertion of chest drains, arterial and venous cannulation, and phlebotomy) are stressful, unpleasant, and painful. It is now accepted that even the most immature of infants mount physiological responses to procedures, manifest as tachycardia or bradycardia, and hypoxaemic or hypertensive episodes. In addition, there are constant environmental stresses such as excessive noise and light. The provision of adequate analgesia and sedation to sick infants is not only kind but positively beneficial. The agitated and struggling infant on assisted ventilation is more likely to be suboptimally ventilated, develop a pneumothorax or intracranial haemorrhage, self-extubate, or accidentally disrupt intravenous access lines. By carefully tailoring the doses of analgesics or sedatives each infant receives, we may obtain the maximum benefits while minimising the side effects.

Assessment of pain

Pain is difficult to assess, especially in the ventilated infant, where the classic behaviour responses to pain such as crying and distinct facial expressions are obscured by strapping, and the endotracheal tube obscures the baby's face. Blood pressure and heart rate have a poor correlation with the degree of agitation or pain. However, in nonventilated preterm infants, a more objective clinical score has been validated which incorporates body movements as well as facial expression and cry (Neonatal Infant Pain Score or [NIPS]), and a new score has recently been designed for use in ventilated babies.

Management of pain and agitation

Analgesia or a sedative should be administered *before* undertaking procedures (not after several failures!), depending on the procedure and anticipated pain or discomfort.

Morphine

This is widely used as both an analgesic and sedative. Morphine inhibits nociceptive reflexes by mimicking endogenous endorphins. Following a loading dose of 100–200 µg/kg (over 1.5–2 h), a continuous infusion of 10–40 µg/kg per h provides steady levels of analgesia and sedation for the ventilated infant. Morphine infusions reduce the stress response to ventilation in preterm infants. Side effects include respiratory depression, bradycardia, hypotension (histamine release), urinary retention, decreased gastric motility, drug tolerance, and physical dependence. Morphine is metabolised in the liver, and excretion is renal (slower in preterm infants). To avoid withdrawal symptoms, after more than one week of therapy, wean gradually. Long-term follow-up studies up to the age of 5–6 years do not show adverse neurodevelopmental effects in preterm infants who received morphine for sedation during mechanical ventilation.

Diamorphine

Diamorphine is more lipid soluble than morphine, and has a more rapid onset of sedation and less hypotensive effects. Its side-effects profile is similar to morphine. The loading dose is 120 μg/kg (over 2 h) followed by a continuous infusion of 15 μg/kg per h.

Fentanyl

This is a synthetic opioid 80–100 times more potent that morphine. It has a more rapid onset of action (peak effect in 1–2 min when given IV), and a short half-life with very little haemodynamic effect (decreased histamine effect). Following a loading dose of 1–4 μg/kg, a continuous infusion of 1–2 μg/kg per h provides effective analgesia. Side effects include a higher rate of withdrawal symptoms, a more rapid development of tolerance, and chest wall rigidity with rapid, large-dose infusions.

Paracetamol

This is well suited for minor discomfort or pain (as after immunisations) and may be repeated 4–6-hourly at a dose of 10 mg/kg, either orally or rectally.

Ketamine

Ketamine is fast-acting phencyclidine derivative which is both a sedative and potent analgesic. Its effects are apparent within 1–2 min and last 5–10 min. The standard dose is 0.5–1 mg/kg followed by a continuous infusion at 5–20 μg/kg per min. Ketamine increases heart rate, cardiac output, BP, and CBF.

Midazolam

This short-acting, water-soluble benzodiazepine is a commonly used sedative, especially in ventilated infants. It is metabolised in the liver and excreted in the urine. It has a rapid onset (1–5 min), but its half-life in neonates is 6–12 h. Clearance is reduced and half-life increased in neonates compared to older infants. The loading dose is 100–200 μg/kg and the continuous infusion rate is 1–2.5 μg/kg per min. Concurrent administration of fentanyl with midazolam may produce dystonic movements and hypotension.

Chloral hydrate

Chloral hydrate is a hypnotic and sedative agent well tolerated by neonates at 30–50 mg/kg. The parent drug and its active metabolite trichloroethanol have long half-lives and therefore a potential for accumulation with repeated dosage. It has no respiratory depressant or analgesic effects. Side effects include cardiac arrhythmia, gastrointestinal irritability, and paradoxical agitation. Trichloroethanol may compete with bilirubin for hepatic glucuronidation. Toxic effects from prolonged use include hypotension, renal failure, CNS depression, and carcinogenicity.

Massage
The stress response may also be reduced by nonpharmacologic means such as soothing, stroking, or massage.

Muscle relaxation

Routine muscle relaxation is not advocated. However, some critically ill ventilated infants may benefit from paralysis, such as mature infants with ventilator asynchrony or CDH. Complications of paralysis include deterioration of gas exchange; obscuring of seizures, pain, or agitation; tissue oedema; muscle contractures; and myopathy. Muscle relaxants should be given concurrently with analgesics, as infants would still feel pain.

Suxamethonium
This has the most rapid onset of action (1 min) and shortest duration of action (4–6 min), making it ideal for emergencies. It may be used to facilitate intubations. The dose is 2 mg/kg IV or 4 mg/kg i.m. The onset of action is slower (2–3 min) and duration of action longer (10–30 min) when given i.m.

Pancuronium
Pancuronium is metabolised in the liver and excreted in urine (delayed excretion in renal failure). It raises BP, cardiac output, and heart rate. The loading dose is 100 µg/kg IV (effective in 3 min and lasting 60 min). The maintenance dose is 50 µg/kg 4–6 hourly. Hypothermia, acidosis, aminoglycosides, impaired renal function, and hypokalaemia prolong the effects of nondepolarising agents such as pancuronium.

Vecuronium
Vecuronium has few cardiovascular side effects and is metabolised and excreted by the liver (in bile), although renal excretion is important in neonates. The dose is 100 µg/kg IV (effective in 2 min and lasting 30 min) followed by infusion of 1–3 µg/kg per min. When one uses it for long periods, it is wise to stop the vecuronium infusion daily until early signs of muscle activity return before restarting paralysis. This avoids the side effects of drug accumulation. Babies should also be given regular passive movements to reduce the risk of contractures.

Further reading

Alexander SM, Todres ID. The use of sedation and muscle relaxation in the ventilated infant. *Clinics in Perinatology* (1998) **25**:63–78.
Anand KJS, Stevens BJ, Mcgrath PJ. *Pain in Neonates*, 2nd edn. St Louis, MO: Elsevier, 2000.
Berde CB, Sethna NF. Analgesics for the treatment of pain in children. *New England Journal of Medicine* (2002) **347**:1094–103.
Bucher H-U, Bucher-Schmid A. Treating pain in the neonate. In: TN Hansen, N McIntosh (eds). *Current Topics in Neonatology*, No. 1, London: WB Saunders, 1996: 85–110.
Lawrence J, Alcock D, McGrath P et al. The development of a tool to assess neonatal pain. *Neonatal Networks* (1993) **12**:59–65.
Sparshott M. *Pain, Distress and the Newborn*. Oxford: Blackwell Science, 1996.
Stevens B, Grunau R (eds). Pain in the vulnerable population of infants. *Clinics in Perinatology* (2002) **29**:(3).

Related topics of interest

- anaesthesia and postoperative analgesia
- birth injuries
- intubation
- mechanical ventilation
- neonatal surgery
- respiratory distress syndrome.

Seizures

A seizure is a sudden paroxysmal depolarisation of a group of neurones, resulting in a transient alteration in neurological state. This may involve abnormal sensory, motor, or autonomic activity, with or without a change in conscious level. Seizures generally are indicative of another underlying disease process and very few (2–5%) are idiopathic. Seizures are a fairly common occurrence in the neonatal period with an incidence of 1–3 per 1000 live births at term. The incidence may be up to 50 times greater in preterm infants. The incidence of electrographic but clinically silent seizures is unknown, but up to 80% of electrographic seizures may be clinically silent, especially in preterm infants. The primary objective of any intervention is to control the seizures, determine causation, and rapidly correct any treatable causes, as this may improve prognosis.

Seizure types

There are four types of clinical seizures: subtle, clonic, myoclonic, and tonic. Each can be focal, multifocal, or generalised.

Subtle seizures
The most common variety (~50% of all seizures) manifested by apnoea, eye fluttering and deviation, staring, sucking and chewing, cycling, boxing, unstable blood pressure, and tachycardia.

Clonic seizures
Making up 20–30% of all seizures, these are more common in preterm infants and are typified by rhythmic jerky movements (1–4/s) with consciousness usually preserved. They may be focal, suggesting a focal underlying lesion such as cerebral artery infarction (but may also result from metabolic derangements), or multifocal.

Myoclonic seizures
Contributing ~15% of all seizures, these are rapid isolated jerks, especially of the upper limbs, signifying metabolic or major structural derangement. They may be focal, multifocal, or generalised.

Tonic seizures
These constitute approximately 5% of all seizures and are typified by sustained focal or generalised posturing of the body, such as tonic extension of all limbs, pronation of arms, and clenching of fists. Generalised tonic seizures often signify more serious pathology, for example severe IVH.

It is important to distinguish jitteriness and apnoea from seizures. Jitteriness is characterised by a symmetrical tremor of the extremities (spares the face) occurring at a higher frequency (5–6/s) than clonic movements. Jitteriness can be induced by an external stimulus and ceases with gentle restraint. Apnoea may be a manifestation of subtle seizures, especially in term infants and when the apnoea is not accompanied by bradycardia but is associated with staring, eye opening, or deviation of eyes.

Aetiology

Hypoxic-ischaemic encephalopathy (HIE)

This is the commonest cause, accounting for half of the cases of neonatal seizures. Moderate HIE tends to present with subtle and clonic seizures, while severe HIE may present with myoclonic and tonic seizures. The seizures present in the first 24 h.

CNS infection

Prenatal or perinatal infection may account for up to one in five cases of neonatal seizures. The commonest bacterial pathogens are group B streptococcus, *E. coli*, and *Listeria* spp. Herpes simplex encephalitis and other prenatal infections should also be excluded.

Intracranial haemorrhage/infarction

Following birth trauma in term infants, subarachnoid and subdural haemorrhages may cause seizures independently of coexisting asphyxia. IVHs with or without periventricular haemorrhagic infarction can cause generalised tonic seizures. The above causes may account for 10–15% of neonatal seizures.

Metabolic derangements

These may account for one in ten neonatal seizures, the commonest being hypoglycaemia, hypocalcaemia, hypomagnesaemia, and hyper- or hyponatraemia. IMD (such as urea cycle defects, aminoacidurias, and organic acidopathies), though rare, should be considered when there is a positive family history, persistent acidosis, unusual odours, or seizures unresponsive to conventional therapy. Rarely, IMD may present with severe recurrent seizures (myoclonic and clonic), a burst-suppression EEG pattern, and early myoclonic encephalopathy. Pyridoxine dependency is a rare autosomal-recessive defect in gamma-aminobutyric acid (GABA) synthesis, which presents with early onset refractory seizures that are abolished by administering pyridoxine (50–100 mg).

Maternal drug addiction

Neonatal drug withdrawal is an important cause of neurological dysfunction though only one in 20 will develop seizures. Methadone withdrawal seizures may occur as late as three weeks, though most other drugs produce symptoms earlier (<3 days). Cocaine abuse may predispose to prenatal cerebral artery infarction.

CNS malformation

Brain malformations are associated with an increased incidence of seizures. A rare syndrome, early infantile epileptic encephalopathy, may present with severe early tonic seizures and a burst-suppression EEG pattern. It is associated with very poor outcome.

Familial

Benign familial neonatal convulsions is an autosomal-dominant condition presenting with clonic seizures on days 2–3 and resolving within the first six months of life. The infant is normal between seizures, investigations show no abnormalities, and subsequent development is normal.

Miscellaneous

During quiet sleep, some infants may have bilateral synchronous myoclonic jerks, beginning in the first week and resolving within two months (benign neonatal sleep myoclonus). The EEG is normal during and between the events. Normal outcome is expected. Another benign form of neonatal seizures with multifocal clonic seizures has a peak age of onset at five days and resolves by day 15 ('fifth-day fits'). The cause is unknown.

Investigations

Primary investigations
- blood glucose
- U and E, calcium, and magnesium
- blood gases
- blood culture and CSF culture
- cranial ultrasound scan
- EEG.

Secondary investigations
- maternal and neonatal drug screen
- congenital infection screen (maternal and foetal TORCH serology)
- metabolic screen (serum lactate, ammonia, amino acids, and urine organic and amino acids)
- cerebral function monitoring
- therapeutic trial of pyridoxine
- MRI or CT scanning.

Management

The aim is to detect the underlying cause, give appropriate specific therapy, and control the seizures. Although seizures *per se* could cause further neuronal compromise, it is unclear how important this is in the clinical situation, as this has to be balanced against the potential deleterious effects of anticonvulsant therapy. One pragmatic approach is to control frequent (>3 seizures/h) or prolonged seizures (>3-min duration), especially if they adversely affect systemic blood pressure or respiration. As many anticonvulsants cause respiratory depression and impair myocardial function, blood pressure and respiratory activity should be monitored.

Drug therapy

Phenobarbital

This is a very effective first-time monotherapy controlling up to 70% of all seizures. The loading dose is 20 mg/kg IV (may be increased to 40 mg/kg), and the maintenance dose is 5–10 mg/kg per day (given 12-hourly). The half-life is 2–4 days and the serum therapeutic level is 20–40 mg/l (90–180 μmol/l). Phenobarbital is a free-radical scavenger and reduces calcium entry after ischaemia.

Clonazepam

This second-line drug is most useful when seizure control is poor. The loading dose is 100–200 μg/kg (IV over 30 s) followed by an infusion of 10–30 μg/kg per h. Convert to oral once-daily dose when control is achieved. Other benzodiazepines such as lorazepam may also be useful. Diazepam has a very short duration of action and marked respiratory depressive effect, making it unsuitable for long-term therapy.

Phenytoin

This is useful for securing short-term seizure control, but not for long term use, as it causes myocardial depression and has very variable metabolism. The loading dose is 20 mg/kg (IV at <1 mg/kg per min) and maintenance 8 mg/kg/day. Aim for levels of 10–20 mg/l (40–80 μmol/l).

Paraldehyde

The loading dose is 0.4 ml/kg diluted with an equal volume of olive or sunflower oil. Paraldehyde is metabolised in the liver and excreted through the lung (not affected by impaired renal function), and has a half-life of 12–24 h.

Prognosis

The underlying cause determines the prognosis. The prognosis is poor with brain malformations, intractable seizures, generalised myoclonic or tonic seizures, burst-suppression or persistent low-voltage EEG states, and persisting neurological abnormalities on examination.

Further reading

Bernes SM, Kaplan AM. Evolution of neonatal seizures. *Pediatric Clinics of North America* (1994) **41:**1069–104.

Evans D, Levene M. Neonatal seizures. *Archives of Disease in Childhood* (1998) **78:**F70–5.

Levene M. The clinical conundrum of neonatal seizures. *Archives of Disease in Childhood Fetal and Neonatal Edition* (2002) **86:**F75–77.

Rennie JM, Boylan GB. Neonatal seizures. In: TJ David (ed.). *Recent Advances in Paediatrics*, No. 18. Edinburgh: Churchill Livingstone, 2000: 19–32.

Scher MS. Seizures in the newborn infant: diagnosis, treatment, and outcome. *Clinics in Perinatology* (1997) **24:**735–72.

Volpe JJ. *Neurology of the Newborn*, 4th edn. Philadelphia: WB Saunders, 2001.

Related topics of interest

- birth injuries
- childbirth complications and foetal outcome
- germinal matrix-intraventricular haemorrhage
- hypoxic-ischaemic encephalopathy
- periventricular leucomalacia.

Sexual ambiguity

Genetic sex is determined at fertilisation. The foetus develops female *gonadic sex* unless a testis-determining factor (TDF) is present. The SRY gene (sex-determining region Y) on the short arm of the Y chromosome fulfils this role. When a testis develops, it secretes testosterone and Müllerian inhibitor substance (MIS). Testosterone acts on the Wolffian ducts to produce the male internal genitalia, the vas deferens, epididymis, and seminal vesicles. Externally, the androgen target cells convert testosterone into dihydrotestosterone (DHT) with the enzyme 5α-reductase. DHT stimulates the development of the male external genitalia, the penis and scrotum. MIS leads to the regression of the Müllerian ducts that would have developed into the internal female genitalia in the absence of a testis. Thus, a *phenotypic sex* is normally established by the end of embryogenesis, but when this has an uncertain appearance at birth, the baby is considered to have ambiguous genitalia. The *sex of rearing* is determined more by what can be realistically achieved with the anatomy and hormones (and the likely effect of puberty) than by karyotype.

At birth

The parents
The birth of a seemingly well infant but with indeterminate sex can cause unimagined anxiety and distress to the parents, and, if badly managed, can irreparably damage the doctor–parent relationship. The usual cry of 'It's a boy!' or 'It's a girl!' is painfully absent for the parents of most babies with ambiguous genitalia, though some will have a sex assigned by the birth attendant, and this may later prove to be wrong. Therefore, the first issue is to help the parents. Honesty is vital: uninformed guesses about the sex of the baby are devastating if wrong. The discussions with the parents should include the following statements:

- The sex that the baby is destined to be is not yet clear. They should be shown their baby's anatomy and simple drawings of sex-organ development.
- The problem can be solved, and a definite sex assigned.
- In the meantime, the baby should not be named, and the registration of the birth should be delayed until a sex has been assigned.
- Any attempt to assign 'the most likely sex' must be resisted. The baby should always be called 'baby', not 'he', not 'she', and certainly not 'it'!

Parents will want to know how long it will be before a sex can be assigned. It is better to suggest a week or so and to have an answer in 4 or 5 days, rather than to suggest that the information will be available within days, but then have them wait for a week or longer, which parents find unbearable. To avoid confusion, the supervision of all such infants should be under one senior paediatrician, who should be responsible for organising the investigations and communicating the results of the same to parents.

The baby
Assessment includes:

- checking the family history for similar babies, presence of hypospadias or cryptorchidism, and infertile aunts
- checking the history for neonatal or infant male deaths (congenital adrenal hyperplasia [CAH] with salt loss)
- assessment of phallic size, the presence or absence of midline fusion of the labia/scrotum, the position and size of gonads if any are palpable, and the position of the urethral orifice
- physical examination for other congenital abnormalities.

Investigations
These should be performed urgently and the initial investigations should include:

- *chromosomes* that can be sent immediately after birth or from cord blood
- plasma *17-hydroxyprogesterone (17OHP)* to exclude congenital adrenal hyperplasia. As this is raised in all newborns, sampling has to be delayed for 48h (normal value <18nmol/l). It remains elevated in ill and preterm babies, and this may cause diagnostic confusion.

These two investigations may be all that is necessary, because 90% of ambiguous genitalia recognised at birth in the UK are secondary to virilisation of a female (46XX) from CAH, with an autosomal recessive inheritance. The incidence of CAH in the UK is one in 10000, with >95% of cases due to 21α-hydroxylase deficiency (of which there are several allelic forms), wherein very high levels of 17OHP are found. It is also the only life-threatening form, as salt loss and consequent collapse can occur within a few weeks of birth in those with a severe deficiency. The experienced clinician may suspect other problems if characteristic or unusual changes are apparent, and request additional tests.

Classifying the problem

Female pseudohermaphroditism
These infants have a normal female karyotype, ovaries, and müllerian structures, but a masculine external genitalia appearance. The most common cause of this virilisation of a genetically female foetus is congenital adrenal hyperplasia, and in the UK this is nearly always due to a deficiency of 21α-hydroxylase, although 11β-hydroxylase (~5%) and 3β-hydroxysteroid dehydrogenase (3β-HSD) deficiency (<5%) can also cause it. About 50% of 21α-hydroxylase deficiency cases have salt loss. Figure 1 shows the steroid biosynthetic pathways involved, and Table 1 presents some enzyme defects with their clinical outcomes. Other causes of female virilisation are very rare; they include drug ingestion and masculinising tumours in the mother or foetus.

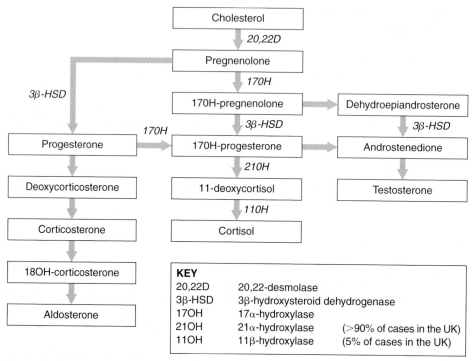

Figure 1 Simplified steroid biosynthetic pathways.

Table 1 Summary of the effects of specific enzyme defects.

Defect	Virilisation in girls	Incomplete masculinisation of boys	Salt loss	Hypertension
20,22D	No	Yes	Yes	No
3β-HSD	Yes	Yes	Yes	No
17OH	No	Yes	No	Yes
21OH	Yes	No	50% Yes	No
11OH	Yes	No	No	Yes

Male pseudohermaphroditism

This is incomplete virilisation of a genetic male with testes. This may be due to the following causes:

Impaired metabolism of androgens by peripheral tissues

- 5α-reductase deficiency is an autosomal recessive defect, in which the internal male organs (testosterone-dependent) develop normally, but the external genitalia (DHT-dependent) are ambiguous, and the phallus is small.
- Testicular feminisation comprises androgen receptor/post-receptor defects in which the end organs do not respond to the androgens; this condition is present as a spectrum of abnormalities from an apparently normal female (but sometimes with bilateral inguinal hernias with a testis in them) to an infertile male.

Impaired testosterone production
This condition is rare.

Abnormal gonadal differentiation

- True hermaphroditism occurs when an individual has both testicular tissue with seminiferous tubules and ovarian tissue with follicles. They may combine as an ovotestis or be separate gonads. Some present at birth with abnormal genitalia, and others only at puberty when secondary sexual characteristics do not develop normally. Eighty per cent are XX, 10% XY, and 10% mosaic.
- Asymmetrical gonadal dysgenesis results in a testis on one side and a streaked gonad on the other.
- XX males frequently have the SRY gene translocated to the paternal X chromosome.

Further reading

American Academy of Pediatrics. Evaluation of the newborn with developmental anomalies of the external genitalia. *Pediatrics* (2000) **106:**134–42.

Levine LS, Pang S. Prenatal diagnosis and treatment of congenital adrenal hyperplasia. *Journal of Pediatric Endocrinology* (1994) **7:**193.

McLaughlin DT, Donahoe PK. Sex determination and differentiation. *New England Journal of Medicine* (2004) **350:**367–78.

Rangecroft L. Surgical management of ambiguous genitalia. *Archives of Disease in Childhood* (2003) **88:**799–801.

Schafer AJ. Sex determination and its pathology in man. *Advances in Genetics* (1995) **33:** 275–329.

Warner GL, Hughes IA. The clinical management of ambiguous genitalia. In: CGD Brook, PC Hindmarsh (eds). *Clincal Paediatric Endocrinolgy*, 4th edn. Oxford: Blackwell Science, 2001.

Related topics of interest

- acute collapse
- congenital malformations and birth defects
- postnatal examination
- prenatal diagnosis.

Shock

Shock constitutes a medical emergency where prompt and appropriate action can lead to a full recovery, but delayed, though appropriate, action may be inadequate to save the patient's life. A state of shock implies a generalised inadequacy of blood flow and tissue perfusion throughout the body, resulting in tissue damage. It can develop insidiously or rapidly progress to an irreversible stage.

Shock may be categorised by its aetiology into septic, hypovolaemic, cardiogenic, anaphylactic, and neurogenic. Despite the varied aetiology, the clinical features are remarkably similar.

Clinical features

- generalised pallor
- ill-looking
- cold peripheries
- poor capillary refill
- weak or impalpable pulses
- tachycardia and hypotension
- cyanosis and mottled skin
- tachypnoea and/or laboured breathing
- metabolic or mixed acidosis
- CNS depression and hypotonia.

Management

Resuscitative measures must be instituted before any detailed examination.

Improve oxygen delivery to tissues
- Administer oxygen by face mask or bagging.
- Intubate and ventilate if there is severe respiratory distress, respiratory failure or marked acidosis.

Improve cardiac performance
- Restore circulating blood volume if hypovolaemic (administer 15–20 ml/kg of 4.5% albumin, FFP, blood, or normal saline and then reassess).
- If not hypovolaemic, give a 10-ml/kg volume challenge (colloid or normal saline) to increase venous return.
- Improve myocardial contractility by:
  —Correcting acidosis: commence artificial ventilation and/or administer $NaHCO_3$ (or THAM) if pH <7.25, and reassess.
  —Administering inotropes: dopamine infusion (5–20 µg/kg per min) preferably via central line, as there is risk of tissue necrosis if given peripherally; adrenaline infusion (0.1–1 µg/kg per min) if in severe shock.

Determine the likely cause by reviewing risk factors

- Suspect *infection* in the presence of preceding temperature instability, fever or hypothermia, long lines, feed intolerance, and respiratory instability (as in apnoea). Promptly institute antibiotics (empirically) following appropriate cultures (blood, urine, and CSF).
- Suspect a *cardiac cause* in the presence of gallop rhythm, pulse differential (brachial/femoral), cardiomegaly, murmur(s), hepatosplenomegaly, lung crackles, or cyanosis. Beware of cardiac tamponade, especially with indwelling central lines and muffled heart sounds. Perform echocardiography and remove central line immediately if tamponade is confirmed. Aspirate pericardial effusion.
- Suspect a *pulmonary cause* in the presence of reduced breath sounds (tension pneumothorax), vomitus or blood in oropharynx (aspiration of vomitus or pulmonary haemorrhage), tachypnoea, and grunting.
- Suspect *anaphylactic reaction* if drugs and/or blood products have recently been administered or are currently being administered. Discontinue any ongoing parenteral medications or blood products and give adrenaline (1:10000 at 0.1 ml/kg IV—minimum 1 ml or 100 μg). You may repeat this after 5 min. Hydrocortisone (5–10 mg/kg IV) may be given in a severe reaction. Observe the patient for recurrence of symptoms over the next 24 h.
- Suspect *intra-abdominal cause* in the presence of abdominal distension and/or bilious vomiting (NEC with or without perforation)—place NG tube and empty stomach to decrease risk of aspiration.
- Suspect *adrenal insufficiency* if hyponatraemic, hyperkalaemic, ± hypoglycaemic and dehydrated.

Investigations

1. Arterial blood
   (a) acid–base balance and blood gases
   (b) FBC and coagulation studies
   (c) U and E, creatinine, and glucose.
2. chest radiograph and abdominal radiograph (with abdominal signs).
3. infection screen (urine, blood, and/or CSF culture). LP may be delayed. Remove intravascular catheters and send tips for culture. Swab any surgical wounds or infected sites.
4. echocardiography (with cardiac signs).
5. cranial ultrasound scan (intracranial haemorrhage).

Useful website

www.emedicine.com/ped/topic2768.htm
Part of the largest and most current online clinical knowledge base available to health professionals.

Further reading

Donn SM, Faix RG (eds). *Neonatal Emergencies*. Mount Kisco, NY: Futura, 1991.

Greene CL, Goodman SI. Catastrophic metabolic encephalopathies in the newborn period: evaluation and management. *Clinics in Perinatology* (1997) **24:**773–86.

Seri I. Neonatal shock: etiology, pathophysiology and management. *Prenatal and Neonatal Medicine* (2001) **6:**15–22.

Related topics of interest

- acid–base balance
- acute collapse
- congenital heart disease
- resuscitation.

Skin disorders

Helen Goodyear

The skin structure of a full-term neonate is the same as that of an adult apart from the neonate's dermis, which is thinner. All four layers of the epidermis are present by 24 weeks' gestation, but the epidermis is much thinner in preterm infants under 34 weeks, particularly the stratum corneum (outer layer). Barrier function is poor, with the potential for high water loss and increased absorption of topical applications.

Physiological skin lesions

- milia
- vernix caseosa
- sucking blisters
- cutis marmorata
- physiological scaling
- lanugo hairs in preterm
- harlequin colour change
- sebaceous gland hyperplasia.

Vesiculopustular lesions

The majority of neonatal skin lesions are vesiculopustular, and lesions fall into four categories—transient rashes, infections and infestations, genodermatoses, and naevoid disorders. The history of the appearance and distribution of lesions is helpful in differentiating between these causes.

Transient rashes

- *Miliaria.* This is due to blockage of the eccrine sweat ducts. If blockage is superficial, clear, thin-walled vesicles (miliaria crystallina) are seen, whereas itchy, red papules (miliaria rubra) are present if blockage is lower down in the epidermis. They are typically seen in the first two weeks of life.
- *Erythema toxicum neonatorum.* This is present in up to 50% of neonates and typically presents in the first 48 h of life. Skin lesions range from erythema to urticarial papules and pustules which contain eosinophils. It may recur beyond the first month of life.
- *Transient neonatal pustulosis.* This is commoner in neonates with black skins. Superficial fragile pustules containing neutrophils are present at birth and rupture easily (sometimes in utero), to leave a pigmented macule with a collarette of scale. Macules may last for three months.
- *Infantile acropustulosis.* This presents in the first three months of life. Recurrent crops of itchy 1–4 mm vesiculopustules containing neutrophils and sometimes eosinophils are typically on the hands and feet. Lesions cease by the second or third year.

- *Eosinophilic pustular folliculitis.* This is a rare condition with male predominance. Lesions may be present at birth and come in recurrent crops of white/yellow pruritic papules which tend to affect the scalp, hands and feet.
- *Neonatal acne.* This is relatively common, particularly closed comedones on the nose, forehead, and cheeks. Open comedones, inflammatory papules, and pustules may occur. It tends to resolve within 1–3 months without scarring.

Infections and infestations
- bacterial—impetigo and staphylococcal scalded skin syndrome
- herpes virus infections—HSV, VZV, and CMV
- fungal—*Candida* and *Pityrosporum*
- parasitic—scabies.

Genodermatoses
- *Epidermolysis bullosa (autosomal dominant and recessive).* This is a group of inherited disorders with an abnormal tendency to blister formation. The severity depends on the level of cleavage in the skin.
- *Incontinentia pigmenti (X-linked dominant).* This usually presents in the first few days of life with vesiculobullous lesions. These last for a few weeks and are followed by warty papules. It is usually lethal in utero in males.

Naevoid disorders
Urticaria pigmentosa (mastocytosis)
Reddish-brown macules which urticate when rubbed may be present shortly after birth. Lesions usually resolve by puberty.

Naevi
- Salmon patches are flat pink lesions present at birth usually on the upper eyelids, glabella or nape of the neck. They gradually fade, although 10–20% of those on the neck may persist.
- Port-wine stain (naevus flammeus) is a deep red/purple lesion present at birth and does not change with time.
- Strawberry marks are usually not present at birth but develop in the first few weeks, initially as a flat lesion and subsequently becoming raised and red.
- Sebaceous naevus is an oval or linear yellow-orange, warty lesion typically affecting the scalp. There is a risk of neoplastic change after puberty.
- Giant pigmented naevus (bathing trunks naevus), an extensive, brown-pigmented naevus, is present at birth and carries a risk of malignant melanoma. Treatment is required in the first week of life.

Congenital ichthyoses
- *Collodian baby.* The baby is red and covered in a shiny, translucent membrane.
- *Harlequin foetus.* Thick plaques with fissures cover the body surface.

It is important to start treatment without delay. Nurse in a high-humidity incubator and apply lightly a greasy emollient such as white soft paraffin and liquid paraffin in a 50:50 mixture every 2h to the skin. Fluid requirements may be as high as 200–250ml/kg and need close monitoring.

Neonatal lupus erythematosus

This presents within the first few weeks of life as an erythematous scaly rash, typically around the eyes, and may be associated with heart block. There may be no history of systemic lupus erythematosus (SLE) in the mother, but there is placental passage of antibodies, most commonly anti-Ro (anti-SSA).

Developmental abnormalities

- *Aplasia cutis.* There is localised absence of skin, most commonly affecting the posterior scalp. An ulcer is present at birth and heals slowly with scarring.
- *Amniotic band deformities.*

Useful website

www.med.jhu.edu/peds/dermatlas
A most useful atlas of dermatology.

Further reading

Eichenfield L, Frieden IJ, Esterly N. *Neonatal Dermatology*. Philadelphia: WB Saunders, 2001.

Harper J, Oranje A, Prose N. *Handbook of Paediatric Dermatology*. Oxford: Blackwell Science, 2000.

Van Praag MC, Van Rooij RW, Folkers E et al. Diagnosis and treatment of pustular disorders in the neonate. *Paediatric Dermatology* (1997) **14:**131–43.

Verbov JL. *Handbook of Paediatric Dermatology*. London: Martin Dunitz, 2000.

Related topics of interest

- congenital malformations and birth defects
- postnatal examination.

Stridor

Stridor is the noise produced on inspiration or expiration due to abnormal narrowing of the upper airway (trachea or larynx). Inspiratory stridor is more common. The aetiology is varied, including both congenital and acquired causes. Persistent stridor in the neonatal period requires investigation.

Aetiology

1. *Subglottic stenosis*. This may result from the trauma of endotracheal intubation, especially if prolonged, or may be congenital. Inspiratory and expiratory stridor is present.
2. *Laryngomalacia*. This is due to floppy aryepiglottic folds. Inspiratory stridor predominates and is worsened by lying in a supine position but is relieved by lying prone. The cry is normal. This is the least serious of causes and generally improves with growth.
3. *Vocal cord palsy*. This is associated with respiratory distress, inspiratory stridor, and difficulties in feeding.
4. *Tracheal compressions*. This may be external (as in vascular strictures from double aorta or anomalous vessels) or internal (as in subglottic haemangiomas and papillomas), producing inspiratory and expiratory stridor. Subglottic haemangiomas commonly coexist with cutaneous haemangiomas.
5. *Miscellaneous*. Laryngeal clefts, webs, and other rarer congenital malformations may also produce stridor, respiratory distress, and feeding difficulties. Some rare disorders; for example, Pelizaeus–Merzbacher disease (an X-linked leukodystrophy) may also be associated with stridor.

Clinical features

*   Very mild stridor may not be associated with obvious physical signs.
*   Moderate to severe stridor is accompanied by tracheal, sternal, and intercostal recession.
*   Severe stridor is not influenced by posture.
*   Tachycardia may be a sign of impending collapse.
*   The obligatory excess respiratory work in moderate to severe stridor may cause failure to thrive.
*   Cutaneous capillary haemangiomas may be associated with subglottic haemangiomas.

Investigation

*   pulse oximetry
*   AP chest radiograph and lateral view of neck
*   barium swallow (vascular rings)
*   fibre-optic laryngoscopy

- microlaryngoscopy
- CT scan (vascular rings).

Management

Laryngomalacia generally improves over time but where there is serious hypoxaemia, surgery may be required (such as supraglottic trimming), but it may be difficult to avoid tracheostomy. Systemic steroids may be used with benefit to treat subglottic haemangiomas and postextubation stridor. Congenital laryngeal and tracheal anomalies may require specialist surgical correction. Vascular rings may require resection or rearrangement. Rarely, tracheostomy may be required.

Useful websites

www.neonatology.com
Neonatology on the web—an extensive resource on neonatology.

www.emedicine.com/ped/topic2624.htm
Part of the largest and most current online clinical knowledge base available to health professionals.

Further reading

Dinwiddie R. *The Diagnosis and Management of Paediatric Respiratory Disease.* Edinburgh: Churchill Livingstone, 1997.

Greenough A, Milner AD (eds). *Neonatal Respiratory Disorders,* 2nd edn. London: Arnold, 2003.

Kirkpatrick BV, Mueller DG. Respiratory disorders in the newborn. In: V Chernick, T Boat (eds). *Kendig's Disorders of the Respiratory Tract in Children,* 6th edn. Philadelphia: WB Saunders, 1998: 328–64.

Richardson ME. *Otolaryngology (Pediatric Volume),* 3rd edn. St Louis, MO: Mosby, 1998.

Zalzal GH. Pediatric stridor and airway management. *International Congress Series* (2203) **1240:** 803–8.

Related topics of interest

- complications of mechanical ventilation
- congenital malfomations and birth defects
- intubation
- respiratory distress.

Surfactant replacement therapy

In 1980, Fujiwara and coworkers were the first to show a benefit from intratracheal surfactant instillation in preterm babies with RDS. They used a modified bovine surfactant; other natural surfactants have been derived from bovine or porcine lungs and human amniotic fluid. Synthetic surfactants are composed mainly of dipalmitoyl phosphatidylcholine (DPPC or 'lecithin'), which lowers surface tension, and a spreading agent such as tyloxapol and hexadecanol or unsaturated phosphatidyl glycerol. Presently, they do not contain surfactant proteins.

Early trials of both natural and synthetic surfactants showed a reduction of about 40% in mortality from RDS and a similar reduction in pneumothoraces compared to control babies who did not receive surfactant. The incidence of IVHs is not greatly affected, but PDA, pulmonary haemorrhage, and apnoea are slightly more frequent in surfactant-treated babies. PDA and pulmonary haemorrhage both result from an early lowering of pulmonary vascular resistance, which increases pulmonary flow and left-to-right shunting through the duct, and so fills up the pulmonary vasculature. Pulmonary haemorrhage—best thought of as pulmonary haemorrhagic oedema—is seen in about 4% of surfactant-treated babies. Delayed ventilator pressure weaning may help reduce the incidence. Apnoea occurs more frequently, as babies come off the ventilator sooner.

It is now clear that:

- Early treatment with surfactant is better than late.
- Natural surfactants are more effective than synthetic ones.
- Surfactant therapy benefits babies with meconium aspiration. It may also be beneficial in congenital pneumonia, CDH, PPHN, and pulmonary haemorrhage; as a transient therapy in infants with congenital deficiency of the surfactant-associated protein SP-B; and in the 'adult' (or 'acute') respiratory distress syndrome (ARDS), where natural surfactants (which contain SP-B and SP-C) may be superior to synthetic surfactants (which do not contain proteins).

The timing of surfactant treatment has been divided into:

- prophylactic surfactant given at birth or before respiratory distress develops
- later treatment (rescue therapy) given as soon as moderate respiratory distress develops in a baby and preset thresholds are passed—for example, a mean airway pressure of $7\,cmH_2O$ or $FiO_2 > 40\%$.

The debate now is whether babies at risk should receive surfactant at birth or just as early as possible during respiratory distress, perhaps even being intubated solely for surfactant administration, and then extubated and put on nasal prong CPAP if their disease is mild. There is little doubt that preterm babies who receive surfactant within minutes of birth benefit more than those who receive it early in the disease even if this is only 1–2 h later. The greatest benefit from prophylactic surfactant treatment in terms of neonatal survival is seen at ≤28 weeks' gestation. Prophylactic natural surfactant reduces the risk of pneumothorax and mortality compared with rescue treatment in infants of under 31 weeks' gestation. However, the cost of giving it at birth to all babies of (say) under 32 weeks is prohibitive because only 20–40% of the more mature babies in this group would go on to need ventilation and surfactant.

They are the most numerous, and also those least likely to die and/or develop chronic lung disease. The clinical benefits and the benefit/cost ratio increase inversely with gestational age.

Guidelines on surfactant administration

Based on the evidence from clinical trials and animal studies, the following guidelines appear most appropriate. *Prophylactic surfactant* is recommended only for infants of under 28 weeks' gestation unless the mother has not received antenatal steroids and the infant requires endotracheal intubation for resuscitation, in which case surfactant should be administered. A surfactant dose of 100 mg/kg should be adequate. *Rescue therapy* is appropriate for infants of ≥32 weeks' gestation when intubation is required ($FiO_2 > 0.4$ and/or RDS on chest radiograph). For infants of 29–31 weeks' gestation early CPAP is recommended with surfactant being administered once intubation is required ($FiO_2 > 0.3$ and/or RDS on chest radiograph). Should intubation be required during resuscitation at birth, surfactant should be administered. For rescue therapy, a dose of 100 or 200 mg/kg may be used, depending on the severity of RDS, and keeping in mind that the higher dose is associated with a reduced need for retreatment. For infants of 25–31 weeks' gestation, surfactant and early CPAP combined are useful in avoiding mechanical ventilation and reducing the risk of CLD. Current evidence shows that the combination of prenatal steroids and prophylactic surfactant is the most effective intervention for babies at high risk of developing RDS.

Synopsis of surfactant therapy

Head-to-head trials have compared natural with synthetic surfactants. Compared to those treated with the synthetic surfactant, babies treated with a natural one had odds ratios (OR) of 0.8 for neonatal mortality, 0.86 for the combined endpoint of chronic lung disease and death, and 0.53 for pulmonary air leaks (not every commercially available surfactant has been evaluated in such trials). Natural surfactants also act more quickly. This is because of the presence of the surfactant-associated proteins SP-B and SP-C that help in the adsorption and spread of the surfactant. SP-A and SP-D are removed during the extraction process. Both play a role in host defence mechanisms, and SP-A is involved in the local recycling of surfactant. To date, head-to-head clinical trials comparing two natural surfactants with each other (such as Survanta vs Infasurf, or Survanta vs Curosurf) have not shown major differences in long-term outcome (such as mortality and chronic lung disease) between these preparations. However, there is suggestive evidence that Curosurf may be superior to Survanta when used as rescue therapy.

The phospholipid content of a normal surfactant pool has been estimated to be approximately 100 mg/kg body weight, and surfactant treatment aims to replenish this deficit. Preterm infants with RDS may have only 5 mg phospholipid/kg. Current evidence suggests that a surfactant dose of 100–200 mg/kg is required to treat RDS, but for prophylaxis, a lower dose may be effective. Manufacturers' dosing and redosing recommendations have ranged from a relatively restrictive use to a more liberal one (such as multiple doses given every 6 h if the baby remains intubated and requiring >30% oxygen). On average, 2–3 doses are given, but in conditions characterised by surfactant inactivation, multiple doses may be more effective. Respiratory disease in term infants causes abnormalities in surfactant metabolism. Meconium displaces and inhibits surfactant, and the increased capillary permeability in pneumonia leads to surfactant inactivation by fibrin. Treatment is aimed at reversing or overwhelming this pathology. Optimal dosing schedules for this have yet to be established, but six-hourly aliquots of 150–200% of the normal dose, starting soon after birth, have been used in some trials.

Further reading

Baroutis G, Kaleyias J, Liarou T et al. Comparison of three treatment regimens of natural surfactant preparations in neonatal respiratory distress syndrome. *European Journal of Pediatrics* (2003) **162:**476–80.

Barrington KJ, Finer NN. Care of near term infants with respiratory failure. *British Medical Journal* (1997) **315:**1215–58.

Findlay RD, Taeusch HW, Walther FJ. Surfactant replacement therapy for meconium aspiration syndrome. *Pediatrics* (1996) **97:**48–52.

Fujiwara T, Maeta H, Chida S et al. Artificial surfactant therapy in hyaline membrane disease. *Lancet* (1980) **1:**55–9.

Halliday HL. Natural vs synthetic surfactants in respiratory distress syndrome. *Drugs* (1996) **51:**226–37.

Kattwinkel J. Surfactant: evolving issues. *Clinics in Perinatology* (1998) **25:**17–32.

Kattwinkel J, Bloom BT, Delmore P et al. Prophylactic administration of calf surfactant extract is more effective than early treatment of respiratory distress syndrome in neonates of 29 through 32 weeks' gestation. *Pediatrics* (1993) **92:**90–8.

Long W (ed.) Surfactant replacement therapy. *Clinics in Perinatology* (1993) **20**(4).

Morley CJ. Systematic review of prophylactic vs rescue surfactant. *Archives of Disease in Childhood, Foetal and Neonatal Edition* (1997) **77:**F70–4.

Ramanathan R, Rasmussen MR, Gertsmann DR et al. A randomized, multicenter masked comparison trial of poractant alfa (Curosurf) versus beractant (Survanta) in the treatment of respiratory distress syndrome in preterm infants. *American Journal of Perinatology* (2004) **21:** 109–19.

Soll RF, Dargaville P. Surfactant for meconium aspiration syndrome in full term infants. The Cochrane Library, Issue 2. Chichester: John Wiley & Sons, 2004.

Soll RF, Morley CJ. Prophylactic versus selective use of surfactant in preventing morbidity and mortality in preterm infants (Cochrane Review). In: The Cochrane Library, Issue 3. Oxford: Update Software, 2002.

Related topics of interest

- mechanical ventilation
- meconium aspiration syndrome
- persistent pulmonary hypertension of the newborn
- pulmonary haemorrhage
- respiratory distress syndrome.

Surgical emergencies

In a minority of deliveries, the newborn infant may require acute life-saving intervention for cardiorespiratory support or immediate and rapid assessment for a variety of congenital anatomical defects that require urgent attention. The greatest assets in dealing with any infant with a problem in the immediate newborn period are anticipation and a team approach. Anticipation of a problem is commonly based on antenatal diagnosis by ultrasonography. When there is ample warning before the delivery, the assembled team can best decide on the timing, route, and site of delivery. Infants with complex congenital defects will require transfer to a tertiary paediatric surgical centre. Maternal transfer to an appropriate maternity unit facilitates the infant's postnatal care. Despite all the advances in antenatal diagnosis, some newborn infants may still be found to have unexpected anomalies requiring urgent surgical attention. In addition, previously well neonates may also develop acute medical disorders requiring urgent surgical attention.

Conditions presenting at birth

Abdominal wall defects
- gastroschisis
- ectopia vesicae.

Management
- Keep the infant warm at all times.
- Cover the defect(s) with dry sterile dressing and/or plastic covering (such as cling film), and keep the infant warm.
- Obtain venous access and administer colloid to support the circulation—if necessary.
- Administer an infusion of 10% dextrose to maintain normal blood glucose.
- Obtain blood from infant and mother for blood grouping and cross-matching.
- Refer to a paediatric surgical service.

Anomalies of the gastrointestinal tract
- oesophageal atresia
- TOF
- small bowel obstruction (such as duodenal or ileal atresia) with or without perforation.

Management
- Withhold oral feeds.
- Obtain venous access and maintain normal blood glucose by administering an infusion of 10% dextrose.
- Use nasogastric suctioning to decompress the stomach and constant oropharyngeal suctioning to clear pharyngeal secretions (oesophageal atresia).
- Obtain maternal and infant's blood for grouping and cross-matching.
- Refer to a paediatric surgical service.

Urological anomalies
- posterior urethral valves
- severe bilateral hydronephrosis
- ureteric rupture and urinary ascites
- bilateral pelviureteric junction/vesicoureteric junction obstruction.

Management
- Confirm prenatal findings with postnatal ultrasound scan.
- Catheterise infants suspected of having posterior urethral valves.
- Obtain urgent MCUG and refer to paediatric urologist.
- For suspected bilateral pelviureteric/vesicoureteric junction and ureteric rupture, refer immediately to paediatric urologist. Commence prophylactic intravenous antibiotics.

Cardiac anomalies
As most of these anomalies are not diagnosed until referral to a specialist paediatric cardiology centre, early referral to such a centre is therefore desirable. A handful of lesions require early surgical intervention if chances of survival are to be enhanced. The main conditions are as follows:

- HLHS
- coarctation of the aorta/interrupted aortic arch
- obstructed total anomalous pulmonary venous drainage
- TGA with intact ventricular septum
- pulmonary atresia with intact ventricular septum
- complex congenital heart lesions
- tricuspid atresia.

It is essential to commence a prostaglandin E_1 or E_2 infusion (start at 5 ng/kg per min increasing to 10–20 ng/kg per min in 5 ng/kg per min increments) in infants suspected of having duct-dependent lesions at the earliest opportunity. Correct metabolic acidosis and commence treatment for heart failure (if present) with diuretics (such as furosemide 1–2 mg/kg per dose). Intubation and mechanical ventilation may be necessary. Once the infant is stabilised, transfer to a paediatric cardiac centre.

Specific disorders
Congenital diaphragmatic hernia
If the condition has been previously diagnosed antenatally, intubate infant immediately at birth and avoid bagging to prevent aeration and expansion of intrathoracic bowel. Proceed to surgery when infant has stabilised. (See 'Congenital diaphragmatic hernia'.)

Torsion of the testes
This is a real emergency as the affected testis must be operated on within a few hours or it becomes nonviable. The affected testis is higher, often larger, and, if recently twisted, very tender. This may occur prenatally, in which case the enlarged bluish testis is nontender. Urgent exploration is required to untwist the testis, if still viable, or orchidectomy, if nonviable, with orchidopexy being performed on the contralateral side.

Conditions presenting later

These are mainly gastrointestinal in nature and are summarised below:

- intra-abdominal perforation with peritonitis
- strangulated hernias (inguinal and femoral)
- NEC
- volvulus.

Occasionally, a variety of other acute medical conditions may arise and require urgent surgical input. These include acute thromboembolic phenomena, accidents with vascular lines (such as snapped central intravascular lines with a retained distal portion), major subdural haemorrhage, serious postoperative wound dehiscence, and serious accidental injuries.

Management

- Commence nasogastric drainage to decompress the abdomen.
- Withhold oral feeds and commence infusion of a dextrose-electrolyte solution to maintain normal blood glucose.
- Administer analgesia as continuous IV infusion whenever infants are, or are likely to be, in pain.
- For suspected intra-abdominal perforation and NEC, commence broad spectrum antibiotics including metronidazole.
- If surgery is likely to result in significant blood loss, obtain infant's blood for grouping and cross-matching.
- Administer colloid to support the circulation (where necessary).
- Commence broad spectrum antibiotics (including metronidazole) when gastrointestinal wall integrity is suspect (eg NEC).
- Unless an expert opinion is already available on site, transfer to an appropriate paediatric surgical service.

Further reading

Belman AB, King LR, Kramer SA (eds). *Clinical Pediatric Urology*, 4th edn. London: Martin Dunitz, 2001.

Black JA, Whitfield MF. *Neonatal Emergencies: Early Detection and Management*, 2nd edn. Oxford: Butterworth-Heinemann, 1991.

Charsha D. *Neonatal Emergencies Series Video*. St Louis, MO: Mosby, 1998.

O'Neill JA Jr, Rowe MI, Grosfeld JL et al. *Pediatric Surgery*, 5th edn. St Louis, MO: Mosby, 1998.

Puri P (ed.). *Newborn Surgery*, 2nd edn. London: Arnold, 2003.

Related topics of interest

- abdominal wall defects
- congenital diaphragmatic hernia
- herniae
- necrotising enterocolitis
- neonatal surgery.

Thermoregulation

Thermoregulation is the ability to maintain a normal body temperature in varying environmental conditions and temperatures. When these protective homeostatic mechanisms are overcome, body temperature rises or falls outside the normal range. The thermal stresses a baby may have to deal with include:

- excessive cooling from evaporation, radiation, convection, and conduction
- excessive heating from high environmental temperatures and humidity, radiant heaters, and overwrapping.

Cooling

There is a clearly established relationship between hypothermia and increased mortality and morbidity, and prompt attention to temperature control is mandatory. Hypoxia reduces the ability of the baby to respond to a cold stress, so the asphyxiated baby and/or the baby with respiratory distress are at particular risk. Evaporation of amniotic fluid from the skin of a newborn baby is a common cause of cooling immediately after birth, even in tropical environments or warm rooms. Such evaporation can drop a term baby's temperature as much as $2\,°C$ in $15\,min$. Rapid drying and wrapping reduce this fall, but many commercially available radiant heaters do not. The use of polyethylene occlusive wrapping of VLBW infants at birth (especially those under 28 weeks' gestation), significantly reduces evaporative heat loss and the postnatal temperature fall. Heat is also radiated from a naked baby, who is a 'hot spot', radiating heat to his cooler surroundings. Significant radiant heat loss occurs from the head, so dressing a baby includes putting a hat on. Convective and conductive heat losses in a dressed baby are minimal, providing bedding and clothes are at body temperature when put on, and the baby is not in a draught, which would also increase evaporative cooling.

Preterm and small-for-dates babies are particularly prone to hypothermia because of their:

- high surface area to body size ratio
- lack of subcutaneous adipose tissue that helps insulate the body
- poor energy stores and limited brown-fat deposits.

Babies respond to cooling with:

- reduction of heat loss by peripheral vasoconstriction and assumption of the foetal position to reduce the exposed surface area
- extra heat production. This involves the release of noradrenaline, which acts locally in the brown-fat deposits to stimulate lipolysis and hence heat production. For this to be successful, there must be adequate oxygenation of the tissues and a good circulation. Glucose will also be metabolised for heat production, and hypoglycaemia must therefore be avoided. Newborn infants cannot warm themselves through shivering.

Thermoneutrality

A baby with a normal temperature who is trying neither to increase heat production nor to increase heat loss is said to be in a *thermoneutral* environment. Incubators should therefore be capable of providing a thermoneutral environment for a range of babies at different ages. The environment must be defined not just in terms of temperature but also humidity, convection (draughts), and surrounding radiant heat sources. A well, week-old, 3.5-kg baby needs lower environmental temperatures than a small extremely preterm one on the first day when temperatures in excess of 37°C and high humidity in a draught-free environment may be necessary if the baby is naked.

Overheating

Larger babies can become overheated under phototherapy lamps, near radiant heaters, and inside closed incubators, or if overwrapped in a warm room. As best their circumstances allow, they will respond to this by:

- Increased heat loss through peripheral vasodilation and increasing the exposed surface area by adopting a 'sun-bathing' posture.
- Sweating. However, term babies are able to achieve only a modest increase in cooling through sweating—much less than children or adults—and preterm babies have even more limited sweating. If the child is overswaddled, the response to heat stress can be very limited and the baby becomes hyperthermic.
- Panting. This limited response to heat stress which persists for some weeks after birth, together with the inability to wriggle free of bedclothes and clothing, contributes to the risk of cot death in overswaddled babies.

Further reading

Gunn AJ, Bennet L. Is temperature control important in delivery room resuscitation? *Seminars in Neonatology* (2001) **6:**241–9.

Lyon AJ, Pikaar ME, Badger P et al. Temperature control in very low birthweight infants during the first five days of life. *Archives of Disease in Childhood, Foetal and Neonatal Edition* (1997) **76:**F47–50.

Okken A, Koch J (eds). *Thermoregulation of Sick and Low Birth Weight Neonates*. Berlin: Springer, 1995.

Polin RA, Fox WW, Abman SH (eds). *Fetal and Neonatal Physiology*, 3rd edn. Philadelphia: WB Saunders, 2003.

Vohra S, Frent G, Campbell V et al. Effect of polyethylene occlusive skin wrapping on heat loss in very low birth weight infants at delivery: a randomized trial. *Journal of Pediatrics* (1999) **134:**547–51.

Related topics of interest

- extreme prematurity
- neonatal surgery
- resuscitation
- transport of sick infants.

Trace minerals and vitamins

Eight trace minerals are nutritionally essential for humans: chromium, copper, iodine, iron, manganese, molybdenum, selenium, and zinc. They play vital roles in several metabolic pathways. Clinical deficiencies have been described for six of the minerals. As accretion of trace minerals occurs during the last trimester of pregnancy, prematurity is associated with low stores at birth and the premature infant is at increased risk of developing trace mineral deficiencies.

Chromium

Chromium is involved in glucose homeostasis, and this is the only biological role postulated for this micromineral. Chromium deficiency has not been described in infants. Human milk has 0.3–0.5 μg chromium/l and the chromium content of preterm human milk is unknown. The recommended enteral chromium intake is 0.1–0.5 μg/kg per day and 0.05–0.2 μg/kg per day (0.2 μg/kg per day in the preterm infant) parenterally. There are no data to justify intakes higher than that received by the breast-fed infant.

Copper

Copper is contained in several enzymes, including cytochrome oxidase, and is required for connective tissue formation, myelinisation, and iron utilisation. The most abundant copper-containing enzymes are the superoxide dismutase enzymes which protect cell membranes against oxidative injury. Caeruloplasmin, representing 60% of the copper in plasma and the interstitial fluids, is a weak oxidase and primarily transports copper from its storage sites in the liver and muscles. The deficiency state (copper <40 μg/dl and caeruloplasmin <15 mg/dl) is associated with hypotonia, osteoporosis and fractures, pallor, sideroblastic anaemia resistant to iron therapy, neutropenia, decreased pigmentation of skin and hair, failure to thrive, diarrhoea, hepatosplenomegaly, skin rashes akin to seborrheic dermatitis, psychomotor retardation, and lack of visual responses. Therapy is with 1% copper sulphate solution, giving 0.6–0.8 mg copper/kg per day. The copper content of early preterm mother's milk is 0.8 mg/l, falling to 0.6 mg/l by four weeks. Formula feeds contain 0.01–1.4 mg copper/l. The recommended enteral copper intake for term and preterm infants is 120–150 μg/kg per day and 20 μg/kg per day parenterally. Withhold copper in the presence of cholestasis.

Iodine

Iodine is essential for normal thyroid function. Iodine deficiency depresses the production of thyroid hormones, especially tetraiodothyronine (T_4). In geographic regions where dietary iodine is <15 μg/kg per day, endemic goitre may occur. Endemic cretinism may result from maternal iodine deficiency, 5–15% of cases of endemic neonatal goitres developing overt cretinism. Preterm infants are more susceptible to both iodine deficiency and excess due to impaired compensatory mechanisms.

Such infants may also absorb excess iodine through their skin from povidone-iodine and alcohol-iodine in skin-cleansing agents. Bovine-milk-based formulas contain 50 μg iodine/l, preterm formulas contain 50–146 μg /l, and breast milk contains 70–90 μg/l. The recommended enteral iodine intake is 30–60 μg/kg per day with a parenteral intake of 1.0 μg/kg per day (both term and preterm infants). Based on these recommendations, an exclusively breast-fed preterm infant should receive iodine supplementation, as their intake would fall below the 30 μg/kg per day lower limit.

Iron

The total body iron is approximately 75 mg/kg, which is the same for term and preterm infants. Iron is present in the foetus as haemoglobin iron, tissue iron (myoglobin and iron-containing enzymes), and storage iron (as ferritin and haemosiderin in the liver and spleen). The iron content of human milk falls from 1 mg/l to <0.5 mg/l during the first 6 months of lactation, but iron levels in preterm breast milk are similar to those in term breast milk. Iron absorption and utilisation is better with human milk than with bovine milk or formula milk. Consequently, exclusively breast-fed term infants do not require iron supplementation for the first six months of life, whereas formula-fed infants are commonly started on iron-enriched formula from birth. VLBW infants remain iron replete until their birth weight has doubled, commonly at age 2 months. The recommended iron supplementation dose is 2 mg/kg per day up to a maximum of 15 mg per day, a dose which should be started at 4–8 weeks in preterm infants and continued for the rest of the first year. If total parenteral nutrition is provided exclusively for the first two months of life parenteral iron will be required at 0.1–0.2 mg/kg per day.

Manganese

Manganese deficiency has not been described in humans. It acts as an activator of the gluconeogenic enzymes pyruvate carboxylase and isocitrate dehydrogenase, protects mitochondrial membranes through superoxide dismutase (a manganese-containing enzyme), and activates glycerol transferase which takes part in mucopolysaccharide synthesis. Preterm infants may be at increased risk of toxicity. The manganese content of human milk is ~5 μg/l formula milks containing 0–340 μg/l. The recommended enteral manganese intake for term and preterm infants, respectively, is 0.75–7.5 μg/kg per day and 1.0 μg/kg per day parenterally.

Molybdenum

In mammals, molybdenum is essential for the function of three enzymes: aldehyde, sulphite and xanthine oxidases. Sulphite oxidase is required for the disposal and excretion of sulphur, while xanthine oxidase is required for the terminal oxidation of purines and their excretion as uric acid. Molybdenum deficiency has not been described in preterm infants. The molybdenum content of human milk is ~2 μg/l, but the molybdenum content of preterm milk is not known. The recommended enteral molybdenum intake for term and preterm infants, respectively, is 0.3 μg/kg per day, and 0.25 µg/kg per day parenterally (but only when on long-term total parenteral nutrition).

Selenium

The only established physiological role of selenium is as an integral part of the selenium-dependent enzyme glutathione peroxidase. Selenium protects cell membranes from peroxidase damage through detoxification of peroxides and free radicals. Selenium and vitamin E have overlapping functions. Deficiency produces myopathy, cardiac failure, and haemolytic anaemia. Clinical selenium deficiency has not been described in the preterm infant, although biochemical deficiency occurs. Low hepatic selenium stores at birth predispose the preterm infant to deficiency. The selenium content of mature human milk is 20 µg/l (falling to 15 µg/l by 3–6 months), while colostrum contains twice as much selenium. Preterm human milk contains 24 µg selenium/l, while formula milks contain 7–14 µg/l. The recommended enteral selenium intake for preterm infants is 1.3–3 µg/kg per day (breast-fed infants receive ~3 µg/kg per day). The recommended parenteral selenium intake is 1.5–2.0 µg/kg per day (2 µg/kg per day for the preterm infant). Parenteral intake should be reduced in infants with renal impairment.

Zinc

Zinc is essential for the human, playing especially important roles in cell growth and development. It is found in 200 metalloenzymes, including RNA and DNA polymerase, alkaline phosphatase, erythrocyte carbonic anhydrase, and several other enzymes associated with haem synthesis, protein metabolism, and carbohydrate and energy metabolism. It is essential for cell division and for insulin activity. The normal plasma zinc level is >70 µg/dl. Zinc is better absorbed from human milk than from bovine or formula milk. Colostrum has a high zinc content. The zinc content of formula milk is higher than that of human milk (0.5–2.5 mg/l). Excretion is via faeces except in the parenterally fed infant, where the primary excretory route is renal.

Clinical zinc deficiency is manifest by decreased appetite, failure to thrive, hair loss, poor wound healing, skin lesions, and depressed immunity. Plasma zinc levels and alkaline phosphatase activity are subnormal. A deficiency state acrodermatitis enteropathica (autosomal recessive) due to defective zinc absorption leads to a scaling pustular/erythematous rash around the mouth, ears, fingers, toes, and anogenital region; diarrhoea; and failure to thrive, along with low plasma zinc. Therapy is with zinc sulphate, 1–3.5 mg zinc/day. The recommended enteral zinc intake is 1 mg/kg per day (720–1400 µg/kg per day for preterm infants), and 400 µg/kg per day parenterally.

Vitamins

Vitamin A

This is required for synthesis of rhodopsin and other retinal pigments and also maintenance of epithelial membranes. It is degraded by light and is stored in the liver with tightly regulated excretion bound to retinol-binding protein. Deficiency may predispose to chronic lung disease, susceptibility to infection, xerophthalmia, and blindness. An excess produces irritability, brittle bones, dry skin, loss of hair, and raised intracranial pressure. The recommended intake of vitamin A in term infants is 333 IU/kg per day and 1500–2800 IU/kg per day (450–840 μg/kg per day) in preterm infants.

Pyridoxine (B$_6$)
Pyridoxine serves as a cofactor for several reactions involved in the synthesis, inter-conversion (transamination and decarboxylation), and catabolism of amino acids. Deficiency causes convulsions, weakness, anaemia, and dermatitis. The recommended oral intake is 150 μg/100 kcal, the parenteral intake being 1.0 mg/kg per day (term infants) and 0.18 mg/kg per day (preterm infants).

Vitamin C
Vitamin C has a role in collagen synthesis and amino acid metabolism, catecholamine synthesis, carnitine synthesis, and iron absorption, and it protects against hyperphenyl-lalaninaemia and hypertyrosinaemia in the newborn period. A supplement of 200 μg/day is recommended.

Vitamin D
Natural vitamin D (D$_2$ from plants or D$_3$ synthesised in skin) is converted to 25-hydroxyvitamin D (25-OHD) in the liver, and then in the kidney into the active metabolite 1,25-dihydroxyvitamin D (1,25-(OH)$_2$ D), which increases calcium and phosphorus absorption from the gut. Preterm infants have lower stores of vitamin D at birth and a greater need for skeletal mineralisation. With adequate phosphorus and calcium, 400–600 IU vitamin D per day should suffice.

Vitamin E
'Vitamin E' is the generic term for a number of tocopherol compounds. The vitamin is an antioxidant which inhibits the naturally occurring peroxidation of cell membrane polyunsaturated fatty acids by scavenging free radicals. The physiological effects of vitamin E include facilitation of normal phagocytosis, haem synthesis, and prevention of anaemia. The proposed pharmacological effects have included the prevention of retinopathy of prematurity, IVH, and CLD, but these have not been unequivocally proven. High doses produce toxicity and may be associated with sepsis and NEC. Preterm infants should receive 5–25 IU/day oral vitamin E.

Vitamin K
Vitamin K is required in the synthesis of clotting factors II, VII, IX, and X by the liver. A single dose of 1 mg i.m. (0.5 mg for preterm infants) protects against haemor-rhagic disease (vitamin K deficiency bleeding [VKDB]). If given by mouth for VKDB, two oral doses of 2 mg in the first week is enough for formula-fed babies, but for those exclusively breast-fed, a third dose of 2 mg is given at one month of age.

Folic acid (pteroylglutamic acid)
Folic acid is a water-soluble vitamin that functions as a coenzyme donor and acceptor of one-carbon units in nucleotide and amino-acid metabolism. It is required by

enzyme systems which synthesise RNA, DNA, and some amino acids (such as serine). It is absorbed from the proximal small intestine but is not stored to any great extent, making a daily intake necessary. Preterm infants are more susceptible to deficiency due to their more rapid postnatal growth and limited hepatic stores. Deficiency produces neutrophil hypersegmentation, megaloblastic changes, poor growth (disturbed DNA synthesis may alter cell division in several tissues), and, in severe cases, macrocytic anaemia and hypotonia. The human milk content of folate increases with advancing lactation, averaging 50 µg/l (range 26–141 µg/l). The folate content of formula milk and human milk fortifiers is considerably greater than this. The recommended dietary allowance for folic acid is 25 µg/day/six for infants from birth to 6 months. For VLBW infants, an enteral intake of 25–50 µg/kg per day is recommended until 40 weeks postconceptual age, whereupon 4 µg/100 kcal (the minimal recommended intake for term infants) should suffice. Preterm infants fed on preterm formulas and term formula-fed infants on at least 150 ml/kg per day should meet their daily requirements. However, preterm infants fed human milk may benefit from folate supplementation of at least 50 µg/day. The recommended parenteral folic acid intake is 56 µg/kg per day for preterm infants and 140 µg per day for term infants.

Further reading

Greene HL, Hambidge KM, Schandler R et al. Guidelines for the use of vitamins, trace elements, calcium, magnesium, and phosphorus in infants and children receiving total parenteral nutrition: Report of the Subcommittee on Pediatric Parenteral Nutrient Requirements from the Committee on Clinical Practice Issues of the American Society of Clinical Nutrition. *American Journal of Clinical Nutrition* (1988) **48**:1324–42.

Groh-Wargo S, Thompson M, Cox JH, Hartline JV (eds). *Nutritional Care for High-Risk Newborns* 3rd edn. Chicago: Precept Press, 2000.

Litov RE, Combs GF. Selenium in pediatric nutrition. *Pediatrics* (1991) **87**:339–52.

Morgan JB, Dickerson JWT (eds). *Nutrition in Early Life*. Indianapolis, IN: Wiley, 2003.

Tsang RC, Lucas A, Uauy R et al (eds). *Nutritional Needs of the Preterm Infant: Scientific Basis and Practical Guidelines*. Baltimore, MD: Williams & Wilkins, 1993.

Zlotkin SH, Atkinson S, Lockitch G. Trace elements in nutrition for premature infants. *Clinics in Perinatology* (1995) **22**:223–40.

Related topics of interest

- chronic lung disease
- fluid and electrolyte therapy
- neonatal surgery
- nutrition.

Transfusion of blood and blood products

Sick preterm infants frequently require blood transfusions in the first weeks of life due to significant cumulative losses from repeated blood sampling. In preterm infants, the amount of blood loss may easily equal or exceed the infant's circulating blood volume. Older preterm infants often require transfusion at a later time for anaemia or prematurity. Large acute blood losses or cumulative chronic losses in the mature infant may also require transfusion to replace the blood volume. In the immediate newborn period, transfusions aim to bring the haemoglobin back to the original normal level while in the later period the haemoglobin is maintained at 12–14 g/dl (PCV≥40%). While blood transfusion has been made considerably simpler and safer, it still carries some risks for the infant.

Indications for early transfusion

- exchange transfusion
- significant anaemia at birth
- significant acute haemorrhage
- iatrogenic blood losses (cumulative sampling losses for diagnostic purposes)
- prenatal haematological disorders (such as rhesus isoimmunisation).

Indications for late transfusion

- severe NEC
- severe sepsis
- surgery with significant blood loss
- symptomatic anaemia of any cause (producing tachycardia, apnoea, feeding difficulties, and poor weight gain).

Requirements for neonatal blood transfusion

- The blood used should have been screened for infection with CMV, HIV, HBV, and HCV.
- Blood and blood products should also be free from bacterial infection (approximately 16% of transfusion fatalities reported by the US FDA between 1986 and 1991 were due to bacterial contamination).
- Use of small subunits derived from one pack (octopus or satellite units) is encouraged to reduce donor exposure.
- For massive transfusions (such as ECMO or exchange transfusion), fresh whole blood less than 48 h old or reconstituted whole blood (washed packed red cells and fresh-frozen plasma) is required.
- In the immediate newborn period, maternal blood is required to ensure compatibility.

Potential complications

- haematomas from extravasation of blood during transfusion
- metabolic acidosis from large transfusions with stored blood (blood pH falls with storage)
- hypocalcaemia and hypomagnesaemia (citrate binding in CPD or CPDA-1 units)
- hypernatraemia (high sodium of blood stored in CPD)
- hyperkalaemia (serum potassium rises in stored blood)
- heart failure from rapid or large-volume transfusions
- transfusion reaction due to incompatible blood
- sensitisation to red cell antigens (older infants)
- hypothermia from transfusing blood directly out of the refrigerator (4–6 °C), and also apnoea, hypotension, and hypoglycaemia
- mechanical haemolysis due to passage of erythrocytes through fine cannulae (or peristaltic infusion pump!)
- transmission of infection (HIV, CMV, HBV, HCV, malaria, syphilis, and other bacterial infections). A recent estimate of the risk of infection from a repeat whole-blood donor gave a risk of one in 64000 for HBV, one in 103000 for HCV, and one in 493000 for HIV (US data)
- transfusion-associated graft-versus-host disease (TA-GVHD)—rare but rapidly fatal with a mortality over 90% (may be prevented in infants receiving large transfusions by irradiating the blood prior to transfusion, an action which inactivates the T lymphocytes responsible for TA-GVHD).

Transfusion reactions

There are two important serologic differences between infants and older children or adults. First, infants have IgG antibodies derived from the maternal circulation, which gradually decline during the first few months of life. Second, infants have a poor response to antigenic challenges such as allogenic red cell antigens. Thus, when transfused with red cells that differ from their own, infants do not respond by making alloantibodies until after the third month of life. Any antibodies detected in a newborn's blood sample are maternal in origin. Therefore, if an infant's initial antibody screen is negative, blood of an appropriate blood group can be issued to the infant without the need for further typing or cross-matching for the first three months of life.

Transfusion reactions are therefore relatively rare in the newborn period, but when they occur, they may be life-threatening. A transfusion reaction may be immediate or occur after several days or weeks. Immediate reactions include fever (often due to antileucocyte antibodies), allergic reactions (anaphylaxis or urticaria), acute haemolysis, and a haemorrhagic state. Delayed reactions include the development of haemolysis and sensitisation to red cell antigens, making later cross-matching more difficult and predisposing the infant to more transfusion reactions. An acute haemolytic reaction due to incompatible blood is serious, as it can result in acute renal failure and DIC. Symptoms include fever, bleeding, and shock. The transfusion must be discontinued, the blood bank notified, and the blood pack returned to the blood bank along with 3–5 ml of the infant's blood (clotted sample), and BP and urine output should be monitored. Treat shock, if present, appropriately (see 'Shock'). The

Table 1 Donor recipient blood group compatibility.

Infant's blood group	Compatible donor red cells	Compatible donor plasma
O	O	AB, O, A, B
A	O, A	AB, A
B	O, B	AB, B
AB	O, A, B, AB	AB

vast majority of these reactions are due to clerical errors and can therefore be avoided by careful double-checks. Note that acute haemolytic transfusion reactions *do not* occur in the very young infants. They also do not manifest delayed haemolytic transfusion reactions as they do not produce antibodies to allogenic erythrocytes. Isohaemagglutinins (the naturally occurring antibodies against other blood groups), which are responsible for acute haemolytic transfusion reactions, are detectable in under 50% of infants at age 6 months.

Special considerations

Occasionally, strongly held parental beliefs against the transfusion of blood or blood products, make for potentially difficult management, particularly in the very preterm infant. Where possible, it is desirable to be mindful of the parents' wishes, as the parents will assume the care of the infant following discharge from the unit. Blood sampling for diagnostic purposes should be reduced to the minimum. Erythropoietin administration reduces the need for late transfusions. Where the need for a blood transfusion is overwhelming and parents still object to a blood transfusion, it may be necessary to initiate legal proceedings, making the infant a ward of court.

Other blood products

Human albumin
This may be used to support the circulating blood volume at 10–20 ml/kg (4.5% albumin), or for dilutional exchange (20–30 ml/kg). In oedematous states, 25% salt-poor albumin may be used to increase the plasma oncotic pressure. Some 4 ml of 25% salt-poor albumin provides 1 g of albumin. It should be noted, however, that the use of human albumin for hypovolaemia or hypoalbuminaemia in critically ill patients may carry an increased risk of mortality.

Fresh-frozen plasma (FFP)
FFP may be used for supporting the circulating blood volume (10–20 ml/kg), treating haemorrhagic states (such as DIC and vitamin K deficiency), and for dilutional exchange (20–30 ml/kg).

Cryoprecipitate
This is used to replace clotting factors and correct bleeding states including fibrinogen deficiency (or fibrinogen <1 g/dl). It may therefore be used in haemophilia A, von

Willebrand's disease, and dysfibrinogenaemia. A unit or bag is sufficient for an infant. An average of 80 units of factor VIII activity is present in each 5–10-ml bag.

Platelet concentrate

One unit of platelets (30–50 ml/unit) raises the platelet count by 50000. One recent guideline suggests giving platelet transfusions (as one unit of platelets, or up to 20 ml/kg) to *all bleeding neonates* with a platelet count of $<100 \times 10^9$/l, *all nonbleeding neonates* with a platelet count of $<30 \times 10^9$/l, and *nonbleeding neonates* with a platelet count of 30–49×10^9/l who meet the following criteria: <1000 g and age <7 days, clinically unstable, have recent major haemorrhage (such as pulmonary haemorrhage or grades 3–4 IVH), require surgery or exchange transfusion, or have a coagulopathy. For infants with neonatal alloimmune thrombocytopenia, human platelet antigen-compatible platelets should be transfused to *all infants* whose platelet count is $<30 \times 10^9$/l, and *bleeding infants* whose platelet count is 30–99×10^9/l.

Safety of blood and blood products

All blood products carry the theoretical risk of transmitting infection (and currently in the UK, new variant Creutzfeldt–Jakob disease [nvCJD]). Up to the beginning of 2004, there had been 143 recorded deaths from nvCJD. The issue of plasma product safety arose when three of the first 23 nvCJD victims were identified as blood donors. At the end of 2003, a possible first report of nvCJD transmission from person to person via blood transfusion was made in the UK. This risk may be reduced by using plasma products from populations not affected by nvCJD (as in the USA).

The UK Blood Transfusion Services and the National Institute of Biological Standards and Control prepare detailed professional guidelines to secure the safety of blood and blood products. Blood centres are required to:

- screen donors
- test donated blood for HIV, HBV, HCV, and syphilis.

Plasma collected for the manufacture of blood products is treated similarly:

- Donors are screened for viruses (including HCV) each time they donate.
- Plasma is not released until the donor returns to give blood and is screened for a second time.
- The products themselves are virally inactivated.

Useful websites

www.bcshguidelines.com
The British Committee for Standards in Haematology—provides up to date advice on the diagnosis and treatment of haematological disease.

www.transfusionguidelines.org.uk
This site contains the full text of guidelines covering donor selection, collection, testing, processing and clinical use of blood products and tissues. These guidelines are produced by experts from UK hospitals, universities and transfusion services, and are updated annually.

Further reading

Boulton F. Transfusion guidelines for neonates and older children. *British Journal of Haematology* (2004) **124:**433–53.

Cohen AC, Manno C. Transfusion practices in infants receiving assisted ventilation. *Clinics in Perinatology* (1998) **25:**97–111.

Dolan G. Blood and blood product transfusion. In: JS Lilleyman, IM Hann (eds). *Paediatric Haematology*, Edinburgh: Churchill Livingstone, 1992: 431–56.

Hann IM, Gibson BES, Letsky EA (eds). *Foetal and Neonatal Haematology*. London: Baillière Tindall, 1991.

McClelland DBL (ed.). *Handbook of Transfusion Medicine*, 2nd edn. London: HMSO, 1996.

Murray NA, Roberts IAG. Neonatal transfusion practice. *Archives of Disease in Childhood Fetal and Neonatal Edition* (2004) **89:**F101–7.

Nathan DG, Orkin SH, Look T et al. *Nathan and Oski's Hematology of Infancy and Childhood*, 6th edn. Philadelphia: WB Saunders, 2003.

Quirlo KC. Transfusion medicine for the pediatrician. *Pediatric Clinics of North America* (2002) **49:**1211–38.

Vengelen-Tyler V (ed.) *Technical Manual of the American Association of Blood Banks*, 12th edn. Arlington, VT: American Association of Blood Banks, 1995.

Related topics of interest

- anaemia
- bleeding disorders
- blood pressure
- chronic lung disease
- neonatal surgery
- shock.

Transport of sick neonates

Of the approximately 150 million infants currently born each year worldwide, the vast majority have no access to the level of neonatal care that they may require. Some infants may therefore require transfer to centralised or regional centres for specialised care. These include preterm infants, newborns with cardiac or surgical problems, and those with complex congenital malformations. In the UK, approximately 1% of all births (7000 infants annually) may require transfer in the neonatal period. Furthermore, one in ten attempts to transfer may be unsuccessful (the majority being for infants of birth weight under 1500 g). Infants declined admission to centres offering a more appropriate level of care have a higher morbidity and mortality. However, interhospital transportation of high-risk infants is also fraught with potential dangers and complications that may further increase morbidity or mortality. Infants transferred under controlled conditions with skilled assistance have a reduced morbidity and mortality and have reduced requirements for intensive care. When time permits, the transfer of the pregnant mother to a more appropriate perinatal centre is associated with a more favourable neonatal outcome. However, transfer in utero with a mother in early labour is associated with increased risk of obstetric and maternal complications, including the unplanned delivery of an infant during transit. Neonatal transportation is therefore a serious undertaking whose success requires skilled personnel, appropriate equipment, and good communication and organisation. The goal of neonatal transport is to provide outborn infants with the same quality of care during transit that they would receive in a level III neonatal unit

Equipment for neonatal transport

The equipment used for neonatal transport should meet the needs of very-low-birthweight infants as well as of the large term infants with surgical or medical problems. It should be easy to operate, light, robust, and securely mounted to the transport system. There should be a reliable battery providing ample backup power for all vital equipment.

1. *Transport incubator.* This should be double-walled and able to provide a stable thermal environment despite variations in external temperature.
2. *Ventilator.* This should be simple to use yet reliable and preferably designed for transport use. It should allow visualisation of the ventilator settings being used and the oxygen concentration being delivered.
3. *Drug and fluid administration equipment.* The 50-ml syringe pump devices are probably the most appropriate—three to six may be needed.
4. *Pulse oximeter.*
5. *Oxygen analyser.*
6. *Suction devices.* These should preferably be battery operated and have adjustable pressure.
7. *Emergency equipment.* For intubation, needle aspiration of the chest and chest drain insertion, along with Heimlich valves, hand ventilation, cannulation for IV access, a portable cold-light source, and standard resuscitation drugs.

8. *Medications.* Because some neonatal units may not have the following medications available at all times, it is preferable for the transport team to carry their own supplies. These include plasma, surfactant, dobutamine, dopamine, morphine, pancuronium, midazolam, and PGE_1 or PGE_2.
9. *Mobile telephone.* This may be very helpful in case of difficulties in transit.

Stabilisation before transportation

The cornerstones of ideal neonatal transportation are the maintenance of an optimal temperature and normal or near normal physiological parameters, and the minimising of unexpected adverse events. For a smooth transfer requiring minimal intervention en route, the infant *must be* stabilised before departure. Stabilisation is the correction or treatment of processes that, left unaltered, may lead to a deterioration in the infant's status. Infants transferred after adequate stabilisation have a lower morbidity and mortality. Stabilisation should assess the adequacy of gas exchange and oxygenation, circulation (perfusion and blood pressure), thermoregulation, acid–base balance, and metabolic control.

Checks before departure

- Secure airway and check position of ET tube by radiographs.
- Assess adequacy of ventilation by the transport equipment by performing arterial blood gases prior to departure. If surfactant has been administered, wait for at least 30 min before performing arterial blood gases, to determine the need to reduce ventilatory support before the transfer.
- Assess adequacy of intravascular access sites and set up 'reserve' access sites if necessary.
- Check that blood pressure and blood glucose are satisfactory.
- Ensure that the infant is well covered, insulated, and warm, leaving only part of the face exposed for monitoring.
- Ensure that analgesia and sedation will be adequate during transport.
- Collect all the relevant maternal, including infant historical data and results of recent laboratory and radiological investigations.
- In order for the receiving team to be prepared for the infant, inform your intended destination of your departure, specifying any preparations which may be required in advance.

During transportation

- Use full remote monitoring of temperature, heart rate, oxygen saturation, and blood pressure.
- Avoid opening the incubator and exposing the infant to cold air.
- Ensure that ambulance cabin heating and lighting are adequate.
- Depending on the duration of the trip (for example, if it is ≥ 2 h) or the occurrence of adverse events, additional monitoring (such as blood-glucose measurements) may be required.

Checks on arrival

- Take the infant's temperature and rewarm the patient if hypothermic.
- Perform arterial blood gases and adjust ventilation and/or correct significant metabolic acidosis accordingly.
- Check blood pressure and augment it if necessary.
- Check blood glucose and correct hypoglycaemia if present.

Transport of infants under 1000 g birth weight

As these infants have a greater morbidity and mortality, their safe transport requires greater vigilance and proficiency of the transporting team. Most of these infants will require assisted ventilation during transfer, and they are more likely to deteriorate during transportation. They are more vulnerable to cold stress, hypoglycaemia, and ET tube blockage (due to narrow ET size of 2–2.5 mm). For the transfer of extremely preterm infants (22–24 weeks' gestation) when the outcome appears unfavourable, it may be preferable for the baby to stay with its parents and not die in transit or in a distant hospital away from them.

Transport of surgical newborns

Four out of five infants requiring surgery in the newborn period are stable term infants and most commonly have an abnormality of the gastrointestinal tract. The essentials of successful transfer remain the same but with the following additional requirements:

- Stabilisation before transport is vital. This will include placement of a nasogastric tube for decompression of the stomach (especially in the presence of intestinal obstruction), prevention or correction of hypothermia, provision of intravenous fluids to prevent hypoglycaemia and replace abnormal fluid losses, securing the airway (ventilation may be required in ~15% of cases), and adequate dressing for exposed viscera (as in gastroschisis).
- All the relevant records, including results of laboratory investigations and radiographs, should accompany the infant.
- A maternal blood sample (10 ml clotted blood) should be forwarded to facilitate cross-matching.
- Where necessary, obtain consent for the operation from the *mother* (if parents are not married, father's consent may not be valid). Consent (even if only verbal) should normally be obtained by the person performing the procedure.
- Administer vitamin K (i.m.).

Transport of newborns with cardiac disorders

In addition to the details already given above, infants suspected of having duct-dependent lesions should be commenced on PGE_2 (5–20 ng/kg per min for stable unventilated infants and 50–100 ng/kg per min for sick, ventilated infants). The lowest possible supplemental oxygen concentration should be used in infants with suspected duct-dependent lesions. Metabolic acidosis should be corrected, inotropes commenced in hypotensive infants, and diuretics in infants with congestive cardiac failure. Unstable infants should be intubated for transfer.

Air transport

Though less common in the UK due to the distances involved, air transport may be essential when long distances are involved, a rapid response time is required, adverse traffic and road conditions exist, and international transfers are required. Commonly, helicopters are used for distances of 30–400 miles and fixed-wing aircraft for distances of over 400 miles. It is even more important to stabilise the infant before transportation by air, as the incidence of complications may be greater (20–40%). Special problems peculiar to air transport may be encountered, particularly vibration and decompression. Air collections (as in pulmonary air leaks) enlarge and may cause clinical deterioration. The risk of hypothermia is increased (temperature falls by $2\,^{\circ}C$ for every rise of 1000 feet).

Avoiding adverse events

- Check transporting equipment daily to minimise unexpected equipment failure or gas cylinders running out during transportation.
- Inexperienced staff should not be assigned to transport sick infants unless accompanied by more experienced staff.
- Regular audits of transport and review of the conduct and outcomes of transport facilitate remedial steps to avoid future recurrence of adverse events.
- The continuing education and training of all members of the transport teams is essential, especially when new members join the team.
- The transport crew should know how to get to the intended destination and the ambulance fleet should be reliable.

Dealing with parents

The birth of a sick infant is accompanied by considerable parental anxiety and distress. This is amplified if the newborn infant requires transfer to another unit away from the parents. Parents should be given accurate information they can easily understand on the condition of their infant and the need for transfer. They should be reassured that transfer is in the best interests of their baby, and the mother should 'rejoin' her infant at the earliest opportunity.

Useful website

www.emedicine.com/ped/neonatology.htm
Part of the largest and most current online clinical knowledge base available to health professionals.

Further reading

Barry PW, Leslie A. *Paediatric and Neonatal Critical Care Transport*. London: BMJ Books, 2003.

Das UG, Leuthner SR. Preparing the neonate for transport. *Pediatric Clinics of North America* (2004) **51:**581–98.

Field D (ed.). Neonatal transport. *Seminars in Neonatology* (1999) **4**(4).

Jaimovich DG, Vidyasagar D. *Handbook of Pediatric and Neonatal Transport Medicine*, 2nd edn. Philadelphia: Hanley & Belfus, 2002.

Mir NA (ed.). *Manual of Neonatal Transport*. Manchester: E Petch Printers, 1997.

Related topics of interest

- acute collapse
- neonatal surgery
- surgical emergencies
- thermoregulation.

Vomiting

Vomiting occurs at certain periods in almost all infants in the neonatal period. Minor vomiting during or after feeds is physiological and universal. However, when it becomes persistent, projectile, and large in volume, a pathologic cause is more likely. Bilious vomiting should always be regarded as abnormal.

Aetiology

- excessive feeding
- gastrooesophageal reflux
- necrotising enterocolitis (NEC)
- sepsis (including UTI)
- oesophageal anomalies (such as pharyngeal cleft)
- intestinal obstruction (especially if vomiting is bilious)
- gastric outlet obstruction (especially pyloric stenosis—incidence three in 1000, male:female ratio 4:1)
- drug-induced—some enteral medication (such as chlorothiazide), increasing the risk of vomiting as may the administration of several medications at the same time along with feeds
- metabolic disorder (inherited metabolic disease [IMD]) as in galactosaemia (urine reducing substances positive)
- feed intolerance (as in cow's milk protein intolerance)
- gut malrotation
- hiatus hernia
- hydrocephalus.

Investigations

- U and E
- abdominal radiograph
- oesophageal pH monitoring
- barium swallow and follow-through examination (oesophageal anomalies and gut malrotation)
- abdominal ultrasound scan (gastric outlet obstruction)
- arterial blood gases (alkalosis with pyloric stenosis and persistent acidosis with IMD)
- infection screen (blood, urine, with or without CSF culture)
- metabolic screen (urine amino and organic acids, plasma amino acids, NH_3, and lactate).

Management

A pragmatic approach should be adopted in managing vomiting. The above list of investigations is certainly not necessary for every vomiting infant. Vomiting is often transient, and attention to the frequency and volume of feeds may be sufficient to improve the symptom. If reflux is suspected, 24-h oesophageal monitoring should be performed. Alternatively, a barium swallow may be performed. Although this is less sensitive, it has the advantage of simultaneously excluding gut malrotation and gastric outlet obstruction. Where such a facility is not available, a trial of antireflux therapy and feed thickeners may be diagnostic and curative. Avoid administering emetic drugs before feeds and spread out oral medication administration over the day, discontinuing any unnecessary medications. Feed intolerance is not as common as imagined, especially in the newborn period. It should be considered, however, when simple remedies have failed to improve the vomiting in the presence of a relevant family history. A soya-based formula (such as Wysoy, Farley Health Products), or one of the elemental formulae (such as Pregestimil, Mead Johnson) may then be tried.

Where the vomiting is persistent with mild to moderate abdominal distension, stop oral feeds and obtain an abdominal radiograph. If this is satisfactory but vomiting recurs on introducing feeds, commence an IV dextrose-electrolyte infusion and rest the gut for 1–3 days before trying enteral feeding again. This is more likely to occur in the growth-restricted infant. The serum electrolytes may occasionally give an indication as to the cause of vomiting (uraemia of renal failure, hyponatraemia in adrenal insufficiency, hypokalaemia in paralytic ileus, or hypochloraemic alkalosis in pyloric stenosis). When vomiting is projectile, perform a test feed (peristalsis may also be visible in pyloric stenosis). Presentation may occur as early as the first week. If a test feed is inconclusive but the clinical picture is highly suggestive of pyloric stenosis, proceed to an abdominal ultrasound examination or barium swallow ('string sign' seen in pyloric stenosis). Low-grade pyrexia may suggest infection and the need for an appropriate infection screen, including urine microscopy.

Bilious vomiting, even with an unremarkable abdominal radiograph, should be regarded as abnormal and a surgical opinion sought. Similarly, an infant with a tense, tender, and silent abdomen probably has a 'surgical abdomen' (NEC, intestinal obstruction, and/or perforation) and requires a surgical review.

Further reading

Black JA, Whitfield MF. *Neonatal Emergencies: Early Detection and Management*, 2nd edn. Oxford: Butterworth-Heinemann, 1991.
Klaus MH, Fanaroff AA. *Care of the High-Risk Neonate*, 5th edn. Philadelphia: WB Saunders, 2001.
Puri P (ed.). *Newborn Surgery*, 2nd edn. London: Arnold, 2003.

Related topics of interest

- abdominal distension
- gastrooesophageal reflux
- Hirschsprung's disease
- infection—general
- necrotising enterocolitis.

Index

Page numbers in *italics* indicate figures or tables.